# BSAVA Manual of Canine and Feline Musculoskeletal Imaging

Editors:

## Frances J. Barr
**MA VetMB PhD DVR DipECVDI MRCVS**
Division of Companion Animals
University of Bristol
Langford House, Langford
Bristol BS40 5DU

and

## Robert M. Kirberger
**BVSc MMedVet(Rad) DipECVDI**
Diagnostic Imaging Section, Department of
Companion Animal Clinical Studies
Faculty of Veterinary Science
University of Pretoria
Private Bag X04
Onderstepoort 0110
South Africa

D1560716

Published by:

**British Small Animal Veterinary Association**
Woodrow House, 1 Telford Way, Waterwells
Business Park, Quedgeley, Gloucester GL2 2AB

A Company Limited by Guarantee in England.
Registered Company No. 2837793.
Registered as a Charity.

Figures 2.1, 2.8, 2.18, 2.22, 7.5, 7.10, 8.2, 8.6, 9.6, 9.7, 9.8, 9.10, 9.11,
9.12, 9.13, 9.19, 9.25, 9.27, 10.6, 10.9, 10.10, 14.5, 14.10, 14.11, 14.12,
14.13, 14.14, 14.17, 15.2, 15.12 and 15.20 were drawn by S.J. Elmhurst
BA Hons (www.livingart.org.uk) and are printed with her permission.

Figures 5.1, 5.12, 5.13 and 5.14 were drawn by Vicki Martin and are
printed with her permission.

A catalogue record for this book is available from the British Library.

ISBN-10 0 905214 86 2
ISBN-13 978 0 905214 86 3

The publishers and contributors cannot take responsibility for information
provided on dosages and methods of application of drugs mentioned in
this publication. Details of this kind must be verified by individual users
from the appropriate literature.

Typeset by: Fusion Design, Wareham, Dorset, UK
Printed by: Replika Press Pvt. Ltd, India

# Other titles in the BSAVA Manuals series:

*Manual of Advanced Veterinary Nursing*
*Manual of Canine & Feline Abdominal Surgery*
*Manual of Canine & Feline Behavioural Medicine*
*Manual of Canine & Feline Clinical Pathology*
*Manual of Canine & Feline Dentistry*
*Manual of Canine & Feline Emergency and Critical Care*
*Manual of Canine & Feline Endocrinology*
*Manual of Canine & Feline Gastroenterology*
*Manual of Canine & Feline Haematology and Transfusion Medicine*
*Manual of Canine & Feline Head, Neck and Thoracic Surgery*
*Manual of Canine & Feline Infectious Diseases*
*Manual of Canine & Feline Musculoskeletal Disorders*
*Manual of Canine & Feline Nephrology and Urology*
*Manual of Canine & Feline Neurology*
*Manual of Canine & Feline Wound Management and Reconstruction*
*Manual of Canine & Feline Oncology*
*Manual of Exotic Pets*
*Manual of Ornamental Fish*
*Manual of Psittacine Birds*
*Manual of Rabbit Medicine and Surgery*
*Manual of Raptors, Pigeons and Waterfowl*
*Manual of Reptiles*
*Manual of Small Animal Anaesthesia and Analgesia*
*Manual of Small Animal Cardiorespiratory Medicine and Surgery*
*Manual of Small Animal Dermatology*
*Manual of Small Animal Diagnostic Imaging*
*Manual of Small Animal Fracture Repair and Management*
*Manual of Small Animal Ophthalmology*
*Manual of Small Animal Reproduction and Neonatology*
*Manual of Veterinary Care*
*Manual of Veterinary Nursing*
*Manual of Wildlife Casualties*

**Forthcoming titles:**
*Manual of Canine & Feline Abdominal Imaging*
*Manual of Canine & Feline Thoracic Imaging*

For information on these and all BSAVA publications please visit our website: www.bsava.com

# Contents

# Contributors

**Graeme Allan** BVSc MVSc MRCVS FACVSc DipACVR
Veterinary Imaging Associates, PO Box 1041, Newtown, NSW 2042, Australia

**Frances Barr** MA VetMB PhD DVR DipECVDI MRCVS
Division of Companion Animals, University of Bristol, Langford House, Langford, Bristol BS40 5DU, UK

**Darryl N. Biery** DVM DipACVR (honorary DipECVDI)
1141 Mews Lane, West Chester, PA 19382, USA

**Steven J. Butterworth** MA VetMB CertVR DSAO MRCVS RCVS
Weighbridge Referrals, Kemys Way, Swansea Enterprise Park, Swansea SA6 8QF, Wales

**Eithne J. Comerford** MVB PhD CertVR CertSAS MRCVS
Division of Companion Animals, University of Bristol, Langford House, Langford, Bristol BS40 5DU, UK

**Jeremy V. Davies** BVetMed PhD DVR DipECVS DipECVDI MRCVS
Davies Veterinary Specialists, Manor Farm Business Park, Higham Gobion, Herts SG5 3HR, UK

**Ruth Dennis** MA VetMB DVR DipECVDI MRCVS
Centre for Small Animal Studies, Animal Health Trust, Lanwades Park, Kentford, Newmarket, Suffolk CB8 7UU, UK

**Ingrid Gielen** DVM MSc PhD
Department of Medical Imaging, Faculty of Veterinary Medicine, Ghent University, Salisburylaan 133, 9820 Merelbeke, Belgium

**Christopher R. Lamb** MA VetMB DipACVR DipECVDI MRCVS ILTM
Department of Veterinary Clinical Sciences, The Royal Veterinary College, University of London, Hawkshead Lane, North Mymms, Herts AL9 7TA, UK

**Johann Lang** Dr.habil Dr.med.vet DipECVDI
Division of Clinical Radiology, Department of Clinical Veterinary Medicine, University of Bern, Länggassstrasse 128, Postfach, CH-3001 Bern, Switzerland

**Robert M. Kirberger** BVSc MMedVet(Rad) DipECVDI
Diagnostic Imaging Section, Department of Companion Animal Clinical Studies, Faculty of Veterinary Science, University of Pretoria, Private Bag X04, Onderstepoort 0110, South Africa

**Hester McAllister** MVB DVR DipECVDI MRCVS
Department of Veterinary Science, Faculty of Veterinary Medicine, University College Dublin, Belfield, Dublin 4, Republic of Ireland

**Fintan J. McEvoy** MVB PhD DVR DipECVDI MRCVS

Department of Small Animal Clinical Sciences, Royal Veterinary and Agricultural University, Dyrlaegevej 32, Frederiksberg C, Copenhagen, DK-1870, Denmark

**Robert G. Nicoll** BSc(Vet) BVSc DipACVR

Veterinary Imaging Associates, PO Box 1041, Newtown, NSW 2042, Australia

**Gerhard Steenkamp** BSc BVSc MRCVS

Department of Companion Animal Clinical Studies, Faculty of Veterinary Science, University of Pretoria, Private Bag X04, Onderstepoort 0110, South Africa

**Emma Tobin** MVB MVM CVR DipECVDI

Department of Veterinary Science, Faculty of Veterinary Medicine, University College Dublin, Belfield, Dublin 4, Republic of Ireland

**Henri van Bree** DVM PhD DipECVDI DipECVS

Department of Medical Imaging, Faculty of Veterinary Medicine, Ghent University, Salisburylaan 133, 9820 Merelbeke, Belgium

# Foreword

This *BSAVA Manual of Canine and Feline Musculoskeletal Imaging* marks another new venture for the BSAVA and its hugely popular Manual series. One of the first BSAVA Manuals was the *Manual of Small Animal Diagnostic Imaging* and although it remains a necessity for any practice, it became clear that any improvements and expansion were impossible to contain within one book. As a consequence this manual and its sister manuals on thoracic and abdominal imaging have been devised.

Like all BSAVA Manuals, this book provides an invaluable source of information for those in general veterinary practice where radiographs are taken on a daily basis. However, as advancements have been made in other imaging techniques, they too are included. The Manual layout is easy to follow and is complemented by clear illustrations and radiographs. The reader will easily find advice on how to obtain the best radiographs possible, how to recognize the various radiological features of disease, and when to consider alternate imaging techniques.

Without exception, the authors are renowned in their field, and the use of both specialist imagers and orthopaedic surgeons lends a unique clinical insight into imaging. The editors and authors have produced a manual that will undoubtedly be in every practice and used almost every day. Congratulations to all those involved – the editors, authors and the BSAVA Publications team!

**Carmel T. Mooney MVB MPhil PhD DipECVIM-CA MRCVS**
**BSAVA President 2005–2006**

# Preface

'The rise, the progress, the setting of imagery should, like the sun, come natural to him'

**Keats**

The original *BSAVA Manual of Small Animal Diagnostic Imaging*, edited by Professor Robin Lee, has for many years been an invaluable source of information for veterinary undergraduates as well as an important presence on the practice bookshelf. However, diagnostic imaging has rapidly developed and expanded over the last 10–20 years. Ultrasonography as an imaging modality has been available for some years, but as technology improves and the body of experience and knowledge grows, the range of potential applications widens. CT and MR are advanced cross-sectional imaging modalities which the general public are increasingly aware of, and thus we all need to be aware of the situations in which such modalities may be usefully applied. Despite the explosion in 'other imaging modalities', radiography remains as the day to day diagnostic imaging modality of choice in many practices. It became clear to us that the original concept of the *BSAVA Manual of Small Animal Diagnostic Imaging* should be retained – but expanded and improved upon. As the amount of knowledge is vast it could not all be accommodated into one manual, thus the concept of the *BSAVA Manual of Canine and Feline Musculoskeletal Imaging* was born, to be followed in due course by its sister manuals of Thoracic Imaging and Abdominal Imaging. Current small animal imaging textbooks tend to either include horse radiology or vast amounts of ultrasonography. These BSAVA manuals will be ideal for those practitioners who do not have an interest in all the species or differing imaging modalities. It also prevents the practitioner having to buy a text that includes the thorax or abdomen if he/she rarely makes radiographs of these body regions.

This manual is extremely practical to use being structured along anatomical lines, with chapters considering each joint, the long bones and the skull and spine. There are additional general chapters considering the soft tissues, bone and joints which are common to all regions of the musculoskeletal system. We have concentrated on radiography and radiology. It is of vital importance that radiographs are of good technical quality so as to maximize the diagnostic information available. So each chapter contains sections on radiographic technique, as well as normal radiographic anatomy, before considering the radiological features which may be associated with injury or disease. A vital part of this new BSAVA Manual is the illustrations; we have kept part of the concept of the original manual with clear line drawings, but added a wide range of radiographs to complement the text. Although radiography and radiology are central, each chapter considers alternative imaging techniques and the situations in which they may be particularly useful, in order to guide the reader appropriately when further diagnostic information is needed.

A panel of renowned authors from all over the world have contributed to this manual, making its content internationally applicable. The clinical questions posed by our patients are the same wherever we work! We deliberately chose both specialist imagers and specialist orthopaedic surgeons as contributors, believing that the variation in background and clinical expertise would strengthen the manual. This manual is therefore not only designed for the veterinary undergraduate or general practitioner, either with or without a special interest in diagnostic imaging, but also for the orthopaedic surgeon as well as specialist radiologist.

Finally, as editors, we have enjoyed working on this manual, and we very much hope you find it useful. We are very grateful to all our authors for their hard work and for adhering so well to the timetables set for them. We also thank Samantha Elmhurst for her drawings, and the editorial team at Woodrow House for keeping all of us 'on track'.

**Frances Barr**
**Robert Kirberger**

**December 2005**

# Soft tissues

### Frances Barr

## Indications

Indications for radiography of the peripheral soft tissues of the body are numerous, and may include:

- Localized or diffuse soft tissue swelling
- Atrophy of one or more muscle groups
- Changes in texture of soft tissues on palpation
- Pain on palpation of soft tissues
- One or more discharging sinus tracts.

## Radiography and normal anatomy

### Radiographic technique

Radiographic examination of peripheral soft tissues requires minor modification of the techniques employed to evaluate skeletal structures. Use of a high detail film screen combination allows the production of images of optimal resolution. It is rarely necessary to use a grid except when undertaking radiography of soft tissues exceeding 10 cm or so in thickness (such as the peripheral soft tissues of the thoracic and abdominal cavities, or the soft tissues of the thigh in larger dogs). It is vital to select appropriate exposure factors; too high an exposure will result in 'burning out' of the soft tissues, which become invisible or difficult to see. Use of a spot light to examine these areas of the radiograph may help in evaluation of soft tissues, but it is preferable to reduce the exposure factors so that the soft tissues are clearly seen. It may on occasions be necessary to take more than one radiograph of a region; one for evaluation of soft tissues and one for assessment of skeletal structures.

Having selected appropriate exposure factors, the X-ray beam should be centred on the area of interest and collimated accurately. Careful collimation of the X-ray beam is important since it minimizes the amount of scattered radiation produced, and thus enhances image quality and radiation safety for personnel. It also minimizes the volume of tissue that is irradiated, which improves patient safety.

It is good radiographic practice to take orthogonal views of each area under examination (i.e. two views at 90 degrees to each other) in order to allow accurate localization of any lesion.

The production of the image on a radiograph depends on the differential absorption of X-rays by different tissues. The inherent characteristics of tissue which influence X-ray absorption are:

- Physical thickness
- Density
- Atomic number.

Gas has a low density and so absorbs X-rays poorly. Consequently, areas of gas on an image appear dark grey or black. Bone and other mineralized materials have a high atomic number and therefore absorb X-rays well. Accordingly, mineralized tissues appear pale grey or white on a radiograph. Soft tissues in general have an intermediate atomic number and density, resulting in an intermediate shade of grey on a radiograph. It is very important to recognize, however, that fat and other soft tissues have small, but characteristic, differences in X-ray absorption. Fat is relatively radiolucent in comparison to other soft tissues and thus appears slightly, but noticeably, darker on the X-ray image (Figure 1.1). Fluid and soft tissues other than fat have a very similar radiopacity. It is not therefore usually possible to distinguish between adjacent soft tissue or fluid structures unless they are outlined by fat, gas or mineralized material, or contrast techniques are used.

It can sometimes be helpful to take radiographs of the contralateral limb in order to compare the soft tissues of the normal and affected limb.

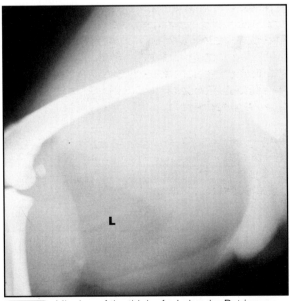

**1.1** ML view of the thigh of a Labrador Retriever. A relatively radiolucent mass (L) is a lipoma.

## Contrast studies

### Sinography and fistulography

Sinography is indicated when a discharging sinus is present and it is considered to be important to establish the extent and direction of the sinus tract(s) within the soft tissues. The technique may also be used to delineate foreign material within, or at the source of, the sinus tracts. Less commonly, the technique is applied to the investigation of a fistulous tract, to determine the direction and termination of the tract. There is often confusion between the terms 'sinus' and 'fistula':

- A sinus is defined as a tract leading from a focus of infection to a hollow organ or the body surface (typical of foreign body reactions)
- A fistula leads from a hollow organ or body cavity to another hollow organ or body cavity, or to the body surface.

In general, any water-soluble, iodinated contrast medium may be used, although the ionic forms tend to be more irritant than the non-ionic forms. If there is any possibility that the tract communicates with the epidural or subarachnoid space, it is important to use a non-ionic contrast medium. A narrow gauge catheter is inserted into the opening of the sinus or fistula, and held securely in place by a purse string suture. Alternatively, a small balloon catheter may be used. The patient is positioned for radiography, and the X-ray tube appropriately centred and collimated. The contrast medium is then injected through the catheter until resistance is felt, or until a sufficient volume has been introduced to delineate the tract, and a radiograph taken immediately. The patient is then repositioned for the orthogonal view, and a little more contrast medium injected before taking the second radiograph (Figure 1.2).

Interpretation of the resulting radiographs must be undertaken with caution. The contrast medium may not demonstrate the full extent of the network of tracts. In addition, filling defects in the contrast medium due to air bubbles or purulent debris may mimic foreign material. Ultrasonography has now replaced sinography

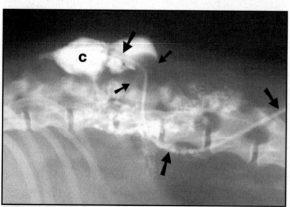

**1.2** Sinogram of a Shih Tzu with a discharging tract in the thoracolumbar region. Small arrows indicate the air-filled balloon of the catheter, whilst the larger arrows show the catheter filled with contrast medium. Contrast medium (C) fills a large subcutaneous cavity dorsal to L1 and L2, with extension of contrast medium into tracts ventrally and caudally.

in many cases since it may be used to localize pockets of fluid and, in many cases, to identify and localize a foreign body. However, sinography remains superior to ultrasonography in demonstrating the precise direction and termination of tracts.

### Lymphangiography

Lymphangiography is rarely used in veterinary medicine, but may occasionally be considered in the investigation of lymphoedema. Subcutaneous injection of methylene blue distal to the site of interest should result in uptake by the lymphatic vessels, which can then be identified and cannulated in large dogs. Water-soluble iodinated contrast medium can then be injected directly into the lymphatic vessels and radiographs of the region taken.

### Peripheral angiography

Selective or non-selective angiography can be performed. Selective angiography involves catheterization of an appropriate artery or vein close to the suspected lesion, followed by the injection of a bolus of water-soluble iodinated contrast medium. Non-selective angiography entails the injection of a bolus of contrast medium into a peripheral vein remote from the lesion and relying on the circulation to distribute the contrast medium around the body. Selective techniques are technically more demanding but tend to produce excellent vascular opacification in the region under investigation.

Radiographs are normally taken towards the end of the injection of contrast medium, so it is important to pay due regard to radiation safety. The person injecting the contrast medium should stand as far from the primary X-ray beam as possible, using extension tubing to facilitate this, and wear appropriate protective clothing.

The indications for peripheral angiography include any situation in which it is important to define the arterial supply or venous drainage of a mass or an extremity. If the vessels do not fill as expected, this may be due to traumatic disruption, or occlusion by thrombi, adhesions, ligatures or neoplasm. However, it is important also to consider potential technical problems, which may include injection of an inadequate volume of contrast medium, spillage of contrast from the catheter, or taking the radiograph too soon or too long after the completion of injection.

## Alternative imaging techniques

### Ultrasonography

Ultrasonography is now increasingly widely used in the evaluation of peripheral soft tissues. It allows differentiation between fluid and soft tissue, and demonstrates the internal architecture of soft tissues. High frequency transducers enable excellent image resolution. Doppler techniques may be used to show the direction, nature and velocity of blood flow in a region, and power Doppler can demonstrate overall perfusion of a tissue or organ by highlighting smaller blood vessels. Detailed consideration of soft tissue ultrasonography is beyond the scope of this book but common applications are:

- Ultrasonography may be used to evaluate the larger tendons; e.g. the tendon of origin of the biceps, and the Achilles tendon (see Chapters 7 and 11). The normal tendon is echogenic, with an orderly striated appearance in longitudinal section and a stippled appearance in transverse section. Disturbances in the normal orderly arrangement of fibres due to partial or complete tears, together with hypoechoic patches due to haemorrhage, inflammation or granulation tissue, provide evidence of tendon damage (Figure 1.3)
- Muscles are relatively hypoechoic when compared with the tendon, but also have a striated appearance provided by the bundles of muscle fibres and intervening fibrous tissue. Disruption of this pattern is indicative of disease or injury
- Ultrasonography can provide useful information about peripheral masses, including the presence or otherwise of fluid-filled foci, the vascularity of the tissue, and the invasion of adjacent structures

- Foreign material can be very difficult to locate in peripheral soft tissues. Radiographs can, of course, demonstrate radiopaque foreign bodies (e.g. bullets, teeth, some types of glass). However, many foreign bodies are vegetable in nature and of very similar opacity to soft tissues. Ultrasonography can often be used to find these; foreign material tends to be echogenic, often casts an acoustic shadow and may be surrounded by a variable amount of fluid. Ultrasound-guided retrieval of foreign material with forceps may be possible
- Ultrasound-guided aspiration or biopsy of soft tissues is widely used. It might be argued that ultrasound guidance is superfluous when the tissue involved is superficial and often palpable. However, ultrasound guidance can be very helpful in locating small pockets of fluid for aspiration or drainage, avoiding necrotic foci within large masses and thus obtaining a useful tissue sample, and avoiding major blood vessels.

## Magnetic resonance imaging and computed tomography

Magnetic resonance imaging (MRI) and computed tomography (CT) are not yet widely used for evaluation of peripheral soft tissues in small animals. There are potential applications, including the assessment of the extent of a neoplasm for the purposes of treatment planning, detailed evaluation of periarticular soft tissues, or the detection of occult lesions (e.g. small brachial plexus tumours).

## Abnormal radiological findings

### Changes in soft tissue mass

#### Diffuse increase
A diffuse increase in the thickness of soft tissues may be difficult to appreciate without comparison with the normal contralateral limb. When the thickened tissues are of a homogenous soft tissue radiopacity, this may be due to subcutaneous administration of fluids, oedema, lymphoedema, cellulitis or infiltrative neoplasia.

Thickening due to muscular hypertrophy may be distinguished from other causes of diffuse thickening since small amounts of fat in the fascial planes delineate the muscle bellies. Muscular hypertrophy is usually a response to exercise, but the uncommon condition of feline hypertrophic muscular dystrophy leads to progressive muscular hypertrophy.

A diffuse increase in the mass of the soft tissues due to subcutaneous fat deposition results in a characteristic radiographic appearance; a layer of relatively radiolucent fat lies between the skin and the muscle.

Increased thickness of soft tissues due to subcutaneous emphysema is also readily recognized, since radiolucent accumulations of gas separate the skin from the underlying fat/muscle, and may dissect along fascial planes (Figure 1.4).

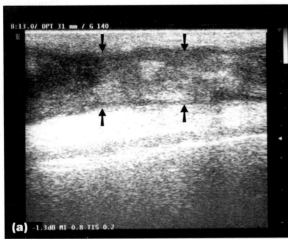
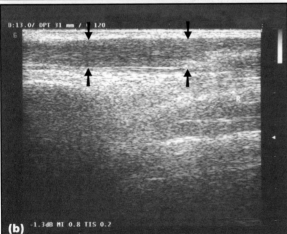

**1.3** **(a)** The left damaged Achilles tendon of a 6-year-old Border Collie is thickened, irregular in outline and shows marked heterogeneity of echogenicity. No normal fibre alignment is apparent. **(b)** The normal right Achilles tendon in the same dog shows orderly fibre arrangement. Arrows indicate the margins of each tendon.

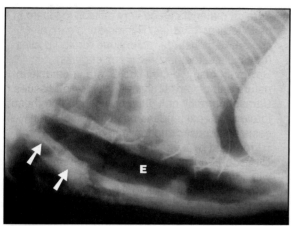

**1.4** Lateral view of the thorax of a cat that has been attacked by a dog. There is extensive subcutaneous emphysema ventrally (E) and two sternebrae have been avulsed cranioventrally (arrowed).

### Localized increase

Any mass (e.g. neoplasm, abscess, cyst, granuloma, seroma, haematoma) may result in a localized thickening of soft tissues (Figure 1.5). Less commonly, arteriovenous anomalies produce a mass, comprising a network of abnormal vessels. Small focal accumulations of gas within a mass may indicate an abscess, or a previous needle aspiration or surgical procedure. Areas of mineralization within the mass are less helpful discriminatory features since these may be found in chronic abscesses, resolving haematomas, granulomas and in neoplasms.

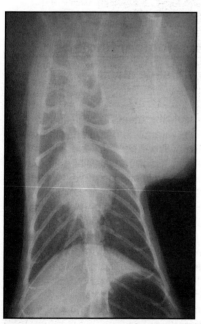

**1.5** DV view of the thorax of a cat with an axillary fibrosarcoma.

### Decrease

A decrease in the thickness of soft tissues is usually due to muscle atrophy. Atrophy may arise due to disuse, may be neurogenic in origin, or may occur as a long term sequel to myositis. Weight loss may, of course, also result in decreased soft tissue thickness due to loss of subcutaneous fat, and later muscle.

## Changes in soft tissue radiopacity

### Artefacts

It is important to recognize artefacts so that they can be distinguished from pathological changes. Common artefactual causes of increased radiopacity include the following:

- Skin folds, such as in the inguinal and axillary regions, result in linear increases in radiopacity (Figure 1.6). Skin folds may be exaggerated in certain breeds of dog, such as the Bulldog or Shar Pei
- Nipples result in rounded areas of increased radiopacity overlying the ventral abdominal and thoracic walls, while the prepuce produces an elongated region of increased radiopacity overlying the caudoventral abdomen
- Skin or subcutaneous nodules of any nature may result in a focal increase in radiopacity. If noted on a radiograph, it is helpful to check the patient for a corresponding superficial nodule. Such nodules become visible radiographically only if they are surrounded by air to provide contrast, and so are less likely to be visible if situated on the dependent side
- Wet hair from blood, saliva or other fluids results in streaks of increased radiopacity overlying the patient. A similar effect may be seen if the patient is lying on wet bedding
- Dirt in the hair coat, between the digits, or in a wound results in streaky or focal increases in radiopacity
- Iodine-containing scrubs and washes cause a marked increase in radiopacity of the skin surface and should be avoided prior to radiography. Similarly, spillage of contrast medium on to the hair coat will produce radiopaque streaks.

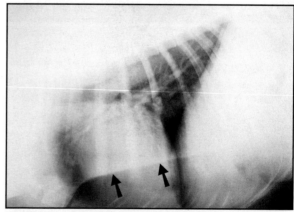

**1.6** Lateral view of the thorax of a dog. The arrows indicate an axillary skin fold.

### Calcification

Regions of calcification have increased radiopacity in comparison to the surrounding soft tissues. The site and pattern of calcification may help to distinguish the cause in some instances, but in other cases the finding is non-specific.

*Calcinosis circumscripta:* Calcinosis circumscripta, also known as tumoral calcinosis, results in focal deposition of calcium within the soft tissues. It is a condition of unknown aetiology, which is usually seen in young (<2 years of age) large-breed dogs, especially the German Shepherd Dog. The lesions are usually solitary and well marginated, with a characteristic radiographic appearance of stippled calcification (Figures 1.7 and 1.8). The lesions may be found in any soft tissue but particularly in the distal limbs, over prominences in the limbs, in the neck or in the tongue. Boston Terriers and Boxers are predisposed to lesions in the cheek and pinna, respectively. Larger masses may suffer mechanical damage but otherwise the condition is rarely of clinical significance.

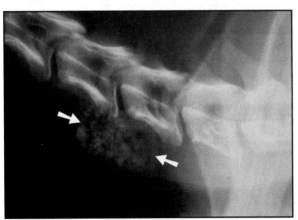

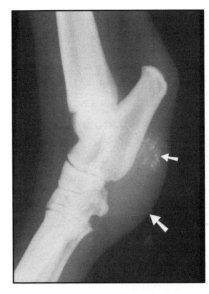

**1.9** ML view of the hock of a cross bred dog. There is a soft tissue swelling on the plantar aspect of the hock (large arrow) with speckled mineralization in the proximal part (small arrow). This proved to be a granuloma.

**1.7** Lateral view of the neck of a German Shepherd Dog. There is a region of stippled mineralization due to calcinosis circumscripta (arrowed) ventral to vertebrae C4 and C5.

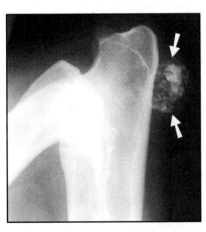

**1.8** ML view of the elbow of a German Shepherd Dog with calcinosis circumscripta caudal to the olecranon (arrowed).

*Metastatic mineralization:* Metastatic mineralization occurs in normal tissues as a result of a systemic disturbance in calcium or phosphorus levels. Mineralization of the footpads and of the walls of peripheral blood vessels, for example, has been described in animals with chronic renal disease. Soft tissue mineralization or ossification (see below) has also been reported in association with hypervitaminosis A (Figure 1.10) and hypervitaminosis D.

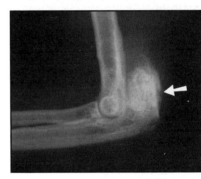

**1.10** ML view of the elbow of a cat with hypervitaminosis A. Note the extensive mineralization of soft tissues in the region of insertion of the triceps (arrowed).

*Chondrocalcinosis:* Synonyms for this condition include pseudogout and calcium pyrophosphate deposition disease (CPDD). This is a rare condition of older animals, with an unknown aetiology that produces mineral deposits within or around the joints.

### Ossification

Ossification within the soft tissues also results in an increase in radiopacity, but may be distinguished from calcification by the presence of a clear trabecular structure in ossified material. Clearly, fracture fragments are a common explanation for ossified structures in the soft tissues. These may be dispersed from a major long bone fracture, or may be fragments that have avulsed with an attached tendon or ligament. There are also situations where abnormal ossification occurs within soft tissues.

*Calcinosis cutis:* Calcinosis cutis produces granular deposits of calcified material within the skin and/or linear streaks of calcification in the subcutaneous fascial planes. It most commonly occurs in dogs with hyperadrenocorticism (canine Cushing's syndrome), but has been reported also in animals with primary or secondary hyperparathyroidism.

*Dystrophic mineralization:* Dystrophic mineralization occurs within necrotic or chronically inflamed tissues, and so may be seen within neoplasms, abscesses or granulomas (Figure 1.9). Resolving haematomas may also mineralize.

*Myositis ossificans:* Myositis ossificans is a benign condition in which bone forms within striated muscle (Figure 1.11). Ossification within muscle and tendon

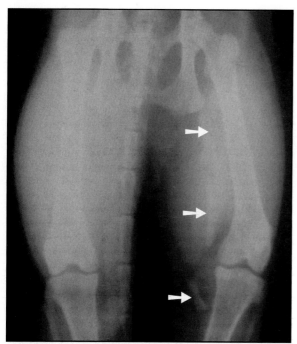

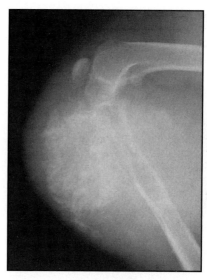

1.12 ML view of the stifle in a Cairn Terrier. There is a large swelling distal to the stifle joint, which is partly soft tissue and partly disorganized abnormal bone. The proximal tibia shows evidence of bone lysis. Histology confirmed that this mass was an osteosarcoma.

1.11 VD view of the pelvis and femurs of a 3-year-old Domestic Short-haired cat with progressive pelvic limb stiffness due to myositis ossificans. The arrows indicate orderly ossification in the soft tissues medial to the left femur and proximal tibia. Note that there is atrophy of the muscles of the left thigh.

after major injury is recognized in both humans and animals. However, myositis ossificans can also occur secondary to chronic disease, or may be idiopathic.

***Fibrodysplasia ossificans:*** Fibrodysplasia ossificans is a rare, progressive condition in cats in which multiple symmetrical formations of bone are seen in the soft tissues. Unlike myositis ossificans, the bone displaces muscle but does not actually involve it.

***Extraskeletal osteosarcomas:*** These are uncommon malignant neoplasms in small animals. Histologically they have a uniform sarcomatous appearance but they produce malignant osteoid or bone, although they are not of osseous origin. Not all extraskeletal osteosarcomas, however, will show radiographic evidence of calcification or ossification. Extraskeletal osteosarcomas have been reported at numerous soft tissue sites, including the limbs and thoracic and abdominal organs.

Radiological detection of ossified material in peripheral soft tissues may also occur in other neoplasms, including primary (Figure 1.12) and metastatic osteosarcoma, and other sarcomas (see Chapter 4).

### Other increases in radiopacity
Microchips (or identichips) are readily recognized as small, well defined, radiopaque capsules. They are usually located in the subcutaneous tissues of the neck or dorsal thorax, but may migrate to other locations.

Surgical implants, including staples, wire and many other orthopaedic implants, have a metallic radiopacity and are thus easily detected radiographically. Foreign bodies are visible radiologically if they are more radiopaque than the surrounding soft tissues.

Thus, metallic or mineralized foreign material (Figure 1.13) is generally visible, and some types of glass may be seen. Vegetable matter is not usually apparent on survey radiographs unless outlined by gas or contrast medium.

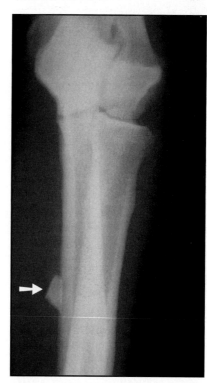

1.13 CrMCdLO view of the elbow and antebrachium of a Labrador Retriever. The arrow shows a rounded, radiopaque object; it was confirmed to be a tooth within a bite wound.

### Decreases in radiopacity

***Fat:*** As already mentioned, fat has a reduced radiopacity compared to other soft tissues. An animal in good body condition will have a thin layer of subcutaneous fat and a little fat within the fascial planes (Figure 1.14). In an obese animal this fat deposition is increased.

A localized mass of fat radiopacity is likely to be a lipoma, or less commonly, a liposarcoma. These may be seen in a subcutaneous location or between muscle bellies (particularly in the thigh) (see Figure 1.1).

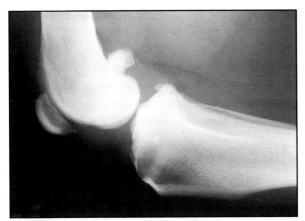

**1.14** ML view of the stifle joint of a Rottweiler. A small quantity of fat highlights the fascial plane just caudal to the joint.

*Gas:* Small bubbles of gas within the soft tissues are suggestive of a puncture wound, previous injection or aspiration, or, rarely, infection with gas-forming organisms (Figure 1.15). Larger accumulations of gas may be seen with extensive wounds, tearing of the pharynx, trachea or oesophagus, or penetration of the thoracic wall (see Figure 1.4). Where gas seems to be contained within tubular structures a hernia or rupture with prolapse of gastrointestinal tract into the soft tissues must be considered.

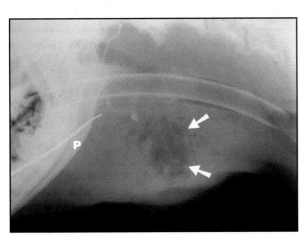

**1.15** Lateral view of the neck of a Labrador Retriever. There is a soft tissue swelling in the ventral pharyngeal region containing gas bubbles (arrowed). A metallic probe (P) shows the position of an oral wound and tract. This proved to be an abscess.

### Fascial planes
The fascial planes within peripheral soft tissues are usually visible due to small amounts of fat (see Figure 1.14). They may become displaced if there is any localized increase or decrease in mass within the soft tissues.

Obliteration of the fascial planes may occur as a result of subcutaneous fluid administration, oedema, lymphoedema, cellulitis or an infiltrative neoplasm. However, it should be remembered that technical imperfections in the radiograph may also obscure fascial planes (e.g. poor selection of exposure factors, movement blur, X-ray film processing faults).

## Changes on sinography/fistulography
When a single tract is present it is usually possible to determine the direction of the tract and its termination. When a network of tracts is present it is more difficult to achieve complete filling of the tracts due to occlusion by purulent material, necrotic debris, fibrous tissue or foreign material. Furthermore, the contrast medium will tend to follow the path of least resistance and may dissect along fascial planes rather than follow the tracts. Given these limitations it is still usually possible to establish the general direction and extent of the network, which will help in surgical planning.

Filling defects within tracts may be caused by foreign material, but also by purulent or necrotic material and air bubbles. It helps to look for a geometric or angular shape delineated by contrast medium (Figure 1.16) as air bubbles and debris often produce small, rounded or irregular filling defects.

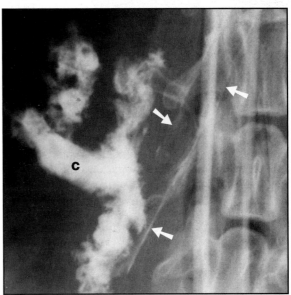

**1.16** Sinogram of a dog with a discharging sinus on the right side of the neck. There is a large subcutaneous accumulation of contrast medium (C) and streaks of contrast medium outline a stick foreign body (arrowed).

## Changes on peripheral angiography

### Arteriovenous fistulae
Arteriovenous fistulae are vascular abnormalities in which there is a direct communication between an adjacent artery and vein, thus bypassing the capillary circulation. These may be small and clinically insignificant, or result in large pulsating masses with serious haemodynamic sequelae. Acquired arteriovenous fistulae usually result from a penetrating wound or blunt trauma, but may also develop secondary to an irritant, infection or infiltrating neoplasia. Acquired fistulae are usually solitary, often large and clinically significant. Arteriovenous fistulae may also be congenital.

Either selective or non-selective angiography is essential to confirm the presence and extent of an arteriovenous malformation. A complex network of distended and tortuous vessels confirms the presence of a vascular malformation (Figure 1.17).

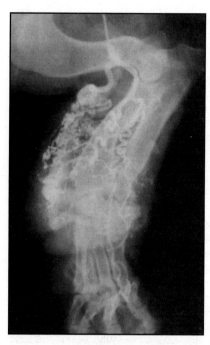

**1.17**

ML view of the forelimb of a Basset Hound. A tortuous network of blood vessels outlined by contrast medium indicates an arteriovenous malformation.

### Vascular occlusion

Partial or complete occlusion of an artery or vein can be demonstrated by peripheral angiography. Occlusion may be due to traumatic disruption of the vessel, external compression (e.g. adhesions, ligature, mass) or an intraluminal mass (e.g. thrombus, neoplastic invasion). If the occlusion is chronic in nature then angiography may demonstrate a network of secondary collateral vessels.

### Vascular supply to masses

It may be important to determine the vascular supply of masses to facilitate treatment planning. Ultrasonography is usually used to assess overall perfusion of a mass but the number and location of major arterial branches supplying a mass may be evaluated angiographically.

## References and further reading

Aron DN, Rowland GN and Barber DL (1985) Report of an unusual case of ectopic ossification and review of the literature. *Journal of the American Animal Hospital Association* **21**, 819–829

Bouyad H, Feeney DA, Lipowitz AJ, Levine SH and Hayden DW (1987) Peripheral acquired arteriovenous fistula: a report of 4 cases and literature review. *Journal of the American Animal Hospital Association* **23**, 205–211

Kuntz CA, Dernell WS, Powers BE and Withrow S (1998) Extraskeletal osteosarcomas in dogs: 14 cases. *Journal of the American Animal Hospital Association* **34**, 26–30

Lamb CR, White RN and McEvoy FJ (1994) Sinography in the investigation of draining tracts in small animals: retrospective review of 25 cases. *Veterinary Surgery* **23**, 129–134

Norris AM, Pallet L and Wilcock B (1980) Generalised myositis ossificans in a cat. *Journal of the American Animal Hospital Association* **16**, 659–663

Scott DW and Buerger RG (1988) Idiopathic calcinosis circumscripta in the dog: a retrospective analysis of 130 cases. *Journal of the American Animal Hospital Association* **24**, 651–658

Warren HB and Carpenter JC (1984) Fibrodysplasia ossificans in three cats. *Veterinary Pathology* **21**, 485–499

# 2

# Bones – general

## Robert M. Kirberger

### Normal bone formation and anatomy

Bone is a dynamic organ that is constantly being renewed and remodelled. It is responsive to mechanical stimuli and to metabolic, nutritional and endocrine influences. It acts as a storage reservoir for calcium, phosphorus and other minerals as well as haemopoietic tissue. Bone is relatively light with a high tensile and compressive strength but with some elasticity.

The bone surface, except where there is articular cartilage, is covered by the periosteum. The periosteum consists of an outer fairly vascular connective tissue layer, which is attached to the underlying cortex by collagenous Sharpey fibres. The inner surface of the cortex is lined by endosteum, which is also made up of connective tissue. Between these two layers and the underlying cortical bone is a layer of osteoprogenitor cells and osteoblasts that are required for osteogenesis.

A long bone can be divided into several regions. The shaft, or diaphysis, has a distinct cortex and medulla (Figure 2.1). The cortex is made up of compact bone and should have smooth outer (periosteal) and inner (endosteal) surfaces, and should remain approximately even in thickness. A clearly defined channel may be seen running at an angle through the cortex, usually from the periosteal surface proximally to the endosteal surface distally (although this direction is reversed in the ulna). This is the nutrient foramen which provides passage for the blood vessels going to and from the medulla. The nutrient foramina are most commonly seen in the long bones of larger dog breeds and must not be mistaken for incomplete fractures. The central medullary cavity has a reduced opacity compared to the cortex, although still usually greater than that of surrounding soft tissues. Towards the end of each long bone is the metaphysis. The distinction between the cortex and medulla becomes less clear here due to thinning of the cortices and a clear trabecular pattern of cancellous bone becomes visible. The main function of the cancellous bone is to support the subarticular bone and transmit mechanical forces to the diaphyseal cortex. Each end of the long bone is termed the epiphysis and has an articular

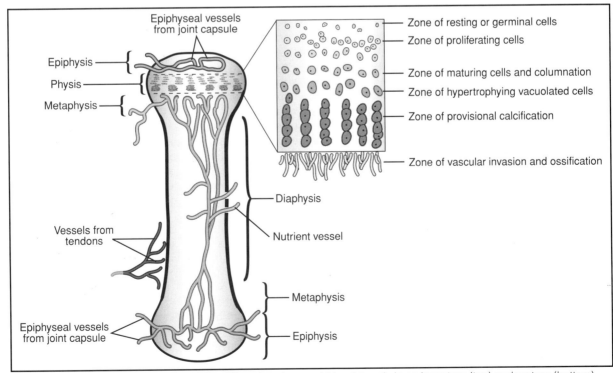

**2.1** Schematic representation of the different regions and blood supply in an immature (top) and mature (bottom) long bone.

surface consisting of subchondral bone covered with cartilage. The latter is radiolucent and thus not visible on radiographs. Between the epiphysis and metaphysis is the physis, or growth plate. In the immature animal the growth plate is active and appears radiographically as a radiolucent band. As the animal matures the physis disappears, although a faint radiopaque line, the physeal scar, may remain visible at the site (for physeal closure times see Chapter 3). Besides long and flat bones there are also short and irregular bones that have a cortex of compact bone with a central cancellous bone component.

Most of the bones of the skeleton start off as cartilage, which is converted to bone by endochondral ossification until in the adult only articular cartilage remains. Flat bones, particularly those of the skull, are formed by intramembranous bone directly from connective tissue. Bone development starts *in utero* with the development of midshaft hyaline cartilage centres, which undergo endochondral ossification to form ossification centres. These are surrounded by perichondral bone, the first compact bone in the fetus. At birth the trabecular bone of the ossification centres has all been resorbed and replaced by bone marrow. However, peripherally in the metaphyseal region the lattice-like trabeculation remains. The physis is responsible for the growth in length of the bone towards the diaphysis. The growth plate has distinct zones characterized by alterations in chondrocyte morphology (see Figure 2.1). Chondrocytes start as resting cells, which then proliferate and mature forming columns. Here the cells hypertrophy, vacuolate and then undergo provisional calcification. Blood vessels and osteoprogenitor cells invade the calcified longitudinal septa and the osteoprogenitor cells differentiate into osteoblasts, which then lay down the bone matrix (osteoid). As the bone matures the osteoid becomes mineralized. Osteoid formation decreases with time and the osteoblasts become entrapped in the new bone to become osteocytes. Osteocytes form the majority of cells in mature compact bone and are interconnected by canaliculi and Volkmann's canals to form the osteon or Haversian system. Osteoclasts are large multinucleated cells that are responsible for bone resorption by eroding mineralized bone. Bone formation and resorption are regulated systemically by parathyroid hormone, calcitonin and vitamin D (see Chapter 3).

At predetermined times after birth secondary ossification centres develop in the epiphyses. The articular cartilage contributes to the growth of the epiphyses by endochondral ossification. There may be additional non-articular protuberances, which form sites of attachment for tendons and ligaments. These secondary centres of ossification are termed apophyses; in the young animal (Figure 2.2) they are separated from the main diaphysis or metaphysis by a radiolucent cartilaginous band but fuse in the mature animal.

Blood supply to bones varies with the type of bone. In the immature long bone the physis is essentially avascular with the epiphysis and metaphysis supplied independently. Epiphyseal blood supply is mainly via the joint capsule and metaphyseal blood comes via the vessels passing through the nutrient foramen (see

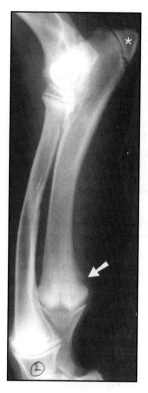

**2.2** ML view of a large-breed dog immature radius and ulna. Note the cutback zone of the distal ulnar metaphysis (arrowed) and the olecranon apophysis (✶).

Figure 2.1). Both vessels send branches towards the physis with the metaphysis being particularly blood rich, making it the preferred location for haematogenous osteomyelitis in the immature animal. The vertebral body can also be considered as a long bone with a central nutrient foramen in the mid-body and numerous smaller vessels supplying the epiphyseal region. The neural arch is a flat bone and, like other flat bones, has an extensive blood supply via numerous small nutrient foramina.

Periosteal blood supply is extensive in immature bones to accommodate the intramembranous bone formation, which increases cortical bone thickness. However, in mature skeletal bone periosteal blood supply is vestigial; blood supply is mainly via the nutrient artery as well as via the metaphyseal arteries, which anastomose with the nutrient artery. This medullary blood supplies the full thickness of the cortex except at sites of fascial attachments where the outer third of the cortex can be supplied by arterioles entering by way of the fascial attachments. Medullary blood supply to the cortex is normally centrifugal with cortical venous drainage taking place via the periosteum and medullary drainage via the nutrient foramen.

Modelling of bone is the process of moulding the bone to its final shape and occurs particularly in growing bones. In the metaphysis the wide physeal region is modelled to the narrower diaphyseal bone by means of active subperiosteal osteoclastic activity. This results in a 'cutback zone', which is often quite irregular and must not be mistaken for pathology (see Figure 2.2). Remodelling of bone is the constant process of bone renewal by resorption and formation of new bone at endosteal and periosteal surfaces as well as at the osteonal surface. In pathological conditions an imbalance occurs between bone resorption and formation.

## Alternative imaging techniques

For information on alternative imaging techniques see Chapters 3 and 4.

## Abnormal radiological findings

Bone has limited response mechanisms when subjected to pathological processes. Bone alignment or length may be altered. More commonly there may be a break in the continuity of the bone (see Chapter 5) or bone mass may be increased or decreased.

### Classification of pathology
Lesion distribution within the skeleton may be:

- Monostotic – involving a single bone (such as an osteosarcoma)
- Polyostotic – multiple bones are involved (as seen with multiple myeloma or haematogenous osteomyelitis; Figure 2.3)
- Focal – may involve a specific bone region (e.g. metaphysis)
- Generalized – involving all bones (as may be seen with metabolic conditions)
- Symmetrical (as may be seen with metaphyseal osteopathy)
- Asymmetrical (as seen with a traumatic premature physeal closure).

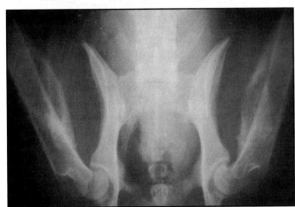

**2.3** Polyostotic bone pathology involving both femoral shafts due to haematogenous fungal osteomyelitis.

Predilection sites for various conditions are common and may be a specific bone or a region within that bone. Some examples are:

- Hypertrophic osteopathy results in periosteal reactions starting distally in the limbs and then extending proximally (see Chapter 4)
- Panosteitis affects the medulla of long bones, often starting in the region of the nutrient foramen (see Chapter 3)
- Growth abnormalities are often most marked at those physes that contribute greatest to the overall length of a bone and the distal radius and ulna will thus be affected first (see Chapter 3)

- Osteosarcoma favours the metaphyseal region of bone due to the good blood supply and high metabolic activity of these regions. Specific bones are more commonly involved and include the distal radius and proximal humerus (see Chapter 4)
- Prostatic neoplasia may metastasize to the caudal lumbar vertebrae (see Chapter 16).

### Aggressive *versus* non-aggressive changes
The exact aetiology of specific radiological changes can rarely be determined from a radiograph alone. However, the type of lesion may assist in shortening the list of differential diagnoses. This is typically done by determining the aggressiveness of a lesion. An aggressive lesion is one with rapid bony change where there is minimal time for the bone to respond and remodel. A non-aggressive lesion is a benign, slow growing, more chronic process with time for bone to remodel. In between these two extremes lies a wide variety of possible radiological changes. Aggressiveness can be characterized by evaluating new bone production, bone loss or destruction, cortical changes and the rate at which change takes place.

#### New bone production
Increased bone opacity may be:

- Artefactual – due to superimposition of structures. This could be one bone abnormally superimposing on another (e.g. often seen with fractures, Figure 2.4) or a superficial soft tissue structure superimposing on bone (e.g. a teat superimposing on the wing of the ileum on a ventrodorsal (VD) abdominal view)
- Real – due to new bone production originating in the medulla, trabecula, endosteum or in the

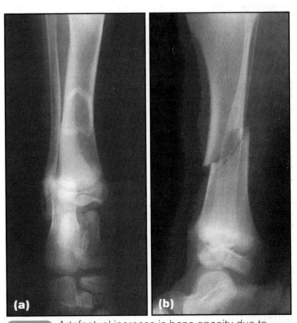

**2.4** Artefactual increase in bone opacity due to superimposition of fracture ends. **(a)** CrCd view of the tibia with two transverse lines of increased opacity in the tibial diaphysis. **(b)** ML view shows slight overriding of the tibia fracture edges.

periosteum individually or together. This may be monostotic or polyostotic. Generalized increased opacity is rare but is seen with osteopetrosis (see Chapter 3).

According to Dobson and Friedman (2002) the radiographic features of localized new bone production in the medullary cavity (osteosclerosis) are dependent upon the nature of the matrix within which mineralization occurs. The matrix may be composed of osteoid, fibrous or cartilaginous tissue. An ivory-like opacity is seen with complete mineralization of the osteoid matrix, as is seen in osteomas (Figure 2.5). Osteosarcoma produces osteoid and the amount of mineralization of the osteoid will determine the opacity of the neoplasm (Figure 2.6). A fibrous matrix results in woven bone production. Initially the lesion will be radiolucent but changes to a more ground glass appearance as bone is produced (Figure 2.7). Mineralization of a cartilage matrix has a stippled appearance which, when replaced by endochondral bone, develops circular or semicircular opacities. This process is typically seen in chrondrosarcomas.

Endosteal and medullary osteosclerosis may occur with chronic osteomyelitis, on the margins of an expansile neoplastic process, with panosteitis, bone infarction and neoplastic new bone formation. Bone infarction in dogs may be associated with primary malignant neoplasia,

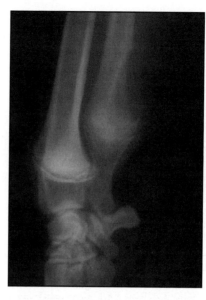

2.7 ML view of a skeletally immature distal radius and ulna with a fibrous cortical defect (ossifying fibroma) of the caudal ulna. The fibrous matrix results in the radiolucent defect which will eventually fill up with bone.

particularly osteosarcoma (see Chapter 4). It has also been described in cats with feline leukaemia. All or most bones distal to the mid-femur are usually affected.

Periosteal new bone formation usually takes place secondary to injury. The reactions are additions to the underlying cortex rather than replacements for it as is seen in shell formation with geographic bone lysis (see below). However, the cortex may also be penetrated by pathological processes originating from the medulla via the enlarged Volkmann canals and Haversian spaces, which may then elevate the periosteum. The periosteal reactions (Figure 2.8) may be classified as continuous or interrupted, which also characterizes their aggressiveness. Types of periosteal reaction, from least to most aggressive, are as follows:

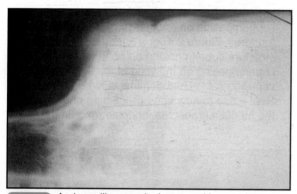

2.5 An ivory-like opacity is seen with complete mineralization of the osteoid matrix as seen in this osteoma of the frontal bone.

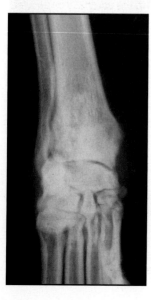

2.6 CrCd view of an early distal radius osteosarcoma. There is mild permeative lysis and early mineralization of the produced osteoid, resulting in patchy areas of increased opacity.

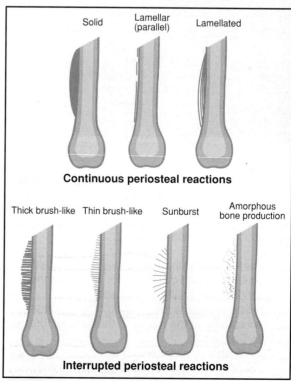

Solid    Lamellar (parallel)    Lamellated

**Continuous periosteal reactions**

Thick brush-like    Thin brush-like    Sunburst    Amorphous bone production

**Interrupted periosteal reactions**

2.8 Schematic representation of periosteal reactions from least to most aggressive.

- Solid periosteal reaction
- Lamellar (parallel) periosteal reaction
- Lamellated periosteal reaction
- Brush-like periosteal reaction
- Sunburst periosteal reaction
- Amorphous bone production.

*Solid periosteal reaction:* The periosteum is slowly lifted over a period of time whilst laying down new bone. A solid periosteal reaction may also develop from a lamellar reaction. The surface may be smooth, undulating or irregular and the opacity of the reaction is indicative of its duration. Solid reactions are indicative of slow growing benign processes (Figure 2.9). Typical causes are fracture callus, chronic osteomyelitis and panosteitis. On the periphery of more aggressive periosteal reactions (see below) the periosteum is lifted more slowly and a triangular solid periosteal reaction is often seen, known as a Codman's triangle. It is usually present on the diaphyseal side of a metaphyseal lesion and acts as a buttress for the cortex which may have been partially or totally destroyed adjacent to it. It is often associated with malignant neoplasia but may also be seen with a variety of other causes.

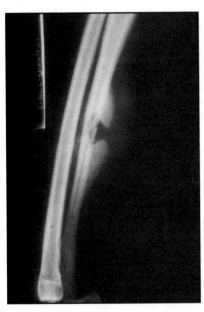

**2.9**

Focal anaerobic osteomyelitis of the caudal ulna with a solid periosteal reaction.

*Lamellar (parallel) periosteal reaction:* The periosteum is lifted by subperiosteal exudate, haematoma or rarely neoplastic cells. The periosteum produces new bone which is seen as a continuous straight or undulating thin line (Figure 2.10). With time the radiolucent space between the thin line and cortex becomes filled with new bone resulting in a solid periosteal reaction. The reaction is usually associated with a benign process.

*Lamellated periosteal reaction:* This reaction is also known as an onion skin periosteal reaction and indicates a fairly slow process but it is more aggressive than the above two reactions. The periosteum is lifted repeatedly over a period of time by sequential insults. The reaction may be seen with osteomyelitis, particularly that of fungal origin, as well as with malignant neoplasia (Figure 2.11).

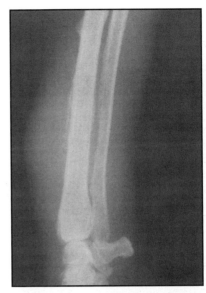

**2.10**

Focal soft tissue swelling and lamellar periosteal reaction cranially on the radius. Radiograph deliberately underexposed.

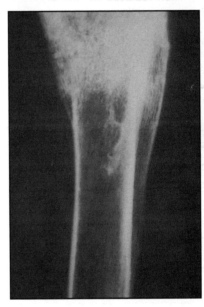

**2.11**

Post-mortem specimen of a proximal femur with fungal osteomyelitis, resulting in a lamellated periosteal reaction.

*Brush-like periosteal reaction:* The periosteum is lifted fairly rapidly over an extensive area of the cortex with osteoblastic activity along the vertically orientated Sharpey's fibres. If the reaction is less aggressive and slower growing, the spicules are thicker and it is known as a thick brush-like or palisade periosteal reaction (Figure 2.12). The thinner the reaction (thin brush-like or spiculated periosteal reaction) the more aggressive the process as there is less time for new bone production. This is more likely to be seen in neoplasia and acute haematogenous osteomyelitis but may also be seen in hypertrophic osteopathy (Figure 2.13).

*Sunburst periosteal reaction:* This reaction is indicative of a highly aggressive process and an osteosarcoma is the most likely cause although other neoplasms may also be involved occasionally. The periosteum is lifted rapidly over a focal area resulting in a dome shape. The Sharpey fibres now have a radiating distribution with the osteoblastic activity along the radiating fibres. Some of the new bone produced may also be neoplastic in origin (Figure 2.14).

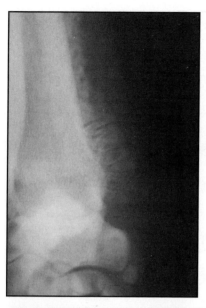

**2.12** Thick brush-like periosteal reaction on the medial surface of the distal radius.

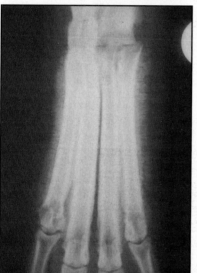

**2.13** Thin brush-like periosteal reaction of the digits in a case of hypertrophic osteopathy.

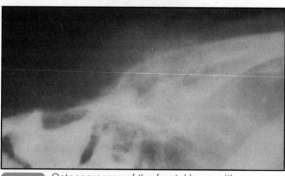

**2.14** Osteosarcoma of the frontal bone with a sunburst periosteal reaction.

***Amorphous bone production:*** This is not a periosteal reaction but neoplastic new bone production seen best beyond the confines of the periosteum which has been destroyed. The amorphous bone may also be more centrally located but is then difficult to distinguish as such. The new bone may have a cotton wool or candyfloss appearance. Amorphous bone is highly suggestive of an osteosarcoma (Figure 2.15).

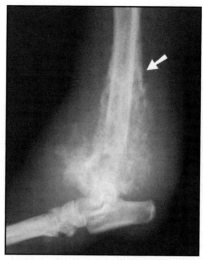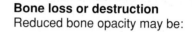

**2.15** Distal tibial osteosarcoma with amorphous bone formation seen cranially and caudally to the tibial shaft. A poorly mineralized Codman's triangle is seen proximally on the caudal cortex (arrowed).

### Bone loss or destruction

Reduced bone opacity may be:

- Artefactual due to:
  - Superimposition of gas
  - Superimposition of a defect in the superficial soft tissues
  - A focal reduction in soft tissue thickness, e.g. distolateral radius (Figure 2.16)
  - Mach effect, which is a curious physiological phenomenon whereby the perception of edges is enhanced through exaggeration of local contrast (Grandage, 1976). Mach lines are optical illusions which mimic hairline fractures where two bones overlap. This is most commonly seen in extremity radiographs that have high contrast. Typical locations are the superimposing tibia and fibula as well as the metacarpal and metatarsal bones.
- Real due to generalized or focal bone loss.

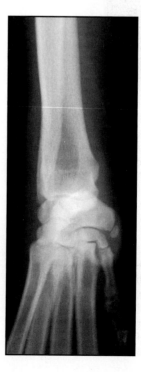

**2.16** CrCd view of the distal radius of a dog with an elongated radiolucency in the distolateral radius adjacent to the ulna, which correlates to the soft tissue depression seen in this region.

Increased osteoclast activity, stimulated by a pathological process (pressure and hyperaemia), results in bone destruction. This becomes radiologically visible only after 30–50% of bone is lost. This process will usually take 7–10 days and the only radiological evidence of possible pathology in this period may be soft tissue changes (see Chapter 1).

A generalized decrease in bone radiopacity is known as osteopenia and is due to a reduction in bone mass. This may be due to osteoporosis or osteomalacia. Osteoporosis is bone atrophy and implies there is less bone than normal but the bone composition is normal. The number of trabeculae will be decreased and the remainder appear coarser and the cortex thinned. This may affect a single bone or limb (e.g. a fracture (Figure 2.17) or primary bone neoplasm resulting in disuse atrophy), or involve the whole skeleton where metabolic disease is more likely. Osteomalacia is a decrease in bone mass with concomitant disturbance in bone composition with insufficient or abnormal osteoid mineralization. Osteomalacia may affect the entire skeleton and is usually also of metabolic origin (see Chapter 3).

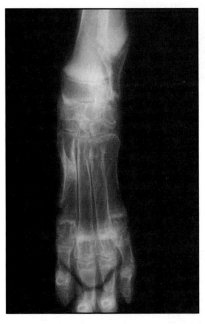

**2.17** Disuse osteoporosis of the pes.

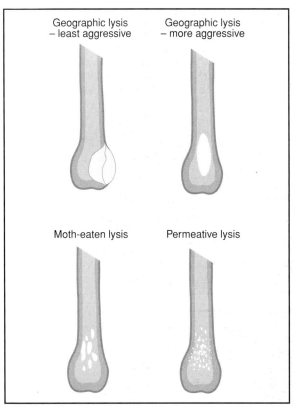

**2.18** Graphic representation of focal bone destruction from least to most aggressive.

Geographic lysis – least aggressive

Geographic lysis – more aggressive

Moth-eaten lysis

Permeative lysis

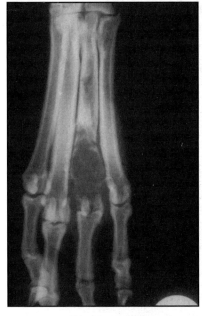

**2.19** Geographic bone lysis of the distal fourth metatarsal bone. Note also the cortical thinning and expansion.

Focal bone loss involves cancellous or cortical bone but is more readily seen in the latter due to the greater contrast. Lysis is a result of increased osteoclastic activity secondary to the pathological insult. Focal bone destruction may be classified (Figure 2.18) as follows:

- Geographic lysis
- Moth-eaten lysis
- Permeative lysis.

***Geographic bone lysis:*** Geographic bone lysis is the least aggressive form of lysis and is generally seen with slower growing lesions. It is usually seen in cancellous bone at the extremities and consists of a single or several large radiolucent areas, cortical expansion and thinning (Figure 2.19). There is usually a sclerotic rim and possibly sclerotic septa, as seen in osteoclastomas and enchondromas. If there is no sclerotic rim and the margin is well defined the lesion is more aggressive and known as a 'punched out' lesion. This is typically seen in multiple myeloma and metastatic bone disease (Figure 2.20). The margin of the lytic area is narrow and the transitional zone between affected and normal tissue is also narrow. A slightly wider and more indistinct margin is an indication of a more rapidly growing and thus more aggressive lesion that is locally infiltrative, such as a fibrosarcoma.

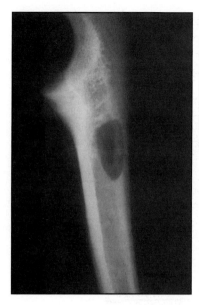

**2.20**
Post-mortem specimen of a metastatic haemangiosarcoma lesion in the ulna showing geographic bone lysis with no sclerotic zone.

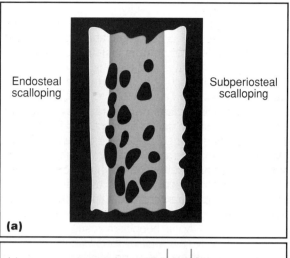

**(a)**

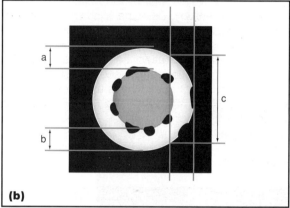

**(b)**

***Moth-eaten bone lysis:*** There are multiple separate foci of lysis, usually a bit larger than 2–3 mm in diameter, with more ill defined and wider margins than geographic bone lysis (Figure 2.21). These are typically seen in the cortex because of greater contrast and are usually endosteal in origin (Figure 2.22). These lesions have intermediate aggressiveness and may be accompanied by visible cortical destruction. The transitional zone between affected and non-affected bone is fairly wide. The lytic areas may eventually coalesce.

***Permeative bone lysis:*** Permeative lysis is the most aggressive form of bone lysis and is seen with rapidly growing lesions. Numerous 1–2 mm diameter lytic areas with poorly defined borders are seen in the cortex and there is a wide indistinct transitional zone (Figure 2.23). Permeative lysis is often associated with cortical scalloping or defects (see below). Osteolytic osteosarcomas and haematogenous osteomyelitis are likely to show permeative lysis.

**2.22** Schematic representation of lysis location in cortical bone destruction (e.g. moth-eaten or permeative) and scalloping. **(a)** Lateral projection of a long bone diaphysis. The lytic areas appear to be in the medulla but are in the superimposed cortex. **(b)** Cross-section of the bone in (a). The lytic areas are actually in the cortex but are superimposed on the medulla. Bear in mind that opacity is influenced by tissue thickness. Thus, as distances a and b combined are about half the distance of c (radiologically seen cortex) they appear relatively radiolucent on the lateral view.

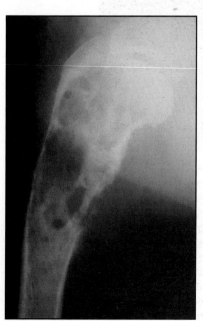

**2.21**
Moth-eaten lysis of the proximal humerus. Endosteal scalloping of the cranial cortex is also seen.

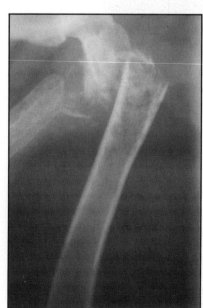

**2.23**
ML view of a proximal femur with an osteosarcoma and pathological fracture secondary to the permeative bone lysis.

## Cortical changes

Cortical changes may also be indicative of the aggressiveness of a lesion. Slow growing processes tend to expand the cortex whilst more rapid changes will erode or destroy the cortex.

*Cortical expansion:* Geographic bone lysis is often seen with an associated expanding cortex that may also be thinned. The expansion results from endosteal resorption due to pressure from an impinging growth or hyperaemia, and is accompanied by periosteal new bone formation (see Figure 2.19). Eventually the whole cortex may be destroyed with only a shell of periosteal new bone remaining. The shell may be thick, thin or lobulated, which indicates a focal variation in growth rate.

*Cortical scalloping:* These are focal erosions of the cortex due to moth-eaten or permeative lysis. Intramedullary neoplasia results in endosteal scalloping, which destroys more and more of the cortex towards the centre of the neoplasm (see Figures 2.21, 2.22 and 2.23). Subperiosteal scalloping is usually associated with haematogenous osteomyelitis where the exudate oozes from the medulla through the Volkmann's canals to the subperiosteum, which is elevated, and stimulates osteoclasts to resorb bone subperiosteally (see Figures 2.22 and 2.24).

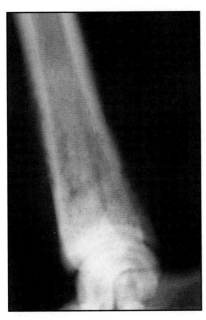

**2.24** Close-up ML view of the distal tibia with mild permeative lysis and marked subperiosteal scalloping of the cranial cortex indicative of osteomyelitis.

*Cortical defects:* Endosteal scalloping may eventually result in a cortical defect which often is associated with a cortical spike (Figure 2.25). This is a sign of a highly aggressive lesion. Cortical defects may also occur with chronic osteomyelitis due to cloaca formation. Here the cortical edges are rounded indicative of a less aggressive and chronic lesion (Figure 2.26).

## Rate of change

Non-aggressive changes will show no or minimal changes on follow-up radiographs taken 10–14 days later, whereas aggressive lesions are likely to show

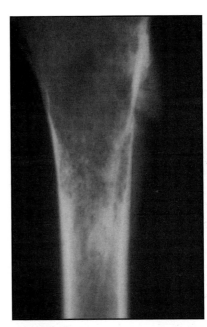

**2.25** Close-up view of a post-mortem specimen of the femur showing endosteal scalloping resulting in a cortical spike proximally. Permeative lysis and a sunburst periosteal reaction are also present.

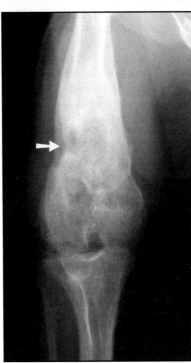

**2.26** CrCd view of a distal femur with chronic osteomyelitis. Note the radiolucent cloaca with a cortical defect with rounded edges (arrowed). A solid periosteal reaction is also present more proximally.

progressing radiological changes. Thoracic radiographs to look for metastasis may also assist in deciding whether a skeletal lesion is a malignant neoplasm.

## Interpreting bone radiographs

A quiet environment, light boxes that can mask peripheral light, and a room that can be darkened are all conducive to optimal radiographic interpretation. A bright light is useful to evaluate overexposed parts of the film and a magnifying glass will assist with evaluation of subtle trabecular patterns and periosteal reactions. An atlas of normal anatomy, radiographs of normal contralateral limbs and a collection of radiographs from normal dogs and cats will all assist in interpreting questionable changes and normal variants.

| Characteristic | Non-aggressive | | | Aggressive |
|---|---|---|---|---|
| Bone destruction | Geographic | Moth-eaten | | Permeative |
| Periosteal reaction | Solid    Lamellar | Lamellated    Thick brush-like | Thin brush-like | Sunburst    Amorphous |
| Edge of lytic focus | Well demarcated & sclerotic margin | Well demarcated | | Poorly defined |
| Transition from lytic region to normal bone | Narrow transition zone | Intermediate | | Wide transition zone |
| Cortical destruction | None to cortical thinning and expansion | Rounded cortical defects | | Cortical spikes accompanied by endosteal or subperiosteal scalloping |
| Rate of change after 10–14 days | None | Mild | | Marked |

**2.27** Range of possible changes to judge whether bone pathology is aggressive or non-aggressive.

The systematic evaluation of a radiograph is essential to optimize recognition of radiological abnormalities. This should include evaluation of the following:

- Radiographic quality and positioning, which needs to be optimal to ensure that maximum information will be obtained from the radiograph
- General bone alignment, shape and length
- Soft tissues surrounding the bone
- Periosteum for new bone formation
- Cortex for lysis and defects
- Endosteum for new bone production
- Medulla and associated cancellous bone for lysis or new bone production or both
- Joints, including the associated soft tissues, the articular cartilage (radiolucent) and subchondral bone
- Physes in skeletally immature patients.

The pathology is described by means of Roentgen signs (size, shape, number, location, margination and radiopacity). This is followed by ascertaining the aggressiveness of the lesion or lesions by integrating the lytic, periosteal and cortical changes described above. Often a range of changes will be present and the most aggressive of these must be used to classify the disease process. Figure 2.27 illustrates how the changes can be integrated.

Finally a list of differential diagnoses in order of probability is composed. Patient signalment, clinical abnormalities and results from ancillary diagnostic techniques are then considered to formulate the most likely diagnosis. A bone biopsy may be required to confirm this diagnosis.

## Differentiating neoplasia from osteomyelitis

For information on how to differentiate neoplasia from osteomyelitits see Chapter 4.

## References and further reading

Dennis R, Kirberger RM, Wrigley RH and Barr FJ (2001) Appendicular skeleton. In: *Handbook of Small Animal Radiological Differential Diagnosis* pp. 1–8. WB Saunders, London
Dobson H and Friedman L (2002) Radiologic interpretation of bone. In: *Bone in Clinical Orthopedics*, 2nd edn, ed. G Sumner-Smith, pp. 175–204. Thieme, Stuttgart
Grandage J (1976) Interpretation of bone radiographs: some hazards for the unwary. *Australian Veterinary Journal* **52**, 305–311
Madewel JE, Ragsdale BD and Sweet DE (1981) Radiologic and pathologic analysis of solitary bone lesions Part I: Internal margins. *Radiologic Clinics of North America* **19**, 715–748
Olsson S-E and Ekman S (2002) Morphology and physiology of the growth cartilage under normal and pathologic conditions. In: *Bone in Clinical Orthopedics*, 2nd edn, ed. G Sumner-Smith, pp. 175–204. Thieme, Stuttgart
Ragsdale BD, Madewel JE and Sweet DE (1981) Radiologic and pathologic analysis of solitary bone lesions Part II: Periosteal reactions. *Radiologic Clinics of North America* **19**, 749–783
Summerlee AJS (2002) Bone formation and development. In: *Bone in Clinical Orthopedics*, 2nd edn, ed. G Sumner-Smith, pp. 1–21. Thieme, Stuttgart
Wilson JW (2002) Blood supply to developing, mature and healing bone. In: *Bone in Clinical Orthopedics*, 2nd edn, ed. G Sumner-Smith, pp. 23–43. Thieme, Stuttgart
Wrigley RH (2000) Malignant versus non-malignant bone disease. *Veterinary Clinics of North America: Small Animal Practice* **30**, 315–347

# 3

# Long bones – juvenile

### Frances Barr

## Indications

Indications for radiography of the long bones are varied and include:

- Pain on palpation of one or more long bones
- Swelling of soft tissues and/or a discharging sinus over a long bone
- Deformity of a long bone or an entire limb
- Trauma
- Evaluation of fracture healing
- Suspected metabolic bone disease
- Suspected systemic disease, which may have skeletal manifestations.

## Radiography and normal anatomy

### Radiographic technique

It is important to take care over radiographic technique in order to achieve images of optimal quality. It is helpful to use a high detail radiographic film/screen combination wherever possible to maximize image resolution. A grid is not necessary in most instances as the volume of tissue involved is not great. However, it is often beneficial to use a grid for radiography of the femur or humerus in larger breed dogs where scattered radiation becomes a significant factor.

As a general rule, the patient should be positioned with the long bone under examination parallel to the X-ray cassette. The X-ray beam should be centred on the region of interest and collimated accurately so that the entire region of interest is included, but no more. Orthogonal projections (i.e. two projections at 90 degrees to each other) are required of each long bone under examination in order to allow full evaluation of the bone and accurate localization of any lesion. It is often useful to take radiographs of the corresponding region of the contralateral limb to allow comparison between limbs. For details of radiographic projections specific to each long bone see Chapter 4.

### Physeal closure

For the normal radiographic anatomy of a long bone see Chapter 2. The approximate ages at which centres of ossification in the long bones become radiographically apparent in dogs and cats are given in Figure 3.1. Physeal closure times vary between species, and even between individuals of the same species. There seems to be more variability in physeal

closure times in the cat than in the dog. Furthermore, physeal closure time has been shown to be delayed in neutered male cats when compared to that of entire cats. One study showed that no physes remained open after 29 months in female cats or entire male cats, while some physes remained open beyond 48 months in neutered males (May *et al.*, 1990). A table of approximate physeal closure times for the long bones of dogs and cats is given in Figure 3.1. For the equivalent data pertaining to the spine and pelvis see Chapters 9 and 15.

### Bone metabolism

In the young growing animal the long bones increase in length by endochondral ossification and increase in diameter by intramembranous ossification. In the normal skeletally mature animal bone production and resorption continues but should remain in balance.

Control of the balance between bone production and resorption is complex. The two hormones primarily involved in maintenance of normal serum calcium levels are parathyroid hormone (PTH) and calcitonin, both of which are secreted by the parathyroid glands. PTH acts on bone to move calcium from skeletal reserves into the extracellular fluids. It does this both by means of the osteocyte–osteoblast pump, which moves calcium from deep within the bone to the surface, and by increased osteoclastic activity leading to bone resorption. Calcitonin acts to inhibit bone resorption stimulated by PTH. The secretion of each of these hormones is influenced largely by serum calcium levels, which in turn are affected by dietary intake and absorption of calcium, and renal excretion of calcium and inorganic phosphorus. Vitamin D is also involved in this process (Figure 3.2). Vitamin D must undergo metabolic activation to 1,25 dihydroxycholecalciferol, first in the liver and then in the kidney. The final stage of metabolic activation of vitamin D in the kidney is partly regulated by serum calcium levels, via PTH, although it may also be influenced by other hormones, including prolactin and oestradiol. In young animals vitamin D is essential for the orderly growth and mineralization of cartilage in the physis, but it is also important in osteoclastic resorption and mobilization of calcium in adults.

Other hormones are also involved in bone metabolism. Glucocorticoids influence serum calcium levels by inhibiting intestinal absorption of calcium and increasing renal excretion of calcium, but also

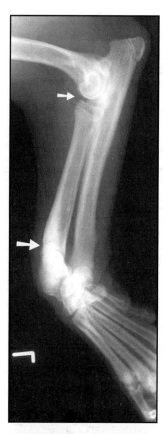

**3.3**

ML view of the antebrachium of a 6-month-old Labrador Retriever with a distal radial physeal disturbance. The humero-radial joint space (small arrow) is widened. There is evidence of an old, healed fracture of the distal radial shaft (large arrow), and the radius distal to this is distorted with no sign of an open physis. There is severe rotation and angulation of the manus.

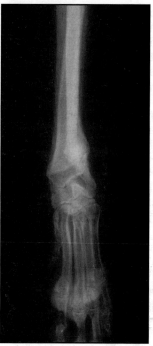

**3.4**

DPa view of the carpus in a cross bred dog with a distal radial physeal disturbance. The distal radial articular surface slopes from proximolateral to distomedial due to asymmetric growth.

- There may be corresponding stretching of the semi-lunar notch of the ulna with widening of the humero-ulnar joint space. Proximal subluxation of the semi-lunar notch of the ulna relative to the humeral condyles and the radial head may be seen. Osteoarthrosis of the elbow joint ensues.
- The distal radial articular surface may have an abnormal slope, leading to angular limb deformity (most commonly carpal varus), but this is variable.

*Ulnar physeal disturbance:*

- The ulna becomes shortened relative to the normal radius (Figure 3.5).
- There may be corresponding distortion and distal subluxation of the semi-lunar notch of the ulna with widening of the humero-ulnar joint space.
- There may be proximal displacement of the ulnar styloid process relative to the accessory carpal bone.
- Non-union of the anconeal process is occasionally seen.
- The radius continues to grow, and as it does the distal diaphysis bows cranially and medially. The caudal cortex of the radius becomes thickened at this point as does the adjacent ulnar cortex.
- Craniomedial subluxation of the distal radius may occur with subsequent development of secondary osteoarthrosis of the radio-carpal joint.
- Lateral deviation, and sometimes also rotation, of the carpus and manus results.

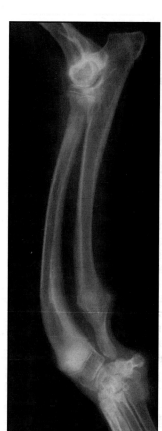

**3.5**

ML view of the antebrachium of a dog with a distal ulnar physeal disturbance. Note the shortening of the ulna with respect to the radius. The radial shaft bows cranially and there is thickening of the caudal cortex. The manus is rotated.

*Other physeal disturbances:* Reduction in growth of the lateral part of the distal femur can lead to a 'genu valgum', or knock-kneed conformation (Figure 3.6), particularly in giant-breed dogs. Premature closure of the proximal tibial growth plate may result in a caudo-distal slope to the tibial plateau with subsequent predisposition to cruciate ligament disease.

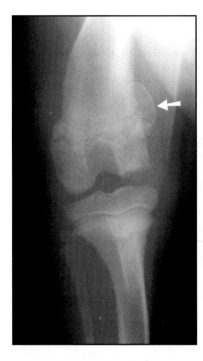

**3.6**

CdCr view of the stifle of a 4-month-old Labrador Retriever kicked by a donkey 1 month previously. There is sloping of the distal femoral articular surface from proximomedial to distolateral, resulting in a varus deformity. The articular surface of the medial condyle is indistinct with ill defined lucency of the subchondral bone. There is associated medial luxation of the patella (arrowed).

## Fractures and avulsions

Fractures and avulsions are considered in Chapter 5 and chapters relating to specific joints.

## Physeal separations

Traumatic separation of the physes is relatively common in immature animals. For further information see Chapter 5.

## Congenital and developmental

### Chondrodysplasia

The term chondrodysplasia covers a large and varied group of conditions, but each involves an abnormality in cartilage development. The epiphyses of the long bones, the vertebral end plates, the physes and metaphyses of the long bones, or any combination of these, may be involved. Radiological features described in association with chondrodysplasias include:

- Slowed growth of long bones, which may appear shorter and thicker than expected
- The physes may appear markedly widened
- There may be retained cartilaginous cores visible in the metaphyseal regions
- Appearance of the secondary centres of ossification in the epiphyses may be delayed
- There may be stippling and distortion of the epiphyses, with later development of secondary osteoarthrosis
- The vertebral end plates may be poorly and irregularly ossified.

It is important to bear in mind that the precise combination of radiological features will vary with the form of chondrodysplasia (some of which are described below). Inherited forms of chondrodysplasia have been described in many breeds of dog (e.g. Alaskan Malamute, Beagle, Bull Terrier, Pointer, Irish Setter, Labrador Retriever, Miniature Poodle, Pyrenean

Mountain Dog, Norwegian Elkhound, Samoyed, Deerhound) and also in cats. Ocular defects have been described in association with the skeletal changes in Labrador Retrievers and Samoyeds. Where the mode of inheritance has been established, a simple autosomal recessive gene is implicated in most cases.

The terminology used in the literature is variable and therefore often confusing. In humans, more than 100 different types of skeletal dysplasia have been described and an internationally recognized system of classification devised. Criteria used for classification include the bones and regions of bones affected, the age of onset, progression, histological features of bone and cartilage, and biochemical characteristics. No such detailed classification currently exists for animals. Some authors in the veterinary literature have therefore used general or descriptive terms for a condition, while others have attempted a match to a corresponding human condition.

The inherited chondrodysplasias described below have been grouped according to the parts of the long bones most prominently affected.

***Epiphyseal:*** Multiple epiphyseal dysplasia has been described in Beagles and Miniature Poodles (Figure 3.7). The main radiological characteristic is the delayed appearance of ossification centres in the epiphyses, which then develop punctate mineralization or 'stippling'. The epiphyses do eventually ossify completely but tend to be deformed in shape so that osteoarthrosis ensues. The bones of the tarsus and carpus, and the vertebrae may also be involved. Riser *et al.* (1980) suggested that the condition in Miniature Poodles should be named pseudoachondroplastic dysplasia, extrapolating from a similar condition in humans, but the term epiphyseal dysplasia is still widely used and is perhaps more descriptive.

An osteochondrodysplasia has been described in Scottish and Highland Fold cats, predominantly affecting the distal limbs and tail. Affected cats show shortening and widening of the epiphyses and metaphyses, and secondary osteoarthrosis (see Chapter 11).

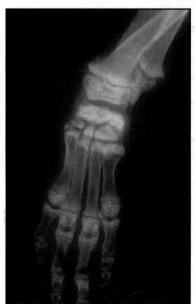

**3.7**

DPa view of the carpus of a Miniature Poodle puppy with epiphyseal dysplasia. Note the stippling of the epiphyses of the long bones and of the carpal bones.

*Physeal:* Enchondrodystrophy in the Pointer leads to disproportionate dwarfism, with female puppies generally more severely affected than males. The first radiological signs are marked widening of the physes. All the physes are affected to some extent, but the most dramatic changes are seen in the distal ulnar, radial and tibial physes. The long bones become shortened and bowed. There is also patchy erosion of articular cartilage with subsequent development of osteoarthrosis. The term enchondrodystrophy is taken from the histopathological description of changes to the cartilage. Similar radiological changes are seen in Alaskan Malamute dwarfism, although articular cartilage erosion and osteoarthrosis is not a feature. Alaskan Malamute dwarfism is also associated with anaemia.

A chondrodysplasia has been described in cats featuring widening of the physes, particularly those of the distal radius, ulna and tibia (Figure 3.8). The long bones are shortened and tend to be bowed.

**3.8**

CrCd view of the antebrachium, carpus and manus of a 5-month-old Domestic Short-haired kitten with a chondrodysplasia. There is marked widening of the distal radial, ulnar and metacarpal physes with metaphyseal flaring, while other visible physes are spared. There is prominent sclerosis on the metaphyseal aspect of each affected physis.

*Metaphyseal:* A chondrodysplasia in the Pyrenean Mountain Dog has been described in which the main radiological abnormalities are seen in the metaphyses of the long bones and in the vertebrae. The metaphyses of all the long bones, but particularly those of the distal radius, ulna, tibia and metacarpals/metatarsals, are widened. Skeletal maturation is delayed but the long bones are nonetheless shortened and bowed. The vertebral end plates are incompletely and irregularly ossified, and the appearance of the secondary ossification centres of the epiphyses may be delayed.

Osteochondrodysplasia in the Deerhound results in short bowed long bones and short vertebral bodies. The physes are irregular in thickness with ragged physeal and metaphyseal junctions. Retained cartilage cores have been seen in the proximal radial and tibial metaphyses. The secondary ossification centres of the epiphyses are present but are often smaller than normal and misshapen. The carpal and tarsal bones may also be small and misshapen.

Oculoskeletal dysplasia in the Labrador Retriever leads to retarded growth of the radius, ulna and tibia, which become shortened and bowed. The distal ulnar

growth plates appear uneven with small retained cartilage cores. There may be delayed development of the epiphyses. Ununited and hypoplastic anconeal and coronoid processes have been described. As the name suggests, there are associated ocular defects. An oculoskeletal dysplasia has also been described in the Samoyed, in which the long bones are shortened and bowed with metaphyseal flaring sometimes evident.

Hypochondroplastic dwarfism in the Irish Setter has been described but the radiological changes are few. The epiphyses, physes and metaphyses appear radiologically normal, but the long bones are shortened with some tendency to bowing of the radius and ulna.

### Osteogenesis imperfecta
This is a rare condition in which the bones are unduly fragile due to a collagen defect. Accordingly multiple fractures, at different stages of healing, may be seen. Skeletal mineralization and physes usually appear radiographically normal. The condition is thought to be inherited, although only small numbers of affected dogs and a single cat have been described in the literature.

### Osteopetrosis
Osteopetrosis is a rare condition in which there is an imbalance in bone turnover. In the congenital form, which is thought to be inherited, there is a decrease in bone resorption, sometimes in combination with accelerated bone formation. Osteopetrosis may also be acquired, but the mechanisms involved are less well understood. Radiologically there is an increase in thickness of cortical bone, which may obliterate the medullary cavity, and an increased opacity of subchondral bone. Despite this increased bone formation pathological fractures may occur. Acquired medullary sclerosis, such as that associated with feline leukaemia virus (FeLV) infection (Figure 3.9) or bone

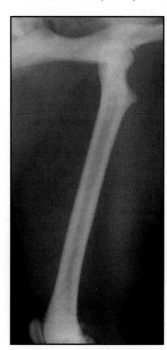

**3.9**

ML view of the femur of a Domestic Short-haired cat with myelosclerosis secondary to FeLV infection. Note the thickening of the femoral cortices and metaphyseal medullary sclerosis.

infarcts (see Chapter 4), may mimic osteopetrosis. There is also progressive diffuse osteosclerosis in Basenjis with anaemia due to erythrocyte pyruvate kinase deficiency.

### Retained endochondral cartilage cores

Retained endochondral cartilage cores are most commonly seen in the distal ulnar metaphyses of young growing dogs, particularly of large or giant breeds, as a 'flame-shaped' radiolucent region with a sclerotic rim (Figure 3.10). Retained cartilage cores are thought to occur most commonly in the distal ulna due to the rapid growth in this region. They may, however, occasionally be found in the distal radius, distal femur or at other sites. The cartilage core usually disappears as the animal matures but remnants may sometimes be seen in the distal diaphyseal region of mature dogs as a mineralized scar.

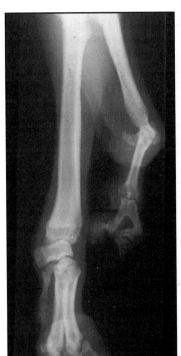

**3.11**
CrCd view of the distal forelimb of an 8-month-old Labrador Retriever with ectrodactyly. The radius and ulna are separated, along with the carpal, metacarpal and phalangeal bones, resulting in a split distal limb. There is radio-carpal bone subluxation and partial metacarpal and phalangeal fusion evident.

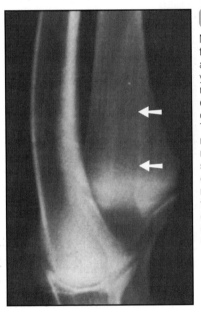

**3.10**
ML view of the distal antebrachium of a young dog with a retained endochondral cartilage core. There is a relatively radiolucent flame-shaped area in the distal ulnar metaphysis with a thin sclerotic rim (arrowed). (Courtesy of M Owen.)

The significance of retained cartilage cores is unclear. They have been associated with physeal disturbances, but equally they may be seen in perfectly normal dogs. It has been suggested that the retained cores in normal rapidly growing dogs have smooth well defined borders, while those associated with growth disturbances tend to have irregular ill defined borders.

### Sporadic anomalies

Other congenital or developmental anomalies of the long bones may occur on a sporadic basis.

***Ectrodactyly:*** The distal forelimb is split, with phalanges, metacarpals and carpal bones divided to become associated with either the distal radius or ulna (Figure 3.11). There may be variable aplasia, hypoplasia or fusion of distal limb bones. This condition is known to be inherited in the cat. It occurs sporadically in the dog with no known breed or sex predisposition.

***Hemimelia:*** One bone of a pair (usually the radius or ulna but occasionally the tibia or fibula) is absent or hypoplastic (Figure 3.12).

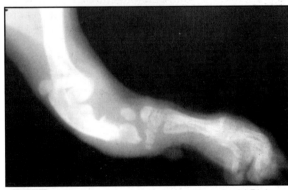

**3.12** ML view of the forelimb of a 9-week-old Bichon Frise puppy with hemimelia. Only a small portion of the distal radius is present, and the ulna is thickened and bowed.

## Infection

### Haematogenous osteomyelitis

Although haematogenous osteomyelitis can occur in animals of any age, it is more common in young animals. Lesions are typically located in the metaphyses of the long bones and are seen at multiple sites (Figure 3.13). Radiological features include:

- Irregular poorly marginated zones of radiolucency in the metaphyses
- Possible associated poorly defined areas of sclerosis
- Soft tissue swelling
- The infection may spread into the diaphysis, resulting in permeative lysis, periosteal new bone formation and subperiosteal scalloping.

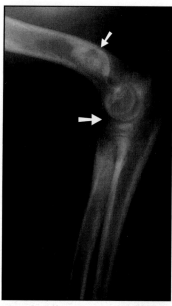

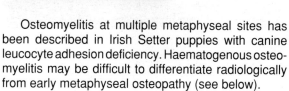

3.13

ML view of the elbow of a young Basenji with systemic *Salmonella* infection and haematogenous osteomyelitis. There is a rounded area of sclerosis in the distal humeral shaft (small arrow) and lysis of the radial head (large arrow) with surrounding sclerosis.

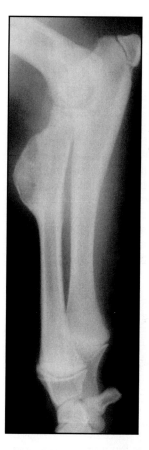

3.14

ML view of the antebrachium in a young Labrador Retriever. There is a smooth broad-based bony lesion on the cranial aspect of the proximal radius, with a relatively radiolucent centre. This proved to be an osteochondroma.

Osteomyelitis at multiple metaphyseal sites has been described in Irish Setter puppies with canine leucocyte adhesion deficiency. Haematogenous osteomyelitis may be difficult to differentiate radiologically from early metaphyseal osteopathy (see below).

### Non-haematogenous osteomyelitis
For information on the radiological features of non-haematogenous osteomyelitis see Chapter 4.

## Neoplasia

### Osteochondroma
Osteochondromas are developmental lesions, which are often considered to be benign neoplasms. They may be single or multiple; multiple neoplasms are also known as multiple cartilaginous exostoses. In dogs the condition is thought to be hereditary. Lesions are typically located in the metaphyseal regions of the long bones or in the flat bones of the ribs, pelvis and vertebrae (see Chapter 16). They usually cease to grow when the dog reaches skeletal maturity, but malignant transformation can occasionally occur. Osteochondromas are often incidental findings, but clinical signs may be seen if the lesion causes compression of adjacent structures (e.g. if located between the radius and ulna). Two radiological forms have been described:

* A smooth bony projection with a wide base and narrower tip. These often have a well defined cortex and medulla, which may be continuous with the cortex and medulla of the parent bone
* An eccentrically located expansion of the bone with a smooth surface and well-defined trabecular pattern (Figure 3.14).

During active growth lesions may appear granular, and may seem separated from the underlying bone due to incomplete ossification. There should be no radiographic evidence of bone destruction or of periosteal new bone formation. In cats, the condition is thought to have a viral aetiology. Lesions may be found in the diaphyseal or metaphyseal regions of long bones, as well as in flat bones. They are less organized in appearance, being poorly defined and irregularly mineralized. Lesions often develop after skeletal maturity and continue to grow.

Osteochondromas may undergo malignant transformation to an osteosarcoma or chondrosarcoma in later life.

### Enchondroma
This is a very rare benign cartilaginous neoplasm, which may be single or multiple. It is characterized by slow expansion within the metaphysis or diaphysis, with thinning of the overlying cortex. Pathological fractures may occur.

### Other neoplasms
For information on the radiological features of other neoplasms see Chapter 4.

## Metabolic disorders
In the normal animal bone production and bone resorption are kept in balance. In metabolic disease this normal balance may be upset, resulting in a shift towards either bone production or, more commonly, towards bone resorption. It is important to recognize when the radiological appearance of the skeletal structures is indicative of a metabolic disturbance to enable the appropriate investigations to be undertaken.

Metabolic bone disease will usually affect the entire skeleton to some extent; however, although some parts of the skeleton may be more severely affected than others, the changes will usually be bilaterally symmetrical. The changes are often more dramatic in young growing animals where bone activity is greater. The physes of the distal radius, ulna and tibia are particularly active so these regions may show radiological changes before other regions. In order to maximize the chance of identifying metabolic bone disease it is important to consider the following:

- **Overall bone opacity.** This will be influenced by technical factors, including exposure factors and film/screen combination. However, the opacity of the bones should usually substantially exceed that of the soft tissues. It is important to bear in mind that 30–50% of bone mineral will have been lost by the time there is a noticeable reduction in radiopacity of skeletal structures
- **Thickness of the cortices of the long bones.** When bone is lost due to metabolic disease there is generally a reduction in thickness of the cortices. There may, additionally, be a 'double cortical line' due to intracortical bone resorption
- **Pathological fractures.** These are common in metabolic bone disease and multiple fractures at varying stages of healing may be seen. Fractures are often folding or compression fractures
- **Physes.** Any increase in thickness of the physes should be noted. There is normally a thin zone of provisional calcification on the metaphyseal side of the physis, which is a fine radiopaque line. This may be absent or interrupted in some instances of metabolic bone disease
- **Metaphyses.** Some irregularity of the margins of the metaphyses is considered normal in young growing dogs, particularly of large breeds. It is important to check for abnormal flaring of the metaphyses, and for changes in the opacity and trabecular structure in this region.

### Nutritional secondary hyperparathyroidism

Nutritional secondary hyperparathyroidism (Figures 3.15 and 3.16) is also termed nutritional osteodystrophy. It is seen in young growing animals, particularly kittens, fed a diet which is low in calcium and/or with an inappropriate calcium:phosphorus ratio. Radiological features may include:

- Reduction in radiopacity of bone so that it approaches the opacity of soft tissues
- Thinning of the cortices of the long bones
- Double cortical line due to intracortical bone resorption
- Multiple folding or compression fractures. Older fractures will show radiographic evidence of healing
- Possible changes in the pelvis and spine (see Chapter 16)
- Radiologically normal physes.

The radiological abnormalities usually resolve once the diet has been corrected but there may be residual bony deformities as a consequence of the fractures.

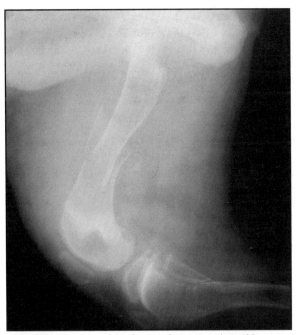

**3.15** ML view of the femur of a young dog with nutritional secondary hyperparathyroidism. Note the thinning of the cortices of the visible long bones, midshaft telescoping femoral fracture and greenstick fracture of the fibula.

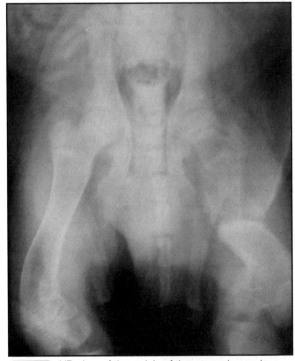

**3.16** VD view of the pelvis of the same dog as in Figure 3.15. Note that the radiopacity of the bones is decreased and approaches that of the surrounding soft tissues. A collapsed pelvic canal is also seen.

### Renal secondary hyperparathyroidism

Renal secondary hyperparathyroidism may occur in an animal of any age as a consequence of chronic renal failure. When seen in immature animals it is usually associated with renal insufficiency due to renal dysplasia. Radiological changes in the long bones are usually similar to those seen in nutritional secondary hyper-parathyroidism, but the most striking abnormalities are often seen in the skull (see Chapter 12). Mineralization of soft tissues may also be seen.

Occasionally renal secondary hyperparathy-roidism gives rise to osteopetrosis rather than osteopenia. The kidneys are important for the final step in the metabolic activation of vitamin D, so renal dysfunction may theoretically lead to signs of vitamin D deficiency (see below). This is not common but has been reported.

### Rickets

Rickets is a rare condition in dogs and cats. It is associated with a deficiency in vitamin D; however, since dogs and cats are able to synthesize vitamin D given adequate exposure to sunlight, dietary defi-ciency is rarely sufficient to cause rickets. An inability to metabolize vitamin D to the active form is more often the explanation, and may be due to congenital defi-ciency of enzymes required for the metabolic pathway, or hepatic or renal disease (see Figure 3.2). Radiologi-cal features include:

- Marked widening of the physes both transversely and longitudinally (Figure 3.17)
- No zone of provisional calcification
- Flaring of the metaphyses with beaked margins
- Since vitamin D influences intestinal absorption of calcium, overall skeletal mineralization may appear reduced and the cortices may be thinned.

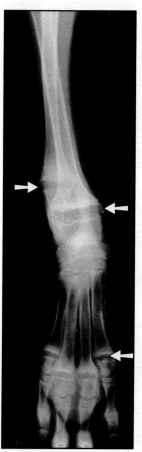

**3.17**

CrCd view of the antebrachium, carpus and manus of a young dog with rickets. There is widening of the physes of the distal radius and ulna, and the distal metacarpi (arrowed), flaring of the metaphyses and marked thinning of the metacarpal cortices.

### Congenital hypothyroidism

Congenital hypothyroidism has been reported in dogs, especially the Boxer, and in cats. It results in disproportionate dwarfism. Radiological findings reported include :

- Delayed and irregular ossification of epiphyses (Figure 3.18)
- Delayed closure of physes
- Thickening of the radial and ulnar cortices with radial bowing
- Subsequent development of secondary osteoarthrosis
- Changes in the skull and spine (see Chapter 16).

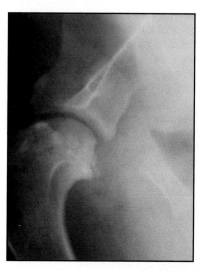

**3.18**

ML view of the shoulder of a 14-month-old Boxer. The caudal proximal humeral epiphysis is incompletely ossified, and the physis is still just visible. The humerus was unusually short. This dog was subsequently shown to be hypothyroid.

Congenital hypothyroidism may be differentiated from the chondrodysplasias by a low serum thyroxine level and a poor response to thyroid-stimulating hormone.

### Pituitary dwarfism

Pituitary dwarfism is seen particularly in young Ger-man Shepherd Dogs and occurs primarily as a result of inadequate GH production, although concurrent hypo-thyroidism may also play a part. Pituitary dwarfism characteristically produces a proportionate dwarfism, which helps to differentiate it from other inherited and metabolic forms of dwarfism described above. Radio-logical features described include:

- Delayed appearance of ossification centres in the epiphyses
- Incomplete ossification of the epiphyses
- Delayed physeal closure.

### Hypervitaminosis A

Hypervitaminosis A is most often recognized in adult cats (see Chapters 8 and 16). Long bone abnormalities have been produced experimentally in puppies and kittens fed a diet with excess vitamin A. Changes described included shortened long bones with prema-ture closure of physes, periosteal proliferation in the metaphyseal region, periarticular osteophytes and pathological fractures.

### Lead poisoning

Lead poisoning in young dogs may result in gastro-intestinal and nervous signs, but radiological changes may also be seen in the long bones. A transverse radiopaque line (2–4 mm thick) is seen in the metaphyseal region of the long bones, particularly in the distal radius and ulna, and the distal metacarpals.

### Mucopolysaccharidoses

This group of metabolic conditions primarily affects cats; dogs are rarely affected. The most striking radiological features are seen in the skull and spine (see Chapters 12 and 16). However, in some forms there is also an epiphyseal dysplasia, leading to secondary osteoarthrosis.

## Miscellaneous

### Bone cyst

Bone cysts are most commonly seen in the long bones of young male large-breed dogs. They have been described most frequently in Dobermanns and German Shepherd Dogs. Bone cysts also occur in cats. They may be located in the diaphysis or the metaphysis, and may affect one (monostotic) or more (polyostotic) bones. The distal radius and ulna are common sites. Bone cysts typically show geographic bone lysis with expansile, relatively radiolucent, lesions with thin cortical margins. There may be thin bony septa visible within the cyst (Figure 3.19). Pathological fractures may occur.

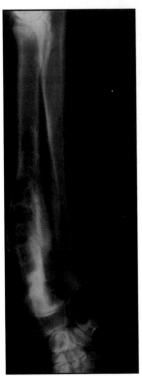

**3.19**

ML view of the antebrachium of a 10-month-old Old English Sheepdog. A multilocular bone cyst is present in the distal radial shaft.

Aneurysmal bone cysts are more often seen in older animals and are associated with a vascular anomaly in the region (see Chapter 4). Osteoclastomas are rare tumours that may mimic a bone cyst. However,

animals suffering from osteoclastoma are generally older than those with a bone cyst. Furthermore, osteoclastomas tend to extend into the epiphysis, while bone cysts are restricted to the metaphysis and diaphysis.

### Panosteitis

Panosteitis is most commonly seen in immature and young adult dogs, particularly male German Shepherd Dogs. However, cases have been described in dogs as old as seven years. Lesions are seen primarily in the medullary cavity of long bones; multiple long bones are commonly affected at different times, most commonly the humerus, radius, ulna and femur. The radiological distribution and appearance of lesions will vary with time, following the shifting and relapsing clinical course of the disease.

- Early lucency around the nutrient foramen is rarely recognized.
- Focal areas of increased opacity within the medullary cavity of long bones; classical 'thumbprint' appearance. These are often near the nutrient foramen (Figure 3.20).
- Opacity may occasionally extend to involve much of the medullary cavity (Figure 3.21).
- Endosteal thickening and irregularity may be noted.
- Occasional smooth solid periosteal reaction, which eventually becomes indistinguishable from the underlying cortex.
- After lesions resolve the medullary cavity may appear unusually empty, with little trabeculation evident. Endosteal roughening and cortical thickening may persist.

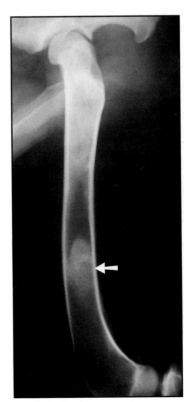

**3.20**

ML view of the femur of a young adult German Shepherd Dog. A focal oval region of increased opacity in the distal femoral shaft (arrowed) is typical of panosteitis. There is a further zone of increased medullary opacity in the proximal femur.

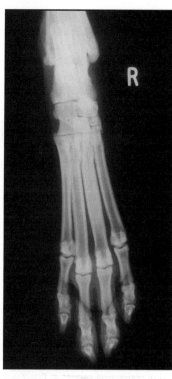

DPl view of the pes of a Mastiff. There is an increased opacity throughout the diaphysis of the third metatarsal due to panosteitis.

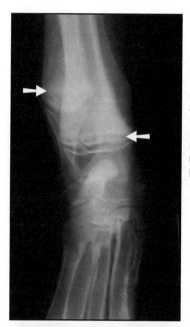

**3.22**

DPa view of the carpus of a 6-month-old German Shepherd Dog with metaphyseal osteopathy. The arrows denote an irregular radiolucent band in the distal radial and ulnar metaphyses, running parallel to the physes.

## Metaphyseal osteopathy

Metaphyseal osteopathy, also known as hypertrophic osteodystrophy, is a condition of unknown aetiology. It has been linked in the past to a deficiency in vitamin C, and hence in older texts may be referred to as 'skeletal scurvy', but this is now known not to be the case. More recent links have been postulated with distemper virus infection. It is seen in young dogs (3–8 months old), often of larger breeds. A predisposition to the condition has been suggested in Great Danes and Weimaraners, but any breed may be affected. Metaphyseal osteopathy presents with acute pyrexia, pain and swelling over the metaphyses of the long bones. Radiological features that may be seen include:

- Soft tissue swelling around the metaphyses
- The earliest feature is an irregular radiolucent line in the metaphyseal region, running parallel to the physis. These changes are most commonly seen in the distal radius and ulna, and the distal tibia, but all long bones may be affected (Figure 3.22)
- Subsequent development of paracortical cuffs of mineralization in the metaphyseal regions. These are linear radiopacities that run parallel to the cortices, but are separated from the cortices by a zone of radiolucency. Their superimposition on the metaphyseal region result in a marked increased metaphyseal opacity (Figure 3.23)
- Eventual uniting of these paracortical cuffs with the cortex, giving the appearance of cortical thickening, which then remodels over time
- Physeal disturbances may be an occasional consequence of metaphyseal osteopathy. This may be due to bridging of the physis by the paracortical cuffs and consequent growth retardation.

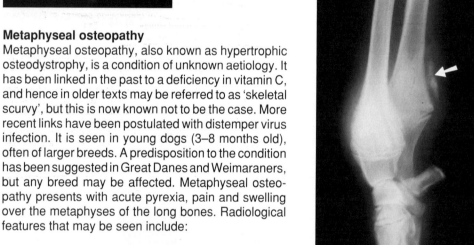

**3.23**

ML view of the carpus of a young Irish Wolfhound with long standing metaphyseal osteopathy. A line of paracortical mineralization is present caudal to the distal ulnar metaphysis (arrowed) and there is roughening of the margins of the distal radial metaphysis indicative of early paracortical mineralization. There is associated increased opacity of the metaphyses. Soft tissue swelling is also present in the region.

In the early stages metaphyseal osteopathy may be difficult to distinguish from haematogenous osteo-myelitis. Once the paracortical cuffs of mineralization develop, a diagnosis of metaphyseal osteopathy can be made with more confidence.

## Craniomandibular osteopathy

Craniomandibular osteopathy affects young dogs, particularly West Highland White, Scottish and Cairn Terriers, although sporadic cases are also seen in other breeds. In West Highland White Terriers the condition has been shown to be inherited as an autosomal recessive gene. The main radiological findings are confined to the skull (see Chapter 12). Occasionally periosteal or paraperiosteal bone formation is seen in the metaphyseal regions, particularly the distal ulna. The metaphyseal lucencies typically associated with metaphyseal osteopathy are not present. This bone formation regresses when the puppy reaches maturity.

### Bone infarction

For information on radiological features of bone infarction see Chapter 4.

### Disuse osteoporosis

Disuse osteoporosis is seen as a consequence of prolonged disuse of a limb. There will be reduced muscle bulk due to atrophy and osteopenia, which starts distally and progresses proximally with time. For further information see Chapter 4.

### Hypertrophic osteopathy

Hypertrophic osteopathy has numerous synonyms, including hypertrophic pulmonary osteoarthropathy and Marie's disease. The skeletal changes generally develop secondary to chronic intrathoracic or, less commonly, abdominal disease. For further information see Chapter 4.

## References and further reading

Bingel SA and Sande RD (1994) Chondrodyplasia in 5 Great Pyrenees. *Journal of the American Veterinary Medical Association* **205**, 845–848

Bohning RH, Suter PF, Hohn RB and Marshall J (1970) Clinical and radiologic survey of canine panosteitis. *Journal of the American Veterinary Medical Association* **156**, 870–883

Breur GJ, Zerbe CA, Slocombe RF, Padgett GA and Braden TD (1989) Clinical, radiographic, pathologic and genetic features of osteochondrodysplasia in Scottish Deerhounds. *Journal of the American Veterinary Medical Association* **195**, 606–612

Carrig CB, MacMillan A, Brundage S, Pool RR and Morgan JP (1977) Retinal dysplasia associated with skeletal abnormalities in Labrador retrievers. *Journal of the American Veterinary Medical Association* **170**, 49–57

Dennis R, Kirberger RM, Wrigley RH and Barr FJ (2001) *Handbook of Small Animal Radiological Differential Diagnosis.* WB Saunders, London

Giger U and Noble NA (1991) Determination of erythrocyte pyruvate kinase deficiency in Basenjis with chronic haemolytic anaemia. *Journal of the American Veterinary Medical Association* **198**, 1755–1761

Gunn-Moore DA, Haggard G, Turner C, Duncan AW and Barr FJ (1996) Unusual metaphyseal disturbance in two kittens. *Journal of Small Animal Practice* **37**, 583–590

Jacobson LS and Kirberger RM (1996) Canine multiple cartilagenous exostosis: unusual manifestations and a review of the literature. *Journal of the American Animal Hospital Association* **32**, 45–51

Johnson KA, Church DB, Barton RJ and Wood AKW (1988) Vitamin-D dependent rickets in a Saint Bernard dog. *Journal of Small Animal Practice* **29**, 657–666

Kramers P, Fluckiger MA, Rahn BA and Cordey J (1988) Osteopetrosis in cats. *Journal of Small Animal Practice* **29**, 153–164

Lamb CR (1990) The double cortical line: a sign of osteopenia. *Journal of Small Animal Practice* **31**, 189–192

May C, Bennett D and Downham DY (1990) Delayed physeal closure associated with castration in cats. *Journal of Small Animal Practice* **32**, 466–467

Morgan JP (1981) *Radiology of skeletal disease – principles of diagnosis in the dog.* Iowa State University Press, Iowa

O'Brien TR, Morgan JP and Suter PF (1971) Epiphyseal plate injury in the dog: a radiographic study of growth disturbance in the forelimb. *Journal of Small Animal Practice* **12**, 19–36

Riser WH, Haskins ME, Jezyk PF and Patterson DF (1980) Pseudoachondroplastic dsyplasia in miniature poodles: clinical, radiologic and pathologic features. *Journal of the American Veterinary Medical Association* **176**, 335–341

Saunders MA and Jezyk PK (1994) The radiographic appearance of canine congenital hypothyroidism; skeletal changes with delayed treatment. *Veterinary Radiology and Ultrasound* **32**, 171–177

Schwarz T, Johnson VS, Voute L and Sullivan M (2004) Bone scintigraphy in the investigation of occult lameness in the dog. *Journal of Small Animal Practice* **45**, 232–237

Smith RN (1968) Appearance of ossification centres in the kitten. *Journal of Small Animal Practice* **9**, 497–511

Smith RN (1969) Fusion of ossification centres in the cat. *Journal of Small Animal Practice* **10**, 523–530

Sumner-Smith G (1966) Observations on epiphyseal fusion of the canine appendicular skeleton. *Journal of Small Animal Practice* **7**, 303–312

Trowald-Wigh G, Ekman S, Hansson K, Hedhammer A and Hard af Segerstad C (2000) Clinical, radiological and pathological features of 12 Irish Setters with canine leucocyte adhesion deficiency. *Journal of Small Animal Practice* **41**, 211–217

Whitbread TJ, Gill JJB and Lewis DG (1983) An inherited enchondrodystrophy in the English Pointer dog. A new disease. *Journal of Small Animal Practice* **24**, 399–411

# 4

# Long bones – mature

## Hester McAllister and Emma Tobin

## Indications

The indications for radiography of the long bones are numerous and include:

- Overt lameness attributed to pain or swelling of a limb on skeletal clinical examination
- Subtle lameness
- Discharging tracts
- Skeletal surveys for metastatic or infectious bone diseases.

Sequential studies are advantageous in:

- Assessing the degree of improvement or deterioration of a disease process
- Healing and callus formation of fractures
- The reassessment of an area that had equivocal initial radiographs.

## Radiography and normal anatomy

For the normal radiographic anatomy of a long bone see Chapter 2.

In the adult dog the epiphysis is continuous with the diaphysis and the physis is completely absent. The growth plates in each long bone close or fuse at different times but are often predictable for each region (see Chapter 3). The site of the closed physis may be present as a 'physeal scar', which is seen as a radiopaque band running across the physeal site (Figure 4.1).

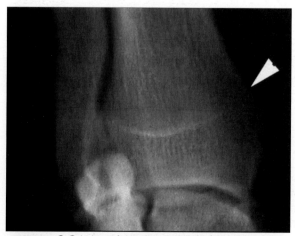

**4.1** CrCd view of the distal radius of a Greyhound. The radiopaque linear band is the physeal scar at the site of the physis of the distal radius (arrowhead).

## Radiographic technique

The implementation of standard protocols for positioning, radiographic exposures and processing techniques are important so that diagnostic radiographs are obtained consistently. Subtle lesions are less likely to be missed if the radiographic technique is of a high standard. Sedation is a prerequisite and if the animal is in pain an analgesic may be required. General anaesthesia is occasionally necessary. Grids are not required for radiographic studies of small dogs (<10 kg) or cats. It is important that there is good corticomedullary definition and that the radiographic quality permits evaluation of the adjacent soft tissue planes.

Larger dogs (10–20 kg) require a higher radiographic exposure and a medium speed rare earth screen film combination provides reasonable bone detail. Dogs greater than 20 kg usually require a grid for studies proximal to the elbow and stifle joints (Figure 4.2a).

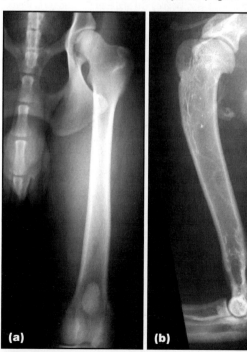

(a)  (b)

**4.2** **(a)** CrCd view of a femur of a 30 kg German Shepherd Dog. A grid with medium speed screens and latitude film have been used. There is good radiographic contrast showing bone and soft tissue detail. **(b)** The high detail screen/film combination on the ML view of the humerus of this cat shows excellent bone and soft tissue detail. The radiopaque streaks in the soft tissues are due to wet fur.

High detail rare earth screens and film or a single screen/film combination provide excellent bone definition in miniature breeds and cats. (Figure 4.2b). Exposure factors should be reduced in cases that have marked muscle wasting and should be increased when soft tissue swelling is present. Correct exposure factors are particularly important when evaluating bones for early signs of osteolysis or periosteal new bone (Figure 4.3). Overexposure will obliterate these early radiographic abnormalities. The use of an exposure chart is useful as it should help to standardize radiographic exposures.

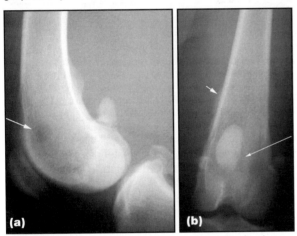

4.3   **(a)** On the ML view there is a subtle circular radiolucent area in the craniodistal aspect of the distal femoral metaphysis (arrowed). **(b)** The CrCd view shows a faint solid periosteal reaction (short arrow) on the distomedial aspect of the femoral diaphysis (long arrow shows the radiolucent defect seen in (a)). This was an early malignant bone neoplasm.

## Standard views

At least two orthogonal views (that is two views taken at right angles to each other) are required to give a three dimensional (3D) representation of the bone. Standard orthogonal views required are a mediolateral (ML) and either a craniocaudal (CrCd) or caudocranial (CdCr) view. Lesion orientated views or oblique studies are occasionally necessary. The central X-ray beam should be located over the mid-diaphyseal region and the adjacent proximal and distal joints should be included. Collimation to the area of interest is important but the adjacent soft tissues should be included on the radiograph. In many instances a comparative study of the opposite limb is helpful. In some cases a horizontal beam craniocaudal or caudocranial technique with the dog in lateral recumbency is a useful adjunct. It permits a more exact perpendicular alignment of the limb bones to the cassettes. It is also advantageous in non-anaesthetized painful animals as there is less manipulation of the limb. However, it can only be used with due regard for radiation safety and ensuring that the beam direction is towards an appropriate barrier.

The overlap of bony structures may cast unusual radiolucencies or radiopacities, which are termed Mach lines. Mach lines or 'edge effects' arise at the margin of a curved bony structure where it is superimposed on an adjacent bone. They are optical artefacts and should not be mistaken for a true pathological finding (Figure 4.4).

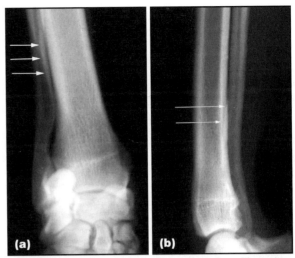

4.4   Mach lines (arrowed) may be **(a)** positive or **(b)** negative, depending on the curvatures of the adjacent bones.

## Humerus

*Mediolateral view:* The animal is recumbent on the affected limb, which is cranial to the sternum. The upper limb is taken caudally and restrained over the thorax by means of a tie and sandbag. The head is extended and a sandbag placed across the neck to keep it in position. The X-ray beam is centred over the middle of the humerus (Figure 4.5a).

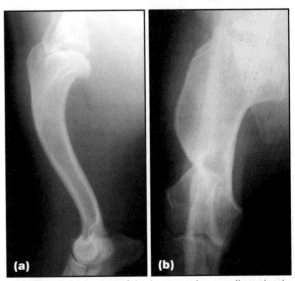

4.5   **(a)** ML view of the humerus in a medium sized terrier dog. **(b)** CdCr view of the humerus in a Basset Hound.

*Caudocranial view:* The animal is placed in dorsal recumbency. A plastic or foam cradle is a useful adjunct to restrain the animal in a comfortable and stable position. The limb under examination is drawn cranially alongside the neck and maintained in an extended position. The limb should be kept parallel to the tabletop and as close as possible to the cassette. The X-ray beam is centred over the middle of the humerus (Figure 4.5b).

**Radius and ulna**

*Mediolateral view:* The positioning of the animal is similar to that for the upper forelimb. The carpus should be elevated by a foam support to ensure the radius and ulna are parallel to the tabletop. It is important that there is no rotation of the limb. The X-ray beam is centred over the middle of the antebrachium (Figure 4.6a).

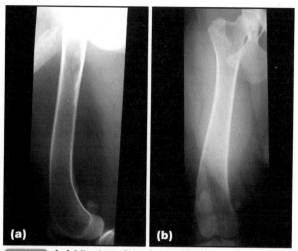

4.7 **(a)** ML view of the femur of a Labrador Retriever; the upper thigh muscles often result in an underexposed proximal femoral diaphysis. **(b)** CrCd view of the femur of a Labrador Retriever.

*Craniocaudal view:* The animal is placed in dorsal recumbency and both legs are extended caudally, parallel to each other and to the tabletop. The stifles should be rotated medially in order to superimpose the patellas on the trochlear ridges. Velcro belts around the thighs help to maintain the limbs in position. In larger dogs ties with small weights anchored around the hocks help to keep the limbs extended. The X-ray beam is centred over the middle of the femoral diaphysis (Figure 4.7b).

**Tibia and fibula**

*Mediolateral view:* The animal is positioned in lateral recumbency and the limbs separated. The upper limb is usually taken caudally, as described for the femoral study. In obese animals and male dogs the abdominal wall or prepuce may be superimposed on the proximal tibial region. In these cases the upper limb should be drawn cranially. The X-ray beam is centred over the middle of the crus (Figure 4.8a).

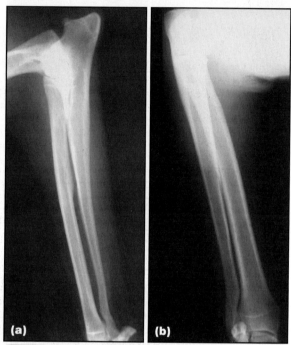

4.6 **(a)** ML view of the radius and ulna of a large-breed dog. **(b)** CrCd view of the radius and ulna of a large-breed dog; note the inadequate extension of the elbow, resulting in oblique positioning of the elbow joint.

*Craniocaudal view:* The animal is placed in sternal recumbency. The limb is extended cranially and held in a straight position with ties or sandbags. A foam support under the axilla helps to keep the dog balanced. It is occasionally useful to move the head slightly away from the midline towards the opposite side of the dog. The X-ray beam is centred over the middle of the antebrachium (Figure 4.6b).

**Femur**

*Mediolateral view:* The animal is recumbent on the affected limb. In order to keep the femur in a true lateral position, the upper limb is taken either cranially or caudally and the tarsus is supported. The recumbent limb is extended in the opposite direction to the upper limb and the hock elevated slightly to bring the tibia parallel with the tabletop so that the femoral condyles are superimposed. The X-ray beam is centred over the middle of the femoral diaphysis. In large-breed dogs there is often underexposure of the proximal femur or overexposure of the distal femur. The use of a silicone wedge with the thick side distally evens out the tissue thickness and results in a more even radiographic contrast (Figure 4.7a).

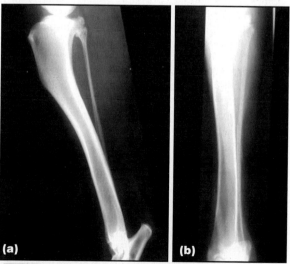

4.8 **(a)** ML view of the tibia and fibula in a Great Dane. **(b)** CrCd view of the tibia and fibula in a Great Dane; note the relative underexposure of the stifle due to the increased thickness of tissues and the greater distance of the stifle from the cassette.

*Craniocaudal view:* The animal is placed in a similar position to that described for the femur. There is some magnification of the limb in this position. In large dogs it is difficulty to obtain optimal images of the stifle and hock on this view due to the relative differences in tissue thickness in these areas (Figure 4.8b).

*Caudocranial view:* The animal is placed in sternal recumbency. The leg under examination is drawn caudally. In large dogs it is often helpful to place the other leg in a semi-flexed position on the tabletop. The stifle is rotated medially and the hock extended and held in position with a sandbag and tie. The X-ray beam is centred over the middle of the crus. Dogs with osteoarthrosis of the hips find this position slightly uncomfortable. In patients with gross soft tissue swelling or limb contracture, a caudocranial study using a horizontal beam provides a diagnostic study with minimal technical difficulties. The potential radiation hazards must be considered with horizontal beam use.

## Normal radiographic anatomy and appearance

### Humerus
The mid-diaphyseal medullary region of the humerus is relatively radiolucent. Further distally it gradually merges with a lacy fretwork of trabecular bone just proximal to the humeral condylar area. The nutrient artery channel is often seen running through the caudal cortex of the mid diaphysis in a caudoproximal to craniodistal direction (Figure 4.9a).

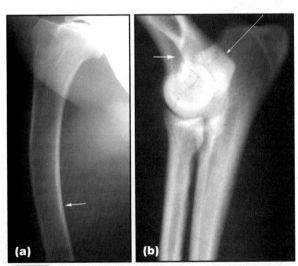

4.9    Normal ML view of the humerus in a dog showing **(a)** the nutrient foramen (arrowed) and **(b)** the supratrochlear foramen (short arrow) and medial epicondyle (long arrow).

*Dogs:* The medial epicondyle projects caudally, forming a right-angled projection just proximal to the elbow joint (Figure 4.9b). On the lateral view the relative radiolucency of the supratrochlear foramen is seen just proximal to the large circular condyles. On the CrCd view the anconeal process engages the supratrochlear foramen, which is a large radiolucent aperture just proximal to the epicondyles.

*Cats:* The supratrochlear foramen is absent in cats. There is a large supracondyloid foramen visible just proximal to the epicondyles on the lateral study. It is visible on the medial aspect of the distal humeral diaphysis on the CdCr view (Figure 4.10). On the CdCr view the anconeal process engages the olecranon fossa, which is seen as a radiolucent area just proximal to the epicondyles and superimposed on the proximal ulna.

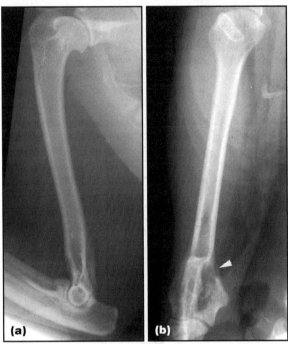

4.10    Normal **(a)** ML and **(b)** CdCr views of the humerus in a cat. The arrowhead indicates the site of the supracondyloid foramen.

### Radius and ulna
The radius is in close apposition to the proximal extremity of the ulna and the two coronoid processes encircle it caudally. The radius has a generalized radiolucency throughout the bone, whereas the ulna often has a slight increase in opacity at its proximal extremity. The distomedial aspect of the radius forms an oblique distal eminence, which is the medial styloid process.

*Dogs:* On the lateral view the olecranon projects caudoproximally. It is pointed and angular and cranially forms a small depression between two rounded prominences located medially and laterally. The ulna gradually narrows as it extends distally and tapers into a slightly bulbous rounded lateral styloid process (Figure 4.11). Occasionally bone modelling due to interosseous ligament traction is quite marked between the mid-diaphyseal region of the radius and ulna (Figure 4.12).

*Cats:* In cats the profile of the proximal extremity of the olecranon is squarer than in dogs. At the distal extremity the lateral styloid process has a comma-shaped distolateral extension that permits pronation and supination (Figure 4.13).

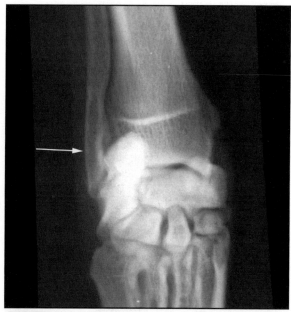

**4.11** CrCd view of a normal lateral styloid process (arrowed) in a dog.

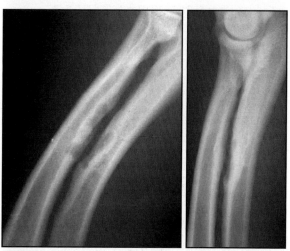

**4.12** Examples of bone modelling in the vicinity of the nutrient foramen on the ML view of the radius and ulna in normal dogs. These are incidental findings.

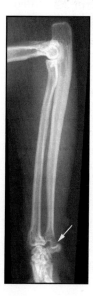

**4.13** Normal ML view of a feline radius and ulna. The lateral styloid process is indicated by the arrow.

## Femur

**Dogs:** On the ML study the femur has a gently curving outline with a slight cranial contour. There are often transverse radiopaque lines visible across the femoral condyles, which represent the proximal aspect of the intercondylar fossa. The extensor fossa may be seen on the cranioproximal aspect of the lateral condyle. The caudodistal aspect of the diaphysis has an irregular profile of varying size, which is the site of origin of the gastrocnemius muscle (Figure 4.14). A nutrient foramen is often visible in the caudal cortex of the mid-femoral diaphysis. The diaphyseal cortex gradually fades out at the level of the trochlear ridges. On the CrCd view three sesamoid bones are superimposed on the distal femur. The patella lies centrally and the fabellae laterally and medially (Figure 4.15a). Occasionally, the fabellae are located at different levels. This often occurs in both limbs (Figure 4.15b). This should be differentiated from a pathological displacement. In addition, on occasions the fabellae may be bipartite or multipartite, often bilaterally and this is usually due to a congenital anomaly and of no clinical significance (Figure 4.15c).

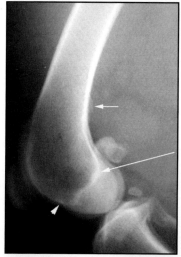

**4.14** Normal radiopaque lines seen on the ML view of the distal femoral condyles caused by the intercondylar fossa (long arrow). Note the prominence on the caudodistal femur (short arrow) associated with the attachment of the gastrocnemius muscle. The extensor fossa is visible (arrowhead).

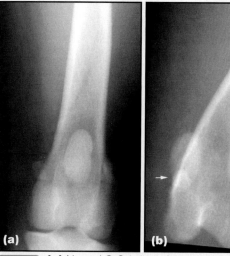

(a) (b)

**4.15** **(a)** Normal CrCd view of the distal femur with the patella and fabellae visible. **(b)** Displaced fabella; the medial fabella (arrowhead) is displaced distally compared with the lateral (arrowed). This was a bilateral finding in this terrier. (continues) ▶

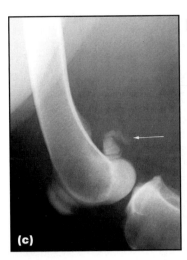

**4.15**

(continued)
**(c)** Multipartite lateral fabella (arrowed) in a Labrador Retriever.

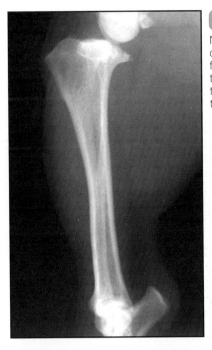

**4.17**

Normal ML view of the tibia and fibula in a small terrier dog. Note the prominent tibial plateau.

*Cats:* The femoral diaphysis is straight with little cranial curvature. Occasionally only one fabella is present (Figure 4.16).

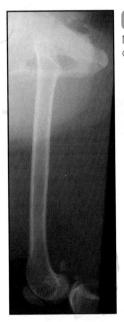

**4.16**

Normal ML view of the femur in a cat. Only one fabella is present.

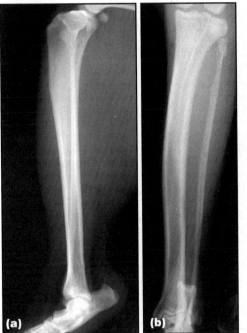

**(a)**    **(b)**

**4.18** Normal **(a)** ML and **(b)** CrCd views of the tibia and fibula in a cat.

### Tibia and fibula

The popliteal sesamoid is sited at the caudoproximal aspect of the tibial plateau lateral to the midline.

*Dogs:* The fibula is orientated in a curved plane with the central third directed towards the tibial diaphysis. Proximally the fibula articulates with the caudo-proximolateral aspect of the tibia. In smaller dogs or dogs with marked limb curvature there is a consider-able variation in the relative alignment of the tibia and fibula (Figure 4.17).

*Cats:* The fibula is a vertically directed bone and runs parallel with the tibia. The fibular head is usually superimposed on the caudoproximal aspect of the tibial diaphysis. At its distal extremity it expands horizontally forming the lateral malleolus (Figure 4.18).

### Breed variations

Chondrodystrophy is an anatomical variation that is a feature of certain breeds, such as Basset Hounds, Corgis and Bulldogs. The limbs are short with marked craniolateral bowing and curvature. The diaphyses are short and wide and proximally form large, flared, elongated articulations (Figure 4.19). Some small dogs, such as Jack Russell Terriers, may show chondrodystrophic features and have considerable variation in the conformation of the long bones (see Figure 4.17). Miniature canine breeds have very fine bones with minimal curvature of the long bone diaphyses.

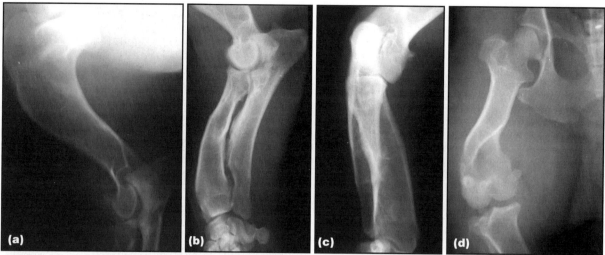

**4.19**   **(a–c)** Normal chondrodystrophic limbs in a Basset Hound. (a) ML view of the humerus. (b) ML view of the radius and ulna. (c) CrCd view of the radius and ulna. **(d)** CrCd view of the femur in a terrier.

## Alternative imaging techniques

### Ultrasonography
Radiography is the mostly widely used technique for the detection of bone abnormalities. In some instances ultrasonography can provide additional information. Because of the reflection and absorption of sound waves the ultrasonographic appearance of bone is a distinct hyperechoic (white) line. Ultrasound examination is useful in assessing the periosteum, the integrity of the cortex and for assisting in the collection of fine-needle aspirates from the diseased bone (Figure 4.20).

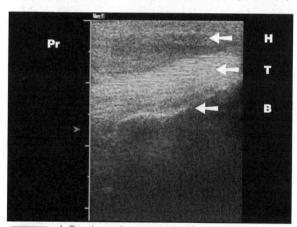

**4.20**   A Greyhound presented with a swelling surrounding the upper thoracic limb. The longitudinal scan of the caudal humerus using a 13 MHz linear array transducer is shown with the proximal limb on the left side of the image. The bone diaphysis (B) is hyperechoic but intact and there is no irregularity, which would occur with periosteal new bone. The triceps tendon (T) is seen as a hyperechoic band with the fibres aligned normally. A resolving haematoma (H) is seen under the skin, which lies at the top of the image.

### Scintigraphy
Bone scintigraphy is very sensitive in detecting active areas of bone turnover. Technetium 99M is labelled with methylene diphosphonate, which binds to hydroxyapatite crystals in bone. There are an increased number of hydroxyapatite crystals in areas of active bone turnover. It can localize active areas of bone turnover 24 hours after an injury has occurred. Scintigraphy is most useful in occult cases of lameness and also in locating metastases on a survey of the skeletal structures (Figure 4.21).

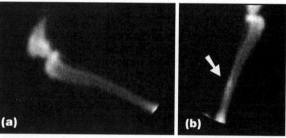

**4.21**   A Greyhound presented acutely lame after a trial. The bone scan shows **(a)** the normal left tibia and **(b)** a focal area of increased radionuclide uptake (arrowed) in the distal third of the right tibial diaphysis. This was a stress fracture.

### Computed tomography
Computed tomography (CT) has the advantage of allowing visualization of the bone in cross-sectional planes (Figure 4.22). It is most useful in imaging complex joints, but may be used for the evaluation of fractures of long bones and also in 3D reconstruction and tumour resection planning.

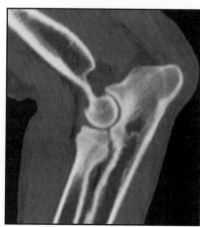

**4.22**   CT of a normal elbow of a Newfoundland dog. (Courtesy of Y Ruel.)

## Magnetic resonance imaging

Magnetic resonance imaging (MRI) is the modality of choice for assessing soft tissue and bone injuries and diseases, as it gives excellent soft tissue and bone anatomical and cross-sectional detail. Like CT it is useful for 3D reconstruction of neoplasms and allows full assessment of disease progression, especially the extent of bone marrow invasion by neoplasms (Figure 4.23).

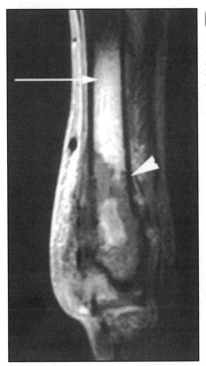

**4.23** MRI study of a dog with an osteosarcoma of the distal radius. The destructive lesion (arrowhead) can be seen in the distal radius and extending proximally into the medullary cavity. There is invasion into the adjacent soft tissue structures. The normal medullary cavity is indicated by the long arrow. (Courtesy of RD Pechman.)

## Abnormal radiological findings

### Trauma

Traumatic injuries are usually manifested by a disruption to the integrity of the bone structure. This may be seen as an interruption and step defect in the cortical outline. The fracture line may be incomplete (greenstick), affecting only one cortical margin. In some cases radiographic signs of a traumatic insult may not be visible immediately. There is a time lag of 7–10 days before periosteal changes become visible radiographically.

### Fractures

A detailed review of fractures and the progression of fracture healing is described in Chapter 5.

***Traumatic:*** A history of external trauma is usually reported. The cortex should be examined carefully for radiolucent defects. Rarely the fragments may be impacted or compressed, in which case the fracture line is radiopaque. The fracture fragments may be single or multiple, in close apposition, impacted, over-riding, avulsed or distracted. Involvement of adjacent joints and presence of foreign bodies are important considerations when assessing the injury (Figures 4.24 and 4.25).

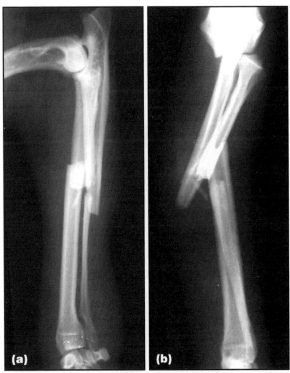

**(a)** **(b)**

**4.24** **(a)** The ML view shows fractures of the radius and ulna of a dog. **(b)** The CrCd view also demonstrates that there is a radial subluxation. This case shows the necessity of taking two orthogonal views, as well as illustrating the importance of including the adjacent joints.

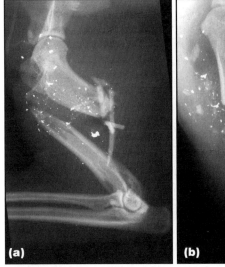

**(a)** **(b)**

**4.25** A 3-year-old cat was presented as non-weight bearing on its right forelimb. The **(a)** ML and **(b)** CrCd radiographs show that there is a comminuted fracture of the humeral diaphysis. The heavy metal opacity remnants of a shattered bullet are visible in the soft tissues. (Note the proximal humeral physis is still visible.)

***Athletic:*** These types of injuries are usually seen in animals that have suffered an injury at speed, at high impact, as a result of torsional stress or as a result of repetitive strain injury. Commonly affected breeds include Greyhounds, Whippets, sight hounds, and sporting and working breeds.

**Pathological:** The common theme with this type of fracture is the lack of a history of trauma. The fracture is often associated with a primary or secondary neoplasm (Figure 4.26). Close inspection of the fracture site may reveal moth-eaten or permeative lysis. Pathological fractures may also occur in animals suffering from osteopenia.

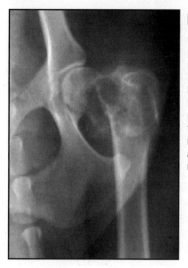

**4.26**

CrCd view of the proximal femur of a middle-aged dog lame on the left hindlimb, showing bone lysis and a pathological fracture through the femoral neck. This was due to a malignant bone neoplasm.

**Idiopathic:** There is a high incidence of lateral humeral condylar fractures reported in spaniels, but also in other breeds such as Pointers, chondrodystrophic breeds and Labrador Retrievers. Incomplete fusion of the condyles is considered a predisposing cause. A clinical history of a fracture occurring with little evidence of a traumatic insult is suspicious. Radiographs of the other elbow should be taken. Special oblique, CrCd or flexed CrCd views are sometimes useful since the fracture line is often difficult to see. CT is the most sensitive method of diagnosis (see also Chapters 5 and 8).

## Complications

- Limb trauma in the young animal may cause premature closure of the physes of the radius, ulna, tibia and fibula, resulting in disproportionate growth (see Chapter 3). There is cortical thickening on the convex side of the bone diaphysis at the site of maximum curvature. This deformity persists in the adult. Valgus or varus deformities occur distally. This deformity may also be observed as a sequel to metaphyseal osteopathy and a retained ulnar cartilage core.
- Disruption to the normal fracture healing process may result in a *delayed union*. The fractured ends form a callus but at a slower rate than usual (see Chapter 5).
- A *non-union* fracture is a feature of fractures of the distal radius, ulna, tibia and fibula, particularly in miniature breeds. Callus formation is present at the fracture ends but fails to bridge the fracture site (see Chapter 5).
- When a fractured bone heals in an abnormal anatomical alignment it is termed a *malunion* (see Chapter 5).

- In young dogs if the fracture fragments involving the paired bones of the antebrachium and crus become united with each other following inadequate reduction, it is termed a *synostosis*. There may be growth restriction of the bone or subluxation.

## Infection (osteomyelitis)

Osteomyelitis is infection of the cortical bone, medullary cavity and periosteum. This can occur either through a direct route, e.g. trauma and secondary infection, or via a haematogenous route.

### Haematogenous

**Bacterial:** Haematogenous bacterial osteomyelitis is rare in the long bones of adult dogs and cats. Discospondylitis is the commonest form of haematogenous osteomyelitis in adult dogs (see Chapter 16). Pathological fractures of the diaphyseal region have been reported secondary to haematogenous osteomyelitis, as the spread is via the nutrient artery in adult dogs. It is prudent to identify the bacteria involved through culture and biopsy of the lesion.

**Fungal:** This type of osteomyelitis is usually spread haematogenously, following inhalation, and is therefore usually polyostotic. These lesions can also be monostotic and are often metaphyseal in location. Fungal infection is more common in dogs than it is in cats. In some countries different types of fungal osteomyelitis are endemic. It is difficult to distinguish radiographically between a fungal osteomyelitis and a neoplasm; therefore a bone biopsy is always warranted.

*Coccidioidomycosis* (Coccidioides immitus): Coccidioidomycosis is found in the southwestern USA, Mexico and Central and South America. The major route of infection is via inhalation, with dissemination to bones developing some months later. The long bones are most commonly affected. Radiographic changes are typically a combination of cortical bone lysis and bony proliferation (Figure 4.27a). Permeative and moth-eaten cortical lysis can be observed, and the lesions are not usually expansile. The zone of transition (the region of transition between the lesion and adjacent normal bone) tends to be shorter and better defined than with osteosarcoma, and the rate of change on serial radiographs also tends to be slower. Thoracic radiographs may reveal a hilar lymphadenopathy.

*Blastomycosis* (Blastomyces dermatitidis): Blastomycosis is most commonly found in the southeastern USA. Most infections are acquired by spore inhalation. Bone involvement occurs in about 30% of cases. Lesions are usually osteolytic with periosteal proliferation and soft tissue swelling. The majority of bone lesions are solitary and occur distal to the stifle and elbow. The transition zone is usually shorter and serial radiographic change tends to be slower than with osteosarcoma (Figure 4.27b).

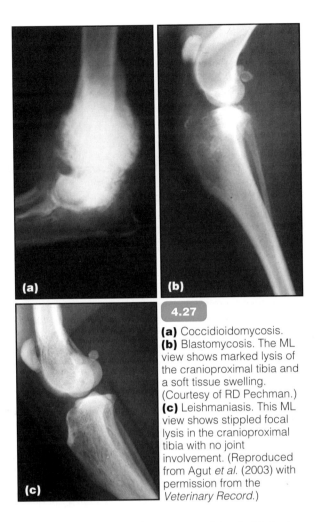

**4.27**

**(a)** Coccidioidomycosis.
**(b)** Blastomycosis. The ML view shows marked lysis of the cranioproximal tibia and a soft tissue swelling. (Courtesy of RD Pechman.)
**(c)** Leishmaniasis. This ML view shows stippled focal lysis in the cranioproximal tibia with no joint involvement. (Reproduced from Agut *et al.* (2003) with permission from the *Veterinary Record*.)

*Histoplasmosis* (Histoplasma capsulatum): Histoplasmosis most commonly occurs in the central zones of the USA. Infection is usually via inhalation but the gastrointestinal route has also been implicated. Cats are as susceptible to infection as dogs. Bone lesions are rare but show a mixed pattern of osteolysis and periosteal new bone formation. The metaphyseal regions adjacent to the carpi and tarsi are most commonly affected.

*Aspergillosis:* This may affect the long bones of adult dogs, particularly the German Shepherd Dog. *Aspergillus fumigatus* is usually associated with localized infection, especially in the nasal cavity. *Aspergillus terreus* and *Aspergillus deflectus* may cause systemic disease and have been reported to cause bone lesions in dogs. Mixed areas of lysis and proliferative bone may be observed and cortical destruction can occur.

*Protozoal:* Hepatozoonosis is a rare protozoal infection that may cause polyostotic aggressive bone lesions. Infections are transmitted via the brown dog tick *Rhipicephalus sanguineus*. The radiographic changes primarily involve the periosteum and can vary from an irregular periosteal proliferation to smooth laminar thickening of the periosteum. Dogs with hepatozoonosis usually have systemic dysfunction.

Another form of protozoal osteomyelitis has been observed with *Leishmania donovani* in Mediterranean countries. Radiographic changes can be mixed with

osteolysis and proliferation and are occasionally polyostotic (Figure 4.27c). In long bones the most common pattern is of a periosteal and intramedullary proliferation, which involves the diaphyses and is related to the nutrient foramen.

### Secondary
The most common cause of secondary bacterial osteomyelitis in the dog and cat is post-trauma or following direct damage to the bone. It may also spread by local extension from an adjoining soft tissue infection. An overwhelming bacterial contamination in combination with severe trauma, surgical intervention or the presence of dead bone, or unstable metallic implants can predispose to osteomyelitis. The most common organisms implicated in osteomyelitis are *Staphylococcus*, *Streptococcus*, *Escherichia coli* and *Enterobacter*. The distribution of secondary bacterial osteomyelitis is usually monostotic. It can be polyostotic but in these cases usually only one limb is affected. Bacterial osteomyelitis often causes swelling, fever and the development of draining tracts. By the time the features of osteomyelitis are identified on a radiograph it has become chronic, as it takes seven to ten days for the first radiographic signs of bone lysis or proliferation to become apparent. Radiographic changes include bone destruction (lysis) and periosteal new bone formation, with or without soft tissue swelling (Figure 4.28). The periosteal reaction is often an aggressive, extensive, pallisading periosteal reaction and may have a mixed osteolytic–osteogenic appearance.

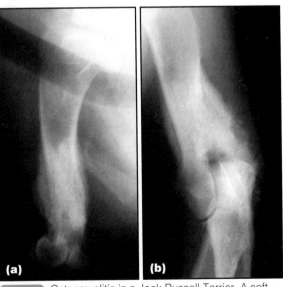

**4.28** Osteomyelitis in a Jack Russell Terrier. A soft tissue swelling has developed at the site of a dog bite. **(a)** ML and **(b)** CdCr views show an aggressive periosteal reaction affecting the distal humerus.

Bone sequestration and involucrum formation may or may not be present. A sequestrum is an isolated bone fragment, which lies within a radiolucent cavity (cloaca), and is surrounded by a sclerotic rim of proliferative bone called the involucrum (Figure 4.29). A sequestrum is usually more opaque than the surrounding bone.

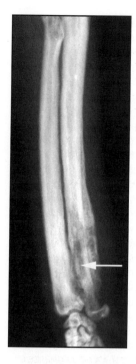

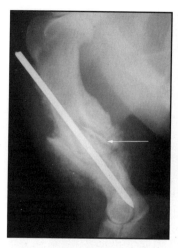

4.29 A cat was presented with a discharge over the lateral aspect of the distal forelimb, following a cat bite. The ML view shows a sequestrum in the distal ulna.

4.30 Humeral fracture in an adult mixed breed dog, repaired using an intramedullary pin. The ML view shows the callus formation is excessive. In the centre of the fracture site is a linear radiopaque fragment (arrowed), which is a bone sequestrum.

Infected non-union fractures may occur when there is reduced or deficient blood supply to the fracture site, complicated by bacterial contamination. Radiological findings of infected non-union fractures usually include areas of callus formation and other areas with an absence of callus and non-reactive bone. Bone healing can occur in the presence of osteomyelitis, in areas not containing residual infection. If the introduction of infection occurs at the time of trauma, the radiological changes associated with osteomyelitis are likely to be confused with the formation of a bony callus. If infection occurs later in the healing process then it may also be camouflaged by the normal elements of the healing process.

The radiological features of bacterial osteomyelitis are not specific. Radiology alone has been shown to have a sensitivity of 62.5% and a specificity of 57.1% in the diagnosis of osteomyelitis. With bacterial osteomyelitis the presence of a sclerotic zone is more likely than in cases of neoplasia. Pathological fractures may occur but are less common than with neoplasia. Positive contrast sinography can be useful in cases of osteomyelitis, which have a draining sinus tract. If the contrast medium tracks to the surface of the bone, this is a good indicator of infected bone.

### Iatrogenic

Iatrogenic infection can occur secondary to orthopaedic surgery and can happen at any age. This is most likely to occur following poor surgical technique. Radiographic changes are similar to those seen in other causes of osteomyelitis (Figure 4.30).

Radiolucent areas surrounding metal implants can be confusing on a radiograph. They are usually either due to implant motion or infection. Those due to motion usually have uniform width and margins, and may be surrounded by a band of sclerosis. The radiolucent areas caused by infection can have an uneven appearance with indistinct bone margins.

### Metallosis

A sterile osteomyelitis, resulting from a reaction to surgical implants (of dissimilar metals) that have been permanently left in bones, is termed metallosis. Areas of radiolucency surround the implant, often having a honeycomb appearance. It may be associated with sinus tract formation. It is quite rare in dogs and cats.

## Neoplasia

### Benign

Benign bone neoplasms are uncommon in the dog and cat. Giant cell tumours (osteoclastoma) are rare neoplasms seen in the epiphyses and metaphyses of long bones, especially the distal ulna. Their radiographic appearance is of an expansile, lytic lesion with a multiloculated septate appearance. They resemble a bone cyst; the differentiating feature is that giant cell tumours usually occur in older patients.

Osteochondroma is a solitary benign lesion; when multiple lesions are present these may be termed multiple cartilaginous exostoses or hereditary multiple exostoses. It is usually recognized in the growing puppy or kitten at a site of endochondral ossification (see Chapter 3). In adults the residual bony prominences are a visual blemish. They are smooth bulbous outgrowths from the proximal or distal diaphysis, which are continuous with the medullary cavity and have a distinct cortical margin (Figure 4.31). They are not

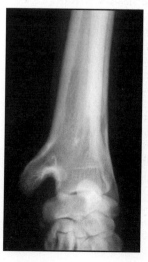

4.31 A 2-year-old Boxer presented with a swelling on the medial aspect of the distal radius. On the CrCd study there was a bony prominence on the distomedial aspect of the radial metaphysis. It was confirmed to be an osteochondroma.

usually clinically significant unless they encroach on an adjacent bone or soft tissue structure. They may undergo malignant transformation into osteosarcoma and chondrosarcoma. In cats, feline leukaemia virus (FeLV) has been associated with osteochondroma formation.

## Malignant

A definitive diagnosis cannot be made from radiographs of suspect bone neoplasms. A bone biopsy is recommended in all cases. It is also prudent to radiograph the thorax to check for metastases.

### Primary monostotic bone neoplasms

*Osteosarcoma:* This is the most common primary monostotic bone neoplasm in dogs. Osteosarcomas account for 80% of malignant bone neoplasms in large-breed dogs and 50% in small-breed dogs. Osteosarcomas or osteogenic sarcomas are malignant neoplasms primarily arising in bone. Seventy-five percent of osteosarcomas occur in long bones, most arising in the medullary cavity, but some originate from the cortical surfaces, periosteum (periosteal, parosteal or juxtacortical osteosarcoma) or in extraskeletal sites. Osteosarcomas cause destruction of the surrounding soft tissue and readily metastasize to the lungs. The most common long bone affected is the metaphyseal region of the distal radius, followed by the proximal humerus, proximal or distal femur, and proximal or distal tibia. Osteosarcomas appear to have a biphasic peak of age occurrence. There is an increase in incidence of osteosarcomas in dogs at two years of age and again eight years of age.

Radiographic changes are variable and may be predominantly lytic, sclerotic or have a mixed pattern (Figure 4.32). An irregular, spiculated periosteal reaction is often observed. An active sunburst periosteal reaction is the classic radiographic feature of osteosarcoma but is not always observed. Larger lesions can cause expansion, thinning and erosion of the cortex.

With osteosarcoma a long and indistinct zone of transition can exist between the centre of the lesion and normal bone. Rarely, an osteosarcoma can invade adjacent bones or cross a joint. Progressive periosteal reaction and cortical lysis is seen if serial radiographs are taken. The presumptive diagnosis for an aggressive, monostotic, metaphyseal lesion should be osteosarcoma, although fungal osteomyelitis must be considered in endemic countries. Thoracic radiographs should be performed as osteosarcomas readily metastasize to the lungs. However, for a definitive diagnosis a bone biopsy is needed. Spontaneous regression of osteosarcoma in dogs has been reported.

*Chondrosarcoma:* This is the second most common primary neoplasm, although it accounts for less than 10% of primary bone neoplasms. Golden Retrievers appear to have a higher risk of developing chondrosarcoma than other breeds. Chondrosarcomas usually occur in flat bones (e.g. pelvis, scapula, skull and ribs) but have been reported in long bones (only 14% of chondrosarcomas). There is no single characteristic radiographic appearance of chondrosarcoma. Chondrosarcomas can appear similar to osteosarcomas but they are often more lytic, expansile and centrally destructive in appearance with a minimal perisoteal reaction. They are slower growing than osteosarcomas, and only metastasize to local lymph nodes and then to the lungs in 20% of cases.

*Fibrosarcoma:* This is another primary bone neoplasm that can have a monostotic distribution. It can be difficult to differentiate a fibrosarcoma from an osteosarcoma, but a fibrosarcoma may be more osteolytic (Figures 4.33 and 4.34). They are slower growing than osteosarcomas and are more likely to invade an adjacent joint space.

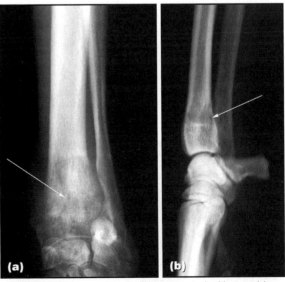

**4.32** Osteosarcoma. **(a)** CrCd view. There is extensive osteolysis of the proximal tibia with cortical discontinuity on the proximomedial aspect of the tibia. **(b)** CrCd study showing signs of an aggressive periosteal reaction, osteolysis, a poor zone of transition and an extensive soft tissue swelling. This is the so-called 'sunburst' appearance.

**4.33** Fibrosarcoma. A dog presented with a sudden history of acute lameness. **(a)** CrCd view. There is a 'moth-eaten' appearance to the bone. A faint vertical radiolucent fracture line is visible (arrowed). **(b)** ML view. The osteolysis (arrowed) is seen in the caudodistal aspect of the radius. ▶

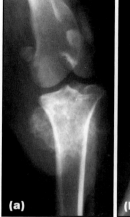
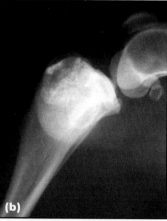

**4.34** Fibrosarcoma. In this case the more productive features that can be associated with fibrosarcoma are demonstrated. **(a)** CrCd and **(b)** ML views. New bone formation encircling the proximal tibia. The cortex is intact and clearly visible.

*Haemangiosarcoma:* This rarely presents as a primary bone neoplasm and may be radiographically indistinguishable from the other sarcomas (Figure 4.35).

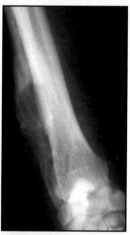

**4.35** CrCd view of a haemangiosarcoma in an adult cross-bred dog. There is a radiolucent expansile lesion in the distal ulna. A smooth periosteal reaction is seen proximally.

*Primary polyostotic bone neoplasms:* Multiple myeloma is the commonest polyostotic primary bone neoplasm. It results from a neoplastic proliferation of plasma cells in the bone marrow. This in turn leads to osteoclastic activity, which results in bone resorption. Radiographs can reveal multiple, focal, lytic lesions in the vertebrae, ribs and long bones (Figure 4.36). Other

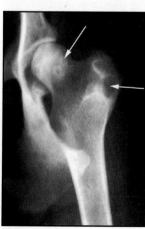

**4.36** Multiple myeloma. VD pelvis; discrete well circumscribed areas of osteolysis (arrowed) are seen in the femoral head and greater trochanter.

neoplasms that produce multifocal bone lysis include lymphosarcoma of bone and polyostotic osteosarcoma.

*Surface osteosarcoma:* There has been a lack of standardization of terminology for primary bone neoplasms, other than central osteosarcoma within the medical literature, with the terms parosteal osteoma, parosteal osteosarcoma, periosteal osteosarcoma, juxtacortical osteosarcoma and surface osteosarcoma all used to describe neoplasms with similar histological and radiological characteristics. There has been corresponding inconsistency in terminology in the veterinary literature.

Thomas *et al.* (1997) suggested that surface osteosarcoma can be classified histologically into three distinct groups:

- Parosteal
- Periosteal
- High-grade surface osteosarcoma.

Parosteal osteosarcoma (also called juxtacortical osteosarcoma) is a slow-growing, low-grade malignant neoplasm, which arises from the surface of the bone (the periosteal connective tissue). It is less common than the central osteosarcoma, which arises from within the bone. Radiographically, parosteal osteosarcomas appear as irregular mineralized masses with smooth borders. The underlying cortex is usually intact but medullary invasion can occur later in the disease. Pulmonary metastases can also occur.

Periosteal osteosarcoma is a more malignant neoplasm carrying a poorer prognosis than parosteal osteosarcoma. It has been described as having an extensive soft tissue component with blotchy or streaky mineralization, which invades the cortex from outside, and thus may be confused with an extraskeletal osteosarcoma.

High-grade surface osteosarcoma is considered even more aggressive in nature, indistinguishable from central osteosarcoma other than by its peripheral location.

*Malignant primary soft tissue neoplasms:* In cases of a malignant soft tissue neoplasm invading bone, a soft tissue swelling with osteolysis and cortical disruption are the main radiographic changes. Slowly developing soft tissue neoplasms may provoke a mild periosteal reaction or minimal change in the bone contour. They are usually sarcomas (i.e. fibrosarcoma, haemangiosarcoma, liposarcoma).

*Secondary or metastatic neoplasia:* Malignant neoplasms may metastasize to bones. The long bones affected are usually the humerus and femur. Metastatic neoplasia tends to be located in the diaphysis because of spread via the nutrient artery, and may be polyostotic.

The radiographic appearance of metastatic bone neoplasia can vary from osteolytic to osteoblastic in nature (Figure 4.37). Scintigraphy may be useful in the detection of metastatic lesions that are not clinically apparent. Detection of malignancy in another organ, along with a diaphyseal polyostotic distribution in an older animal with no exposure to mycotic infections, is highly suggestive of metastatic bone neoplasia. A biopsy is required for a definitive diagnosis.

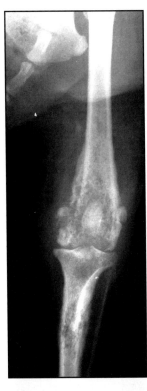

**4.37** Metastatic bone neoplasms. CrCd view; osteolytic areas are seen in the distal femur and proximal tibia. The primary neoplasm was a prostatic adenocarcinoma.

*Malignant transformation:* Malignant transformation (see also Chapter 5) of previous fracture sites to fracture-associated sarcomas has been reported. Possible inciting factors of malignant transformation include:

- Tissue damage, resulting from the initial trauma
- Altered cellular activity associated with prolonged healing of the fracture
- Infection.

Most malignant transformations occur in the diaphysis, as this is the most common site for fracture occurrence (Figure 4.38). The radiological features differentiating osteomyelitis from neoplasia are summarized in Figure 4.39.

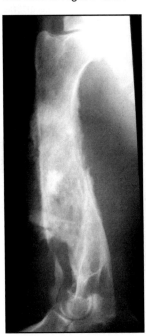

**4.38** Malignant transformation. This dog had a mid-diaphyseal humeral fracture repaired and the implant was removed 6 months postoperatively. Three years later the dog presented acutely lame. The ML view shows a pathological fracture through the mid-diaphyseal region. There is a mottled radiopacity and an aggressive periosteal reaction.

| Factor | Osteomyelitis | Primary malignant neoplasia |
|---|---|---|
| Age | Any | Usually older dogs |
| Species | More common in cats | More common in dogs |
| Breed | Any | Large to giant dog breeds |
| Number of lesions | Polyostotic or monostotic | Usually monostotic unless metastases present |
| Location | Variable:<br>• Metaphyseal (fungal)<br>• Diaphyseal (haematogenous bacterial in older dogs) | Typically metaphyseal. Metastases usually diaphyseal |
| Periosteal reaction | Aggressive, extensive and may be palisading | Irregular, spiculated and may have 'sunburst' appearance |
| Cortical disruption | Localized erosion, which is rarely due to expansion but may be permeative and moth-eaten | Usually expansile lesions with generalized thinning and erosion of the cortex |
| Cortical scalloping | Sub-periosteal indentations, producing rounded cortical defects | Endosteal indentations, which can result in cortical spikes |
| Sequestrum | Sequestrum (piece of dead bone) surrounded by cloaca (radiolucent zone) and involucrum (new bone) | Not a typical feature |
| Bone destruction *versus* production | More productive than destructive | More destructive than productive |
| Transition zone | May have a well defined zone of transition between abnormal and normal bone | Indistinct and long zone of transition between abnormal and normal bone |
| Rate of change | Slow rate of change on serial radiographs | Fast rate of change on serial radiographs |
| History | For fungal osteomyelitis, patients may live in an endemic zone | No history of living in an endemic zone |

**4.39** Factors for differentiating osteomyelitis from primary malignant neoplasia in the long bones of adult dogs.

*Radiation-induced osteosarcoma:* Radiation-induced sarcomas occur following radiation therapy (either orthovoltage or megavoltage radiation treatment). There are several criteria to fulfil in order to reach the diagnosis of a radiation osteosarcoma. The patient must have no radiographically detectable lesion in the affected area prior to irradiation, the neoplasm must have developed in the irradiated field, there is usually a long latent period, and the affected area should have a low incidence of bone neoplasia. The osteosarcoma must be confirmed histopathologically.

## Metabolic disorders

### Hyperparathyroidism
The parathyroid glands produce parathyroid hormone in response to a low serum calcium level, which restores the calcium/phosphate ratio in the blood by resorbing calcium from the skeleton. Primary hyperparathyroidism is uncommon and may occur as a result of hyperplasia or neoplasia of the parathyroid glands.

***Secondary hyperparathyroidism:*** Secondary hyperparathyroidism occurs as a result of renal disease or nutritional deficiency, resulting in a decrease in calcium or excess of phosphates.

*Nutritional secondary hyperparathyroidism:* The reduction in available calcium may occur due to a lack of dietary calcium or an inability to absorb calcium from the intestine: this is called nutritional secondary hyperparathyroidism. This may also occur when there is a reduction in vitamin D, which is necessary for the transport of calcium from the intestine. Calcium resorption is usually from the appendicular skeleton. Nutritional secondary hyperparathyroidism is seen mainly in young animals (see Chapter 3) and is rare in adults. However, the skeletal damage which occurs in the juvenile may persist in the adult, resulting in limb deformities.

*Renal secondary hyperparathyroidism:* This is caused by an inability of the kidney to excrete phosphates. Retention of phosphates results in secondary calcium excretion with resultant reduction in serum calcium levels. The primary areas of pathological change are the bones of the skull (see Chapter 12). It is seen in older dogs with chronic renal disease and, if the animal survives long enough, a generalized osteopenia or reduction in skeletal opacity can occur. Rarely osteopetrosis rather than osteopenia may be seen.

*Pseudohyperparathyroidism:* This occurs due to hypercalcaemia caused by a paraneoplastic syndrome. Osteopenic changes are not usually a major feature of the clinical condition.

### Hyperadrenocorticism
Adrenocorticotrophic hormone (ACTH) is necessary for normal calcium metabolism, including the production of the bone matrix. Hyperadrenocorticism is reported to cause decreased bone formation. It may occur as a result of a pituitary neoplasm secreting ACTH, adrenocortical neoplasms or the administration of excessive glucocorticoids. A generalized osteopenia of the spine and appendicular skeleton may be seen in addition to the more typical radiographic features of 'Cushing's syndrome' in affected dogs. However, the high kilovoltage technique used to radiograph these often obese dogs causes an apparent reduction in the opacity of the skeleton. Radiography is an insensitive method of assessing osteopenia.

## Miscellaneous

### Bone infarcts
Bone infarcts are uncommon and have been associated with skeletal osteosarcoma and fibrosarcoma. They have also been described occurring secondary to a renal adenocarcinoma. If seen in the early stages they appear as an area of irregular decreased opacity with a surrounding sclerotic zone. The changes may be patchy or generalized in one bone or affect several bones (Figure 4.40). Bone infarcts may occur secondary to hip surgery and are also reported to be a potential site of malignant transformation.

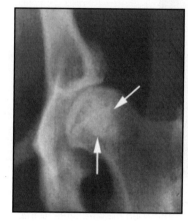

**4.40** Bone infarct: close-up VD view of the left coxofemoral joint showing a triangular radiopacity (arrowed) in the femoral neck. This was determined to be an infarct. The dog had systemic lupus erythematosus. (Courtesy of C Gibbs.)

### Hypertrophic osteopathy
Hypertrophic osteopathy is also called Marie's disease, and was previously known as hypertrophic pulmonary osteoarthropathy. It occurs secondary to a pathological condition, usually a mass lesion in the thorax, but has also been reported in association with abdominal neoplasia. The initial clinical signs include soft tissue swellings affecting all four limbs. A faint periosteal reaction with a brush border effect is the first skeletal radiographic change noted. This progresses to a 'palisade' periosteal reaction (Figure 4.41a) (see Chapter 2). With chronicity, the periosteal new bone becomes rounded and smooth and forms layers aligned parallel with the cortex (Figure 4.41b). In some cases the new bone is located in the soft tissues and is separate from the bone cortex. The new bone formation initially affects the distal

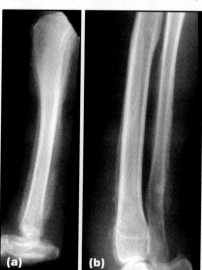

**4.41** Hypertrophic osteopathy ML views. **(a)** Early periosteal reaction along the tibial diaphysis. **(b)** In chronic cases the reaction becomes rounded and smooth with a more lamellar formation, which is visible along the radial diaphysis.

aspects of the limbs and then extends proximally. The medullary cavity is unaffected but the overlying new bone formation simulates an increased opacity within the medulla. If the primary pathological condition is treated the bony changes regress.

## Panosteitis

Panosteitis is usually seen in young dogs (see Chapter 3). However, in some instances it may occur in dogs from 1–2 years of age and has been reported in animals up to 7 years of age. The radiographic features include a patchy increase in opacity in the vicinity of the nutrient foramen (Figure 4.42). Periosteal new bone and endosteal thickening may also be present. The radiographic lesions may persist from an early episode and be seen as an incidental finding (see also Chapter 3).

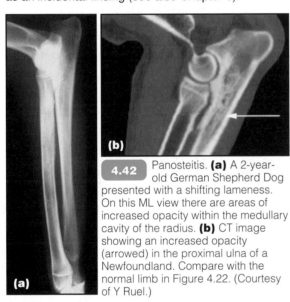

**4.42** Panosteitis. **(a)** A 2-year-old German Shepherd Dog presented with a shifting lameness. On this ML view there are areas of increased opacity within the medullary cavity of the radius. **(b)** CT image showing an increased opacity (arrowed) in the proximal ulna of a Newfoundland. Compare with the normal limb in Figure 4.22. (Courtesy of Y Ruel.)

## Growth arrest lines

Growth arrest lines are occasionally seen as faint linear opacities aligned horizontally in the medullary cavity. They are of no clinical significance (Figure 4.43).

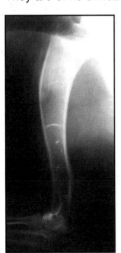

**4.43** Growth arrest lines in a 14-month-old St. Bernard. The radiopaque horizontal bands in the medullary cavity seen on this ML view of the humerus are not clinically significant.

## Osteopetrosis

Osteopetrosis (also known as osteosclerosis fragilis) is a rare condition, which may be congenital or acquired (see Chapter 3). The bones are normal in size and

contour but are more radiopaque than usual. The cortices are thickened and the trabeculae are prominent. The medulla is not visible. The bones become brittle and pathological fractures may ensue (Figure 4.44).

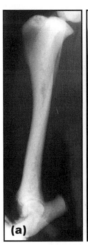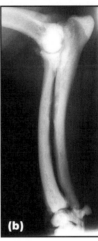

**4.44** Osteopetrosis. The cortices of **(a)** the tibia and **(b)** the radius and ulna are grossly thickened and only faint remnants of the medullary cavities are visible. This abnormality was present in all limbs of this dog.

## Osteosclerosis

Osteoblasts may respond to various insults by producing osseous material in the medullary cavity. It is a rare radiological finding and a bone biopsy is required for a definitive diagnosis. Osteosclerosis has been reported in FeLV-infected cats, producing a widespread increase in opacity throughout the long bones. It may result from myelosclerosis, which is a fibroblastic infiltration of the bone marrow (see Chapter 3).

## Osteopenia

Osteopenia refers to a radiographic decrease in bone opacity (see also Chapter 2). It is reported that a loss of 30–50% of bone mineral is required before it is discernible on radiographs. Overexposure or processing problems may mimic osteopenia. In adults, osteopenia is a rare event. It may occur as a result of non-weight bearing of a limb or a malabsorption syndrome causing a reduction in bone formation. It has also been reported in association with arteriovenous fistulae of the limb. Osteopenia can be divided into osteomalacia and osteoporosis, which are radiographically indistinguishable.

*Osteomalacia:* This is decreased skeletal mineralization with the matrix present. This is an uncommon condition caused by a lack of dietary vitamin D. Radiological features are a generalized reduction in skeletal bone opacity, thin bone cortices and pathological fractures.

*Osteoporosis:* This is decreased skeletal mineralization and decreased bone matrix. It is seen in juveniles with secondary hyperparathyroidism of renal or nutritional origin. It occurs in cats with hypervitaminosis A due in part to disuse. However, the bone proliferation masks a generalized reduction in opacity. The cortex is thin and there is a loss of trabecular bone. Disuse osteoporosis occurs following periods of non-weight bearing and results in a loss of bone mass. It is reported to occur even after two weeks of limb immobilization. If the immobilization is less than twelve weeks then it may be reversible. Pathological fractures may occur. (Figure 4.45).

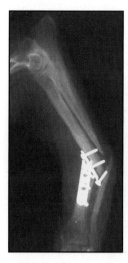

**4.45** Osteopenia. A Yorkshire Terrier had a surgical repair of a fractured radius and ulna one year prior to presentation. The bandage applied at the time had remained in place! Radiographs showed that the implant had failed. Note the generalized reduction in radiopacity throughout the limb but in particular distal to the fracture site.

## Bone cysts

Bone cysts are benign fluid-filled cavities seen in the long bones of immature and young adult large-breed dogs (see also Chapter 3). They are commonly seen in the diaphysis or metaphyseal regions of the radius and ulna but may occur anywhere in the skeleton.

## Aneurysmal bone cysts

Aneurysmal bone cysts are rare. They appear as expansile, osteolytic, multiloculated lesions that are often septate. They are due to vascular anomalies, such as arteriovenous fistulae or vascular defects resulting from trauma or neoplasia. Aneurysmal bone cysts can be differentiated from other bone cysts because they are usually filled with blood and generally occur in the older animal. They have a typical 'soap bubble' appearance created by the compartmentalized cysts, which are lined by trabecular bone and connective tissue (Figure 4.46). Blood flow may be demonstrated within these cysts

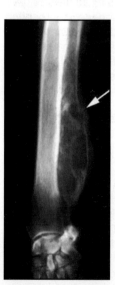

**4.46** Aneurysmal bone cyst. This extensive osteolytic expansile mass has deformed the diaphysis. The cortices are thinned and there is a disruption on the lateral aspect of the ulna (arrowed). (Courtesy of R Pechman.)

using colour flow Doppler ultrasonography. They are difficult to treat and the prognosis is therefore guarded. Malignant transformation is reported.

## References and further reading

Agut A, Corzo N, Murciano J, Laredo FG and Soler M (2003) Clinical and radiographic study of bone and joint lesions in 26 dogs with Leishmaniasis. *Veterinary Record* **153**, 648–652

Barnhart MD (2000) Malignant transformation of an aneurysmal bone cyst in a dog. *Veterinary Surgery* **31**, 519–524

Berry CR, Love NE and Thrall DE (2002) Interpretation paradigms for the appendicular skeleton – canine and feline. In: *Textbook of Veterinary Diagnostic Radiology. 4th edn,* ed. DE Thrall, pp. 135–145. WB Saunders, Philadelphia

Coulson A and Lewis N (2002) *An Atlas of Interpretative Radiographic Anatomy of the Dog and Cat.* Blackwell Science, Oxford

Dennis R, Kirberger RM, Wrigley RH and Barr FJ (2001) *Handbook of Small Animal Radiological Differential Diagnosis.* WB Saunders, London

Denny HR and Butterworth S (2000) *A Guide to Canine and Feline Orthopaedic Surgery, 4th edn,* Blackwell Publishing, Oxford

Dernell WS (1999) Treatment of severe orthopaedic infections. *Veterinary Clinics of North America: Small Animal Practice* **29**, 1261–1274

Dickinson PJ, McEntee MC, Lipsitz D, Keel K and LeCouteur RA (2001) Radiation induced vertebral osteosarcoma following treatment of an intradural extramedullary spinal cord tumor in a dog. *Veterinary Radiology and Ultrasound* **42**, 463–470

Dubielzig RR, Biery DN and Brodey RS (1981) Bone sarcomas associated with multifocal medullary bone infarction in dogs. *Journal of the American Veterinary Medical Association* **179**, 64–68

Emmerson TD and Pead MJ (1999) Pathological fracture of the femur secondary to haematogenous osteomyelitis in a Weimaraner. *Journal of Small Animal Practice* **40**, 233–235

Flecknell PA, Gibbs C and Kelly DF (1978) Myelosclerosis in a cat. *Journal of Comparative Pathology* **88**, 627–631

Kealy JK and McAllister H (2005) *Diagnostic Radiology and Ultrasonography of the Dog and Cat, 4th edn.* Elsevier, USA

Madewell BR, Wilson DW, Hornof WJ and Gregory CR (1990) Leukemoid blood response and bone infarcts in a dog with renal tubular adenocarcinoma. *Journal of the American Veterinary Medical Association* **197**, 1623–1625

Marcellin-Little DJ, De Young DJ, Thrall DE and Merrill CL (1999) Osteosarcoma at the site of bone infarction associated with total hip arthroplasty in a dog. *Veterinary Surgery* **28**, 54–60

Mehl ML, Withrow SJ, Seguin B, Powers BE, Dernell WS, Pardo AD, Rosenthal RC, Dolginow SZ and Park RD (2001) Spontaneous regression of osteosarcoma in four dogs. *Journal of the American Veterinary Medical Association* **219**, 614–617

Morgan JP (1999) *Radiology in Veterinary Orthopedics 2nd edn.* Venture Press, California

Murphy ST, Parker RB and Woodard JC (1997) Osteosarcoma following total hip arthroplasty in a dog. *Journal of Small Animal Practice* **38**, 263–267

Robin D and Marcellin-Little DJ. (2001) Incomplete ossification of the humeral condyle in two Labrador retrievers. *Journal of Small Animal Practice* **42**, 231–234

Schaer M (2003) *Clinical Medicine of the Dog and Cat.* Manson Publishing, UK

Schwarz T, Störk CK, Mellor D and Sullivan M (2000) Osteopenia and other radiographic signs in canine hyperadrenocorticism. *Journal of Small Animal Practice* **41**, 491–495

Sebestyen P, Marcellin-Little DJ and DeYoung BA (2000) Femoral medullary infarction secondary to canine total hip arthroplasty. *Veterinary Surgery* **29**, 227–236

Thomas WB, Daniel GB and McGavin MD (1997) Parosteal osteosarcoma of the cervical vertebra in a dog. *Veterinary Radiology and Ultrasound* **38**, 120–123

Uhthoff HK and Jaworski ZF (1978) Bone loss in response to long-term immobilization. *Journal of Bone and Joint Surgery British volume.* **60-B**, 420–429

Wrigley R (2000) Malignant versus nonmalignant bone bisease. *Veterinary Clinics of North America: Small Animal Practice* **30**, 315–347

# 5

# Long bones – fractures

## Steven J. Butterworth

Radiography remains the mainstay for imaging long bone fractures, partly because it is readily available but also because it generally provides all the information required by a clinician to manage a fracture appropriately. This chapter concerns itself with the radiographic features of long bone fractures, their healing and the complications thereof.

## Indications

- Trauma causing severe lameness associated with pain and swelling.
- To facilitate planning of fracture treatment.
- To evaluate adequacy of reduction and any implant placement post-treatment.
- To document progression of fracture healing.
- To investigate reasons for lack of expected progress following treatment, i.e. fracture complications such as implant failure or infection.
- To investigate the appearance of sinuses following fracture treatment (infection).
- To evaluate malunion.
- To evaluate any long term complications relating to pain at an 'old' fracture site.

## Radiography and normal anatomy

The radiographic techniques required for satisfactory imaging of long bones are discussed in Chapter 3 and appropriate projections are outlined in Chapter 4. Furthermore, normal long bone anatomy and timing of physeal closures are detailed in Chapters 2 and 3.

There are certain normal features that can readily be mistaken for fracture lines, either in normal bones or as additional fissure lines in bones that are fractured:

- Physes
- Nutrient foraminae
- Mach lines (created by superimposition of a cortical margin of one bone, or fragment, on another) (see Chapter 4)
- Overlying fascial planes or skin margins.

Experience and familiarity with the normal radiographic appearance of long bones will help to reduce (eliminate) such misinterpretation (see Chapter 2).

## Alternative imaging techniques

### Computed tomography and magnetic resonance imaging

Although advanced imaging techniques such as computed tomography (CT) and magnetic resonance imaging (MRI) can be used to better define fractures of structures such as the skull or pelvis, their use in the imaging of long bone fractures would be largely of academic interest. One possible exception to this might be in confirming non-union in a situation where the fibrous junction undulates in such a way as to make it impossible to show a conclusive lack of bone union from two-dimensional radiographs. In such cases, CT can be used to confirm the lack of bone union.

### Ultrasonography

Ultrasonography is of little value for imaging fractures of long bones *per se*, although it may be of some use for imaging associated soft tissue structures that might be injured, such as nearby tendons. It can be used effectively to assess fractures of the skull, particularly depression fractures, to evaluate the position of fragments relative to the brain. Ultrasound examination might also be useful to evaluate early callus formation and early osteomyelitis (which results in anechoic subperiosteal fluid). One study looked at whether therapeutic ultrasonography could be used to enhance bone healing but found little difference compared with controls (Lidbetter and Millis, 2002).

### Scintigraphy

Scintigraphy has little value in the imaging of normal fractures. Although it might be of some help in evaluating cellular activity in cases with suspected non-union (see later), there are no clinical reports of it having been used for this purpose in small animal orthopaedics. Scintigraphy has been shown to be useful in the detection of stress fractures in athletic animals. In such cases, an increase in uptake of radioisotope may be seen before radiological evidence of a stress fracture (see later). The technique could also conceivably be used in cases suspected of having pathological fractures associated with neoplasia, to look for bone metastases elsewhere in the skeleton.

## Abnormal radiological findings

### Classification of fractures

A fracture may be defined as a disruption in the continuity of a bone. Most are caused by direct injury in road traffic accidents or falls, the fracture occurring at or near the point of impact. A fracture may also result from an indirect force transmitted through bone or muscle to a vulnerable area of bone, which breaks in a predictable manner; for example, fractures of the tibial tuberosity, olecranon or lateral epicondyle of the humerus.

The aim of fracture classification is to provide a foundation on which to base decisions regarding appropriate management and to document any correlation of fracture type with complications in healing. It also makes it possible to relate the features of a fracture to another clinician who will then have a clear idea of that particular fracture's characteristics, allowing discussion of appropriate fracture management. Fractures may be classified according to:

- Anatomical location
- External wounds
- Extent of bone damage
- Direction of fracture line
- Relative displacement of the bone fragments
- Stability.

### Anatomical location

It is customary to refer to specific fractures of a long bone according to their anatomical location:

- Proximal
- Distal
- Diaphyseal.

The proximal or distal fractures can be further subdivided into articular, epiphyseal, physeal or metaphyseal fractures. Diaphyseal fractures can be further classified according to the direction of the fracture line or the number of fragments (see below). This concept was formalized by the AO/ASIF group so that a 'numerical' reference could be given to any long bone fracture. Firstly, by the bone involved:

1 = Humerus
2 = Radius/ulna
3 = Femur
4 = Tibia/fibula

Secondly, by the zone of the bone involved:

1 = Proximal
2 = Middle
3 = Distal

Thirdly, according to the fracture configuration:

A = Simple
B = Wedge or butterfly fragment
C = Comminuted

For example a simple, transverse mid-diaphyseal fracture of the tibia (see Figure 5.4a) would be classified as 42-A. A fourth tier of classification is then given according to the specific fracture configuration, but the diversity of definitions between regions precludes a concise description and the reader should refer to Brinker *et al.* (1998).

Fractures of the physis are divided into six types (Salter and Harris, 1963). In type I injuries the fracture line travels exclusively through the physis (common in fracture of the proximal femoral physis; Figure 5.1a). In type II the fracture line passes along the physis but then breaks out through the metaphysis (common in fracture of the proximal tibial physis; Figure 5.1b). Type III injuries involve the physis and epiphysis (uncommon but perhaps seen most often in medial humeral condylar fractures of immature dogs; Figure 5.1c). In the type IV injuries the fracture line passes through the epiphysis and metaphysis, crossing the physis (common in fractures of the distal humeral physis and lateral condylar fractures in immature dogs; Figure 5.1d). Type V injuries involve an impaction fracture of part or all of the physis (common in the distal ulnar physis; Figure 5.1e). Finally, type VI injuries involve periosteal bridging of the physis as a result of injury to the adjacent bone; a rare occurrence in small animal orthopaedics (Figure 5.1f).

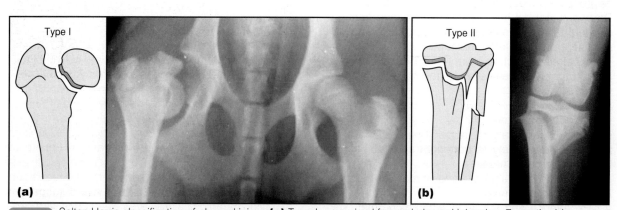

**5.1** Salter–Harris classification of physeal injury. **(a)** Type I: a proximal femoral physeal injury in a 7-month-old Labrador Retriever. The fracture line passes along the line of the physis. **(b)** Type II: a proximal tibial physeal injury in a 6-month-old Boxer. The fracture line passes along part of the physis and out through the metaphysis. (continues) ▶

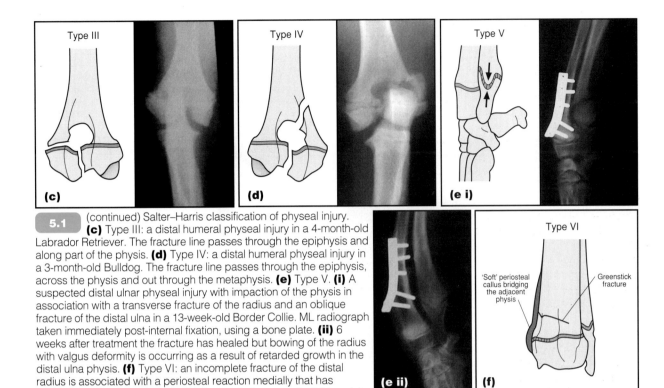

**5.1** (continued) Salter–Harris classification of physeal injury. **(c)** Type III: a distal humeral physeal injury in a 4-month-old Labrador Retriever. The fracture line passes through the epiphysis and along part of the physis. **(d)** Type IV: a distal humeral physeal injury in a 3-month-old Bulldog. The fracture line passes through the epiphysis, across the physis and out through the metaphysis. **(e)** Type V. **(i)** A suspected distal ulnar physeal injury with impaction of the physis in association with a transverse fracture of the radius and an oblique fracture of the distal ulna in a 13-week-old Border Collie. ML radiograph taken immediately post-internal fixation, using a bone plate. **(ii)** 6 weeks after treatment the fracture has healed but bowing of the radius with valgus deformity is occurring as a result of retarded growth in the distal ulna physis. **(f)** Type VI: an incomplete fracture of the distal radius is associated with a periosteal reaction medially that has bridged the distal physis and will influence further growth at this point.

### External wounds

A closed fracture is one in which the overlying skin remains intact. An open fracture is one in which there is a communication between the fracture site and a skin wound. Open fractures are classified as first, second or third degree, according to the severity of soft tissue injury and contamination. In first degree open fractures the skin is punctured by a fracture fragment but there is virtually no soft tissue loss. In second degree open fractures the skin is punctured from the outside and there is generally some loss of soft tissue. In third degree open fractures there is gross contamination and loss of soft tissue or bone.

With long bone fractures, radiography will rarely enable such typing of open fractures, indeed it may not be possible to determine that the fracture is open. Radiographic evidence that the skin has been breached comprises the finding of gas (air) opacities within the soft tissues (Figure 5.2a), complete loss of soft tissues over an area of bone, marked loss of bone mass or the presence of a foreign body (Figure 5.2b). In open fractures, resulting from gunshot injuries, the configuration is dependent on location. The diaphysis tends to shatter, forming a comminuted fracture (Figure 5.2b), whereas the metaphysis tends to puncture with the ballistic energy being absorbed by the surrounding trabecular bone network.

### Extent of bone damage

A complete fracture is one in which the continuity of the bone is totally disrupted and there is usually marked displacement of the fragments (Figure 5.3a).

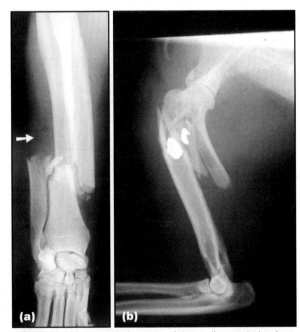

**5.2** **(a)** An open fracture of the radius and ulna in a 3-year-old Boxer. A gas shadow can be seen (arrowed) within the soft tissues proximal to the fracture site. **(b)** An open fracture of the humerus in a 4-year-old Domestic Short-haired cat caused by an air gun pellet.

An incomplete fracture is one in which partial continuity of the bone is maintained, as in greenstick (bending) fractures of young animals (Figure 5.3b) or fissure fractures in mature animals (Figure 5.3c).

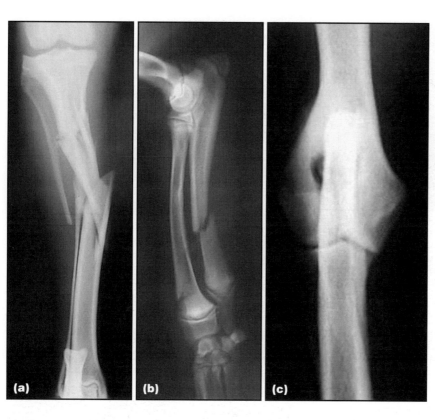

**5.3** **(a)** Complete fracture of the tibia in a 6-year-old Border Collie. **(b)** Incomplete (greenstick) fracture of the distal radial metaphysis with complete fracture of the ulna in a 6-month-old Labrador Retriever. **(c)** Incomplete ossification of the humeral condyle in a 5-year-old Springer Spaniel. The periosteal reaction on the lateral humeral epicondyle suggests an incomplete condylar fracture.

### Direction of fracture line

- A *transverse fracture* is one in which the fracture line is at right angles to the long axis of the bone (Figure 5.4a).
- An *oblique fracture* is one at an angle to the long axis of the bone (Figure 5.4b). A short, oblique fracture line has a length that is less than approximately twice the diameter of the bone. The significance of this is that it is

difficult or impossible to apply interfragmentary compression in a short, oblique fracture using lagged bone screws or cerclage wire. A long oblique fracture has a length that exceeds twice the diameter of the bone and it will be possible to apply interfragmentary compression with such implants.
- A *spiral fracture* curves around the bone. A long oblique fracture will often have a spiral component (Figure 5.4c).

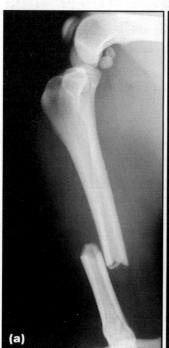
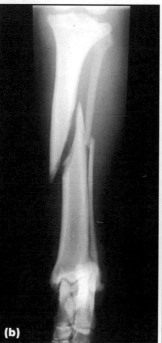
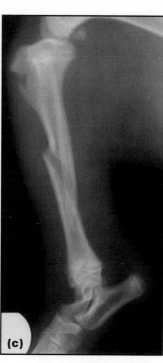

**5.4**

**(a)** A transverse fracture of a tibia in a 4-year-old terrier. **(b)** An oblique fracture of a tibia in a 14-month-old Staffordshire Bull Terrier. Many such fractures will have a spiral element to them. **(c)** A spiral fracture of a tibia in a 15-week-old Cocker Spaniel. (continues) ▶

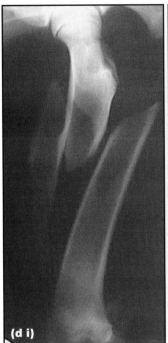
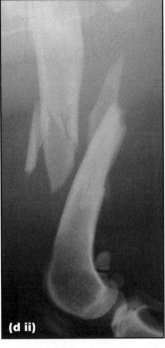
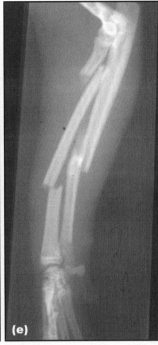

**5.4**

(continued)
**(d)** Comminuted fractures. **(i)** A reconstructable comminuted fracture of a femur in a 7-month-old German Short-haired Pointer. **(ii)** A non-reconstructable comminuted fracture of a femur in a 23-month-old Labrador Retriever. **(e)** A segmental (or multiple) fracture of a radius (with accompanying transverse fracture of the ulna) in a 3-year-old Domestic Long-haired cat.

- A *comminuted fracture* is one in which there are several fragments and the fracture lines communicate (Figure 5.4d). The percentage of bone length involved is often estimated in these fractures. It is also customary to identify the number of fragments, except in highly comminuted fractures where the number is generally not accurately countable. Substantial fragments include the proximal and distal 'segments' and butterfly fragments. The latter are defined as those fragments that are reducible and can be stabilized by application of interfragmentary implants such as lagged bone screws or cerclage wires. Small fragments are those which cannot be reduced and stabilized in this way. This leads to comminuted fractures being classified as either 'reconstructable' or 'non-reconstructable' (Figure 5.4d).
- A *segmental (or multiple) fracture* is one in which the bone is broken into three or more segments such that the fracture lines do not communicate (Figure 5.4e).

### Relative displacement of the bone fragments

- An *avulsion fracture* is one in which a bone fragment is distracted by the pull of the muscle tendon or ligament that attaches to it (e.g. avulsion of the tibial tuberosity; Figure 5.5a).
- An *impacted fracture* is one in which the fractured bone ends are driven into one another (Figure 5.5b).
- A *compression fracture* refers, typically, to a fracture of a vertebra where a compressive force has resulted in shortening of the vertebra.
- A *depression fracture* usually refers to skull fractures in which the affected bone is 'pushed in', resulting in a concave deformity.

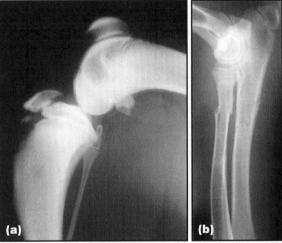

**5.5** **(a)** Avulsion of the tibial tuberosity in a 6-month-old Greyhound. The fragment has become distracted as a result of contraction of the quadriceps muscle group. **(b)** An impacted fracture, with the ends driven into one another, of a radius and ulna in a 6-month-old Great Dane.

### Stability of the fracture

The assessment of a fracture's inherent stability is of particular importance when selecting the appropriate method of fracture fixation. What is the fracture's resistance to shortening, rotation and angulation? Diaphyseal fractures can be broadly divided into stable and unstable fractures.

- Stable fractures are the transverse, blunt (short) oblique or greenstick fractures in which the fragments interlock and resist shortening forces (see Figures 5.3b and 5.4a). The only fixation necessary is to prevent angular deformity and, sometimes, rotation. Depending on the fracture site, this can be achieved either by external coaptation or by application of an intramedullary pin, an external fixator or a plate.

- Unstable fractures are oblique, spiral or comminuted (see Figures 5.4c and d). The fragments do not interlock and a method of fixation is needed that will maintain the length of the bone and prevent angular deformity and rotation. This usually involves application of a plate and screws or an external fixator.

## Pathological fractures

Pathological fractures involve loss of continuity in diseased bone, usually as a result of minimal trauma. The most common causes of such bone fragility are:

- Nutritional – hyperparathyroidism, secondary to feeding of a low calcium diet (e.g. meat) (see Chapter 3)
- Metabolic – renal disease, causing hyperparathyroidism as a result of phosphate retention (see Chapter 4)
- Neoplasia – primary (e.g. osteosarcoma) or metastatic disease (most commonly carcinoma) (see Chapter 4).

For further potential causes of pathological fractures see Chapters 3 and 4. These fractures tend to be simple because the bone tissue is weak. This means that minimal energy is absorbed before bone failure occurs, resulting in a simple fracture configuration (transverse, short oblique) or a 'folding' fracture (Figure 5.6a). The observation of bone lysis within the fracture ends or a periosteal reaction in a case with a fracture of only a few days duration are both suggestive of bone neoplasia (Figure 5.6b). Unfortunately, the abnormal radiolucency may be more easily observed once the fracture has been reconstructed (Figure 5.6c).

## Stress fractures

The only report of 'stress fractures' affecting small animals involved a series of racing Greyhounds with non-displaced fractures of the acetabulum (Wendelberg *et al.*, 1988). Stress remodelling, which is presumed to involve microfracture of cortical bone as a result of chronic stress, is also seen in racing Greyhounds affecting metacarpal or metatarsal bones (Figure 5.7a; see also Chapter 11). Such remodelling has also been noted in some dogs that are lame as a result of an incomplete fracture (which might in itself be, in part, a stress fracture) of the humeral condyle (Figure 5.7b) (Butterworth and Innes, 2001). Such stress remodelling is recognized as a well organized, regular periosteal reaction on the affected metacarpal/tarsal bone or lateral humeral epicondylar crest.

## Post-treatment fracture evaluation

Following a chosen treatment, whether it involves external coaptation, external skeletal fixation or internal fixation, radiographs in two orthogonal planes should be taken. This will allow identification of any errors in fracture alignment, some of which may need correcting (Figure 5.8a) and some of which may be acceptable (Figure 5.8b). Radiography also permits evaluation of implant placement that again might need immediate correction (Figure 5.8c) or give some forewarning of a potential need to remove the implants after fracture healing because of irritation caused by its proximity to a joint (Figure 5.8d). The assessment of post-treatment radiographs should include attention to the following:

- Reduction
- Spatial alignment
- Implants.

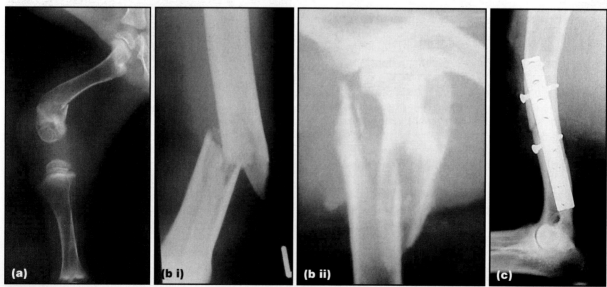

(a)   (b i)   (b ii)   (c)

**5.6**  **(a)** A simple, folding fracture of the femur in a 6-week-old German Shepherd Dog. Note how thin the cortices are. The dog was suffering from nutritional secondary hyperparathyroidism. **(b) (i)** Pathological fracture of the tibia in an 8-year-old Dobermann. Note the subtle lysis of the ends of the two bone fragments. **(ii)** Pathological fracture of the femur in a 6-year-old Dobermann. Note the irregular margins to the fracture ends caused by the pre-existing periosteal reaction. **(c)** Pathological fracture of the humerus in a 10-year-old Labrador X Collie. The region of abnormal radiolucency in the diaphysis at the proximal extremity of the fracture is clearly evident in this radiograph, which was taken after internal fixation.

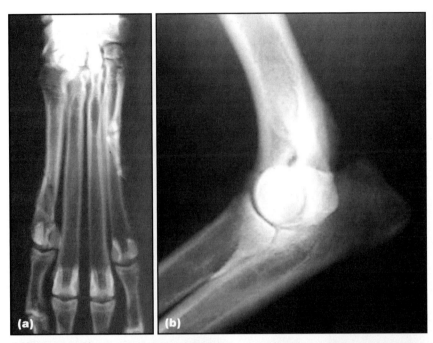

5.7  **(a)** Stress fracture of metacarpal 5 in a racing Greyhound. Note the periosteal reaction present at the time of fracture. (Courtesy of MG Ness.) **(b)** Stress remodelling of the lateral humeral epicondyle in a 5-year-old Springer Spaniel.

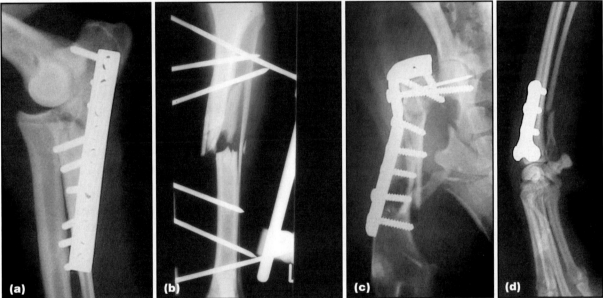

5.8  **(a)** Postoperative radiograph taken following internal fixation of a Monteggia fracture in a 4-year-old Border Collie. The plate is over-contoured, creating elbow joint incongruity, which requires correction. **(b)** Postoperative radiograph taken following external skeletal fixation of an open tibial fracture in a 7-year-old Lurcher. Spatial realignment of the crus is not perfect but is acceptable given the functional appearance of the limb alignment as judged clinically. **(c)** Postoperative radiograph taken following internal fixation of a non-reconstructable, comminuted femoral fracture, which involved the femoral neck, in a 7-year-old Cocker Spaniel. Note the bone screw and K-wire used to stabilize the femoral neck both enter the coxofemoral joint space and need to be replaced and withdrawn, respectively. **(d)** Postoperative radiograph taken following internal fixation of a distal radial fracture in a 15-month-old Toy Poodle, using a T-plate. The plate encroaches on the carpal joint and might cause irritation through this or by lying under the extensor tendons. Implant positioning cannot be improved at this stage, but it is likely implant removal will be necessary after fracture healing if maximal return of limb function is to be achieved.

## Reduction

The proportion of the fracture surfaces that are in apposition is a key factor. In transverse fractures treated with external coaptation or fixation, 50% apposition is generally considered adequate. In fractures treated by open reduction, involving reconstruction and internal fixation, the fracture lines should, ideally, not be visible in either of two orthogonal views (Figure 5.9). This is very difficult to achieve in diaphyseal

fractures but should always be the goal of such treatment, and is imperative in articular fractures. If bone plates are used to treat transverse or short oblique fractures then it is most important not to find a defect in the cortex opposite the plate (the transcortex) as this will cause focal stress on the plate that might well lead to implant failure (see Figure 5.26). In non-reconstructable, comminuted fractures, reduction is not attempted and so is not relevant.

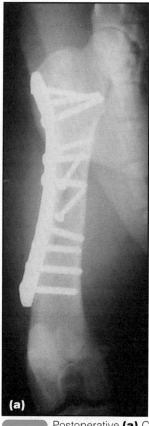
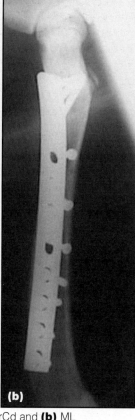

**5.9** Postoperative **(a)** CrCd and **(b)** ML radiographs of reconstructed femoral fracture in a 7-month-old German Short-haired Pointer.

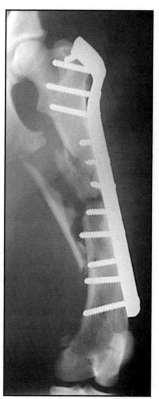

**5.10** Postoperative radiograph of a non-reconstructed femoral fracture, showing bridging fixation using a bone plate, with satisfactory spatial alignment of the bone ends in a 23-month-old Labrador Retriever.

## Spatial alignment

Spatial alignment relates to how the two ends of the bones relate to one another in a three-dimensional sense. If a fracture is reconstructed accurately, then the spatial alignment has to be correct. However, in non-reconstructable, comminuted fractures, where bridging fixation is used, it is important that the two ends of the bone are the correct distance apart and oriented so that joint alignment is correct in terms of angulation and rotation. Such an assessment requires that the joints proximal and distal to the fracture are included in the radiographs (Figure 5.10).

## Implants

It should be ensured that the implants do not compromise joint surfaces or physes, but, if they do, this should be remedied immediately. The stability of the 'construct' used should be checked to ensure it is adequate for its purpose. This would include assessment of the 'size' of the plate used, the configuration of any external skeletal fixator, and the number of plate screws or fixation pins proximal and distal to the fracture. If an implant has been placed in a fracture line then this may be important if loss of purchase for the implant renders the construct inadequately stable, or if it causes loss of reduction of the fracture leading to instability (Figure 5.11). In some cases implants are placed close to joints through necessity and, although, they will not require correction it might well prove necessary to remove them following fracture healing in order to regain optimal limb function (see Figure 5.8d).

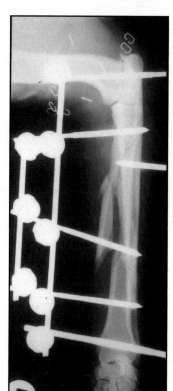

**5.11** Postoperative radiograph of a non-reconstructed open radial fracture showing bridging fixation, using an external skeletal fixator, in an 18-month-old Collie X. Note one of the fixation pins encroaching on a fracture line. Limited purchase and early loosening can be expected for this implant.

## Types of fracture healing

There are essentially three types of fracture healing:

*   Classical
*   Primary
*   Bridging osteosynthesis.

## Classical fracture healing

Classical fracture healing is taken as the pattern of events that follows fracture of a long bone when it is treated conservatively, but is also seen after closed reduction of a stable fracture, which is then supported by external coaptation. At the time a bone is fractured there is also damage to local soft tissues and a haematoma forms at the site (Figure 5.12a), which contains numerous chemical mediators from both the bone itself (e.g. bone morphogenic protein, BMP) and the supporting tissues. These chemical mediators stimulate mitosis and differentiation of mesenchymal cells, and angiogenesis. The source of both cells and new blood vessels includes the periosteum and endosteum but an important extraosseous supply is also derived from the damaged, supporting soft tissues. During this period of early response to fracture the bone ends themselves tend to resorb, for two main reasons. Firstly, the ends of the fragments are deprived of an intrinsic blood supply and so 'die back'. Secondly, increasing the fracture gap reduces the stresses in the interposed tissues caused by movement between the fragments, thus preventing the stresses exceeding the physiological limits of the invading cells.

After invading the clot the mesenchymal cells differentiate into fibroblasts, chondroblasts or osteoblasts, depending on local environmental factors such as movement and blood supply. Under ideal conditions of compression and adequate oxygen tension the cells become osteoblasts and woven bone is produced rapidly. In less ideal conditions of stability and oxygen tension, where osteoblasts would not survive, the mesenchymal cells differentiate into chondroblasts, producing hyaline cartilage that becomes mineralized and converted to bone by the process of endochondral ossification. When the tissue is under tension (e.g. avulsion fractures) the mesenchymal cells differentiate into fibroblasts that produce fibrous tissue. This is an undesirable situation since such tissue does not

enhance stability to allow the invasion of more appropriate cell types, nor does it have the ability to mineralize and become more stable. Thus, the production of fibrous tissue within a fracture gap creates a barrier to healing rather than a contribution to the bone union.

The callus so-formed by the invasion and differentiation of mesenchymal cells can be divided into:

- External – derived from the periosteum
- Internal – derived from the endosteum.

As the callus advances from both sides of the fracture gap it replaces the initial clot and will usually have created a 'bridging callus' by two weeks after injury, although this will only be faintly visible radiographically. At that stage the callus will consist of woven bone over the fracture ends with, in most cases, an area of hyaline cartilage at the level of the fracture gap (i.e. where there is least stability and the callus is thickest, creating a lower oxygen tension within) (Figure 5.12b). In a stable fracture with adequate blood supply, bridging with a bony callus ('clinical union') may be expected within six weeks, but a longer period will be required in less ideal circumstances. The size of the callus is directly related to the stability at the fracture site but is also influenced by the age of the patient. At an unstable site the quantity of callus produced is greater so as to spread the stresses at that site through more tissue, thus keeping the stress at any one point below the maximum that can be tolerated by the cells present. Because callus formation is also a response to periosteal injury, and the fact that immature patients have a more active periosteum, in any given situation of fracture stability an immature patient will produce more callus than a mature one.

Once bridging of the fracture gap with woven bone is complete the callus undergoes compaction and remodelling (Figure 5.12c). Woven bone is converted

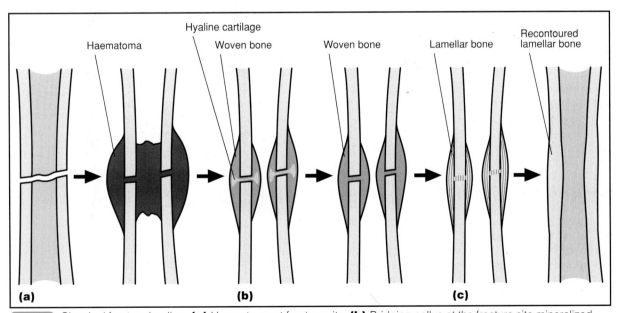

**5.12** Classical fracture healing. **(a)** Haematoma at fracture site. **(b)** Bridging callus at the fracture site mineralized peripherally but with hyaline cartilage at the level of the fracture site. **(c)** Compaction and remodelling of the mineralized callus.

into compact bone by osteoblasts laying down bone on the trabeculae, thus filling in the spaces. As normal structure, and therefore strength, returns to the bone the callus can be reduced in size, according to Wolff's law, and so the remodelling process leads to a gradual flattening of the callus as the bone regains more of its original shape. This remodelling occurs at the same pace as is occurring throughout the skeleton and may take months or years, depending, to some extent, on the age of the patient.

### Primary bone healing

If fracture reduction is accurate and the stability rigid then healing may occur without external callus formation and is termed 'direct' or 'contact healing' (Figure 5.13a). This requires the fracture ends to be perfectly apposed and then compressed together firmly. Since this will eliminate movement at the fracture line, there will be no signal for a callus to be formed. The fracture then heals by the normal process of remodelling, whereby the bone at the ends of the fragments is replaced by new bone through the activity 'cutting cones', forming new osteons that traverse the fracture line. As these bone-filled tunnels are formed across the fracture line so the fragments gradually become reconnected to one another over a prolonged period of time.

Where a small (less than one millimetre) gap exists between bone ends, but stability is sufficient, the gap will become filled with lamellar bone orientated perpendicular to the longitudinal axis. Although the gap becomes filled with bone very quickly, it remains a site of weakness until it is integrated into the normal bone architecture by virtue of the remodelling process. This process is referred to as 'gap healing' (Figure 5.13b).

Although in an ideal situation of compression and stability it might be expected that fracture healing would take place without the formation of callus, in reality some callus will often form in response to the mechanical stimulus of periosteal or endosteal injury,

particularly in skeletally immature patients (see Figure 5.18b).

The advantage of primary bone healing over classical healing is that, because the fragments are extremely stable, the bone as a whole is able to be loaded. This allows early return to limb function during fracture healing, which helps to avoid fracture disease (i.e. joint stiffness, muscle wastage, soft tissue adhesions and disuse osteoporosis). The disadvantage is that, because the process of remodelling takes a long time, the implants used to stabilize the fracture cannot be removed at an early stage.

### Bridging osteosynthesis

The concept of 'bridging osteosynthesis' has developed in an attempt to combine the advantages of classical and primary bone healing, whilst avoiding their disadvantages. It involves the stabilization of the two ends of a fractured bone, relative to one another, without the anatomical reduction of each bone fragment. The site of fracture is left as undisturbed as possible so as to avoid unnecessary removal of fracture haematoma (with its valuable chemical mediators) and also minimize any further compromise of the vascular supply to the region. Thus, the fracture is encouraged to heal by callus formation but in an environment of stability created by bridging of the fracture site, usually with a bone plate or an external skeletal fixator (Johnson, 1998) (± an intramedullary pin) (Figure 5.14) but interlocking nails are also designed for this purpose.

Bridging osteosynthesis carries with it the more rapid return of bone strength seen with classical healing whilst allowing the limb function during healing associated with primary union by virtue of the injured bone being protected. Conversely, it reduces the likelihood of 'fracture disease', which is often associated with methods of treatment relying on classical healing, and avoids the prolonged reliance on orthopaedic implants seen with primary healing.

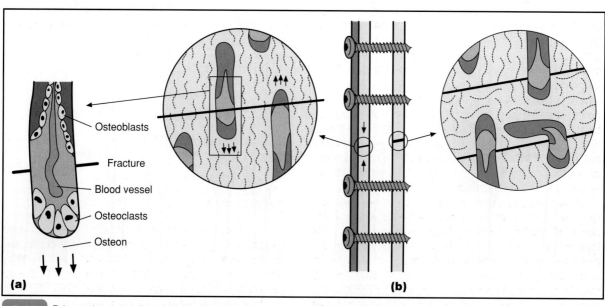

Osteoblasts

Fracture

Blood vessel

Osteoclasts

Osteon

(a)

(b)

**5.13** Primary bone healing. **(a)** Direct or contact healing. **(b)** Gap healing.

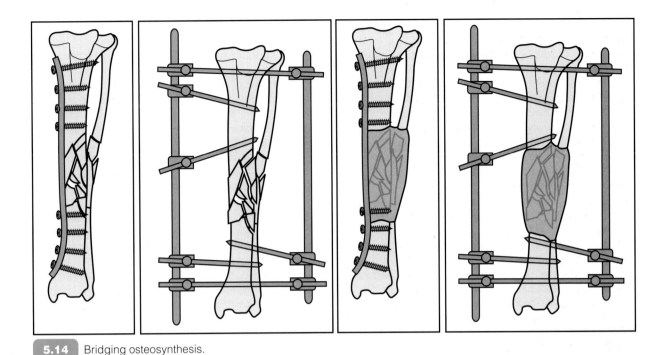

**5.14** Bridging osteosynthesis.

## Radiographic progression of fracture healing

The time taken for a fracture to heal is dependent on a number of factors, including:

- Type of bone involved
- Type of fracture
- Age of patient
- Method of treatment
- Other systemic disease
- Vascular supply.

Cancellous bone has a more abundant blood supply and a greater inherent cellular activity than cortical bone. Therefore, a fracture involving the epiphysis or metaphysis of a bone tends to heal more quickly than one involving the diaphysis. Impacted fractures and long spiral or oblique fractures where the fragment surfaces are in close proximity heal more quickly than those where the fragments are widely separated. Comminuted fractures tend to heal more slowly because of inherent instability and disruption of blood supply to the numerous fragments. On the other hand simple fractures (e.g. transverse fractures), whilst having less disruption to their blood supply when compared with comminuted fractures, may also heal slowly because of relative instability caused by the concentration of stresses over a small area.

Healing is also delayed in the presence of infection (e.g. an open fracture) and may be delayed or not occur in fractures involving diseased bone (i.e. pathological fractures). The initial union and subsequent remodelling of a fracture will be much more rapid in a skeletally immature patient than in one that is middle-aged. It will also be influenced by concurrent systemic diseases, such as hyperadrenocorticism (Cushing's disease), chronic renal failure, or dietary inadequacies such as nutritional secondary hyperparathyroidism. The method of treatment chosen for any given fracture configuration will also influence the speed of healing, depending to a large extent on whether it favours classical healing, primary healing or bridging osteosynthesis. Brinker (1978) defined clinical union as that point in time during the recovery when fracture healing had progressed sufficiently for the fixation device to be removed. Based on the average time taken for a simple fracture in a dog to achieve clinical union Brinker (1978) produced a table illustrating the variation with age and method of fixation (Figure 5.15).

| Age of animal | Time taken to reach clinical union | |
|---|---|---|
| | *External coaptation* [a] *External skeletal fixation* [a] *Intramedullary pinning* [a] | *Plate fixation* [b] |
| <3 months | 2–3 weeks | 1 month |
| 3–6 months | 4–6 weeks | 2–3 months |
| 6–12 months | 5–8 weeks | 3–5 months |
| >12 months | 7–12 weeks | 5–12 months |

**5.15** Time taken to achieve clinical union depending on patient's age and method of management (Adapted from Brinker, 1978). [a] = Classical healing or bridging osteosynthesis. [b] = Primary bone healing.

For the purpose of the discussion below, the radiographic changes relate to healing of a mid-diaphyseal fracture in a young adult dog that is otherwise healthy. The reader will need to adapt the timings of the sequences for dogs that are younger or older, or where fracture healing is compromised by any of the factors listed above.

## Classical fracture healing and bridging osteosynthesis

At the time of fracture the fragment ends will appear clear and sharp. Swelling of the surrounding soft tissues is usually seen, particularly in the distal limb (Figure 5.16a). After 7–10 days the margins of the fragments become less distinct because of demineralization of the edges as part of the 'die back' phenomenon related to loss of blood supply to the bone margins and the need to reduce the level of strain in the tissues between the fragments. At this stage incomplete ('hairline') fractures may be more readily identified. An early, indistinct periosteal reaction may be noted and soft tissue swelling, will generally, have resolved.

After 2–3 weeks a bridging callus will be present and this will be faintly visible radiographically (Figure 5.16b). From 3 weeks onwards the callus will gradually become more opaque radiographically as the cartilage becomes mineralized and converted to bone by the process of endochondral ossification. The maturity of the callus is related to its opacity, which can be compared with the adjacent bone.

By 6–8 weeks there should be a callus of woven bone bridging the fracture and continuous mineralization from proximal to distal should be evident radiographically. To confirm the absence of any remaining cartilage callus requires radiography in at least two planes otherwise the radiolucent line through the callus might be missed. At this stage 'clinical union' will have been achieved (Figure 5.16c). The extent of callus formation is influenced by a number of factors, in particular the stability of the fracture and the age of the patient.

As previously described, instability leads to callus of greater width to distribute stress and strain such that these remain within the tolerance of the tissue involved. Periosteal stripping is more likely in immature patients and this results in the callus extending further proximally and distally. The latter is seen particularly in fractures of the femur where disturbance of the periosteal attachments adjacent to the adductor muscle insertion will often create a bridge of callus on the caudal aspect of the femur, sometimes referred to as 'rhinohorn callus' (Figure 5.17a). Another factor that may influence callus formation is vascularity, or lack of it. Fractures of the femoral neck or proximal femoral physis, and possibly the treatment of such injuries, might be associated with a degree of ischaemia caused by damage to the vascular supply. This might account for a reduction in femoral neck width that is often seen post-healing of the fracture, the so-called 'apple core' effect (Figure 5.17b).

After a bridging mineralized callus of woven bone has been formed, a process of remodelling will begin, as discussed above. During this period, which may continue for months or even years, the callus becomes gradually smaller and is incorporated into the general bone structure with restoration of the bone cortex, medullary cavity and trabecular pattern.

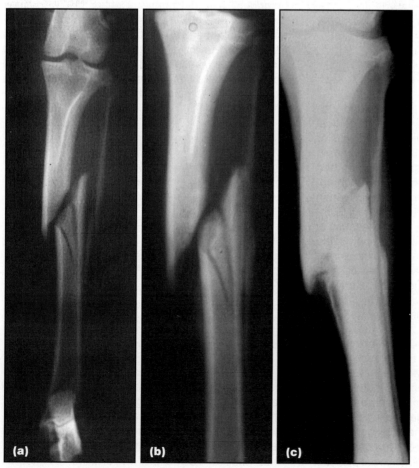

**5.16** Radiographic progression of classical fracture healing and bridging osteosynthesis for a tibial fracture in an adult terrier X treated by external coaptation. **(a)** At the time of fracture the fragments show sharp borders. After 7–10 days the fragment edges become less distinct and an indistinct periosteal reaction may be noted. **(b)** After 2–3 weeks a bridging callus is just visible, which will gradually become more mineralized. **(c)** By 6–8 weeks the callus is mineralized from proximal to distal. The bridging, mineralized callus will remodel over a period of months or years to restore normal bone architecture.

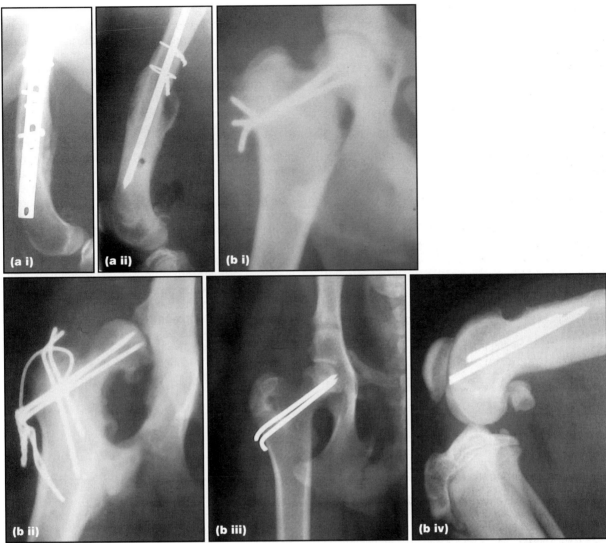

**5.17** Radiographic appearance of primary union by classical fracture healing and bridging osteosynthesis.
**(a) (i)** Radiograph taken 2 months after internal fixation of a reconstructed, comminuted femoral fracture in an 8-month-old Northern Inuit. A spur of callus is seen extending from the proximal segment. This is a result of injury to the attachment of the adductor muscle. **(ii)** Radiograph taken 6 weeks after fixation of a long, spiral femoral fracture in a 5-month-old Boxer. Treatment involved reconstruction of the bone using an intramedullary pin and cerclage wire, followed by the application of a 2-pin unilateral, uniplanar external skeletal fixator with the intramedullary pin 'tied in' to the frame. The external fixator was removed immediately prior to the radiograph being taken. A spur of callus is seen extending from the distal segment as a result of injury to the attachment of the adductor muscle. Note also the pocket of gas, distal and caudal to the fracture site. This was associated with the distal fixation pin track; a mixture of bacteria, including *Clostridium*, were cultured from the site. The infection resolved completely following a 2-week course of broad spectrum antibiotic treatment. **(b) (i)** Radiograph taken 2 months after internal fixation of a Salter–Harris type I injury of the proximal femoral physis in a 5-month-old Labrador Retriever. A limited craniolateral approach was used to reduce the epiphysis and the K-wires were placed in a normograde fashion. A mild 'apple core' effect is noticeable in the femoral neck. **(ii)** Radiograph taken 3 months after internal fixation of a Salter–Harris type I injury of the proximal femoral physis in a 7-month-old Labrador Retriever. A trochanteric osteotomy was used to aid exposure of the fracture and accurate reduction of the epiphysis. A marked 'apple core' effect is visible in the femoral neck and severe acetabular remodelling is evident as a result of postoperative instability. **(iii)** Radiograph taken 2 months after internal fixation of a Salter–Harris type I injury of the proximal femoral physis in a 7-month-old Border Collie. A limited craniolateral approach was used to reduce the epiphysis and the K-wires placed in a normograde fashion. An iliofemoral suture was placed to improve joint stability during the immediate postoperative period. The tunnels the suture was placed through in the ilium and greater trochanter are still evident. A moderate 'apple core' effect can be seen in the femoral neck. **(iv)** Radiograph taken months after internal fixation of a Salter–Harris type I injury of the distal femoral physis in a 5-month-old Border Collie. A mild 'apple core' effect is noticeable on the cranial aspect of the femur.

## Primary bone healing

In an ideal situation of accurate anatomical reconstruction and interfragmentary compression, healing should be by means of remodelling and there should be no requirement for callus formation (Figure 5.18a). However, such injury as periosteal stripping will initiate a reaction that will produce periosteal and endosteal new bone that will form a callus, particularly in skeletally immature patients (Figure 5.18b), which will be radiographically visible within the same time frame as outlined above.

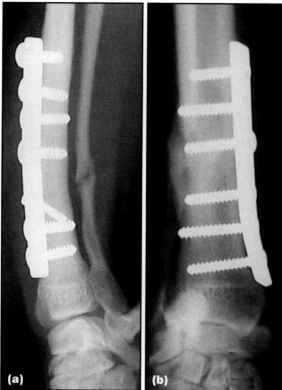

(a)

(b)

**5.18** Radiographic appearance of primary union by primary bone healing. **(a)** Radiograph taken 14 weeks after internal fixation of a transverse radial fracture in a 19-month-old Italian Greyhound. In adult bone, a fracture treated by reconstruction and interfragmentary compression should heal without callus formation and the only radiographic finding should be loss of any faint radiolucent line noted in the bone on postoperative radiographs. The ulna shows non-union, which is not uncommon after healing of the radius under plate fixation. **(b)** Radiograph taken 7 weeks after internal fixation of a transverse radial fracture in an 8-month-old Lurcher. In immature bone, despite the same management, periosteal irritation will produce a visible callus.

## Follow-up radiography

Follow-up radiography for the purpose of monitoring fracture healing may be necessary in some cases. In patients with long bone fractures, completely normal levels of activity should not be resumed until there is good evidence of clinical union. This is the point at which the healed bone and any implants to be left *in situ* are capable of full weight bearing without subsequent failure. Determination of this point in time requires a combination of factors including:

- Radiographic appearance
- Stability on manipulation
- Type of fracture
- Age of patient
- Method of stabilization.

For example, a comminuted tibial fracture in a 2-year-old dog treated using external skeletal fixation will probably have reached clinical union by about 8 weeks. At that stage the radiographic healing will be advanced (see above), stability of the tibia would be good (as determined by manipulation after removal of the connecting bars of the fixator) and the implants

could be removed. If the same fracture was reconstructed perfectly using lagged bone screws and application of a neutralization plate, then the fracture lines should be imperceptible and callus formation minimal. Therefore, if all appears well clinically and radiographically after 8 weeks then it is safe to assume that the bone plate construct will withstand normal limb use. More time might need to be given if, for any reason, implant removal was being considered.

In planning follow-up radiography it is necessary to make an educated guess as to when clinical union will have taken place. This might be four weeks in the case of a 4-month-old puppy with a fracture involving cancellous bone, six to eight weeks in the case of a young adult with a comminuted diaphyseal fracture, or twelve weeks in the case of an aged adult with such a fracture. Unless complications are suspected (e.g. because of worse than expected limb use, deteriorating limb use, evidence of infection) then it is appropriate to take radiographs at the anticipated time of clinical union. The exception to this would be the aged dog, cited above, where radiographs at the half-way stage (approximately 6 weeks) can be recommended as an assurance that all is well.

Evaluation of such films requires assessment of a number of factors (Figure 5.19):

- Reduction
- Spatial alignment
- Implants
- Tissues
- Bone healing.

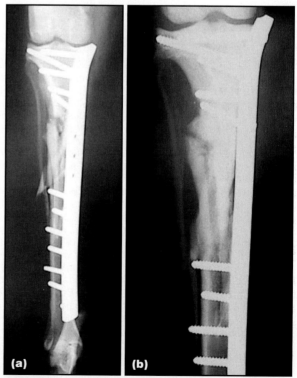

(a)

(b)

**5.19** CrCd views of a non-reconstructable tibial fracture in a 6-year-old Border Collie taken **(a)** immediately post-surgery and **(b)** 9 weeks postoperatively. Good bone union is evident with no evidence of implant failure and exercise restriction is no longer required.

### Reduction

The veterinary surgeon should determine whether reduction has altered when comparing the new radiographs with those taken immediately post-treatment. If reduction has altered, is it related to implant failure and is it of clinical significance (especially likely if articular surfaces are involved)?

### Spatial alignment

The clinician should determine whether the spatial alignment has altered when comparing the new radiographs with those taken immediately post-treatment. If the spatial alignment has altered, is it related to implant failure and is it of clinical significance (i.e. is the degree of malunion likely to be non-functional, see below)?

### Implants

Implants should be examined for evidence of failure in terms of breakage or loosening at the bone-implant interface; details of this are discussed below. Even if fracture healing is complete, the presence of failed implants is likely to cause clinical lameness and, if this is the case, their removal should be recommended.

### Tissues

Bone opacity outside the fracture zone may change during healing. Osteopenia, resulting from disuse is common within 2–4 weeks of treatment when external coaptation is used to treat fractures and is most notable in the distal limb and in areas of cancellous bone. This should be seen rarely when internal fixation or external skeletal fixation is used since reasonable to normal weight bearing through the limb should be achieved relatively quickly. Where the bone extending away from the fracture zone shows increased opacity, infection should be suspected as this will cause such a change as a result of periosteal reaction.

Soft tissue mass might decrease as a result of reduction in swelling, when compared to immediate post-treatment films, or disuse (or neurogenic) atrophy, when compared with the contralateral limb. A diffuse increase in mass (or failure of the post-injury swelling to resolve) is usually indicative of infection and the presence of gas opacities (beyond 7–10 days post-internal fixation, since surgery will allow air to become trapped in the tissues) would endorse such a suspicion. More localized soft tissue swelling may be associated with a loose implant or a sequestrum.

### Bone healing

The extent of healing should be reviewed in line with the expectations detailed above. If this is inadequate then the cause should be considered. Generally, poor healing is associated with instability but slow healing (in the absence of such factors as old age or infection) might require destabilization of, for example, an external skeletal fixator to promote healing by increasing load on the bone.

## Fracture complications

### Delayed and non-union

The term 'delayed union' is, to an extent, subjective and applies when the healing time has exceeded what would be considered normal in that particular case. With time, the fracture might heal or else progress to 'non-union', at which point it is considered healing will not take place, however long the fracture is given. A delayed or non-union may result from one or a combination of factors, including:

- Inadequate stabilization
- Poor vascularity
- Excessive fracture gap (± interposition of soft tissue, a loose implant or devitalized bone fragment)
- Infection
- Systemic or local disease
- Idiopathic factors (generally relating to atrophic non-union).

The radiographic appearance of these types of fracture complication may be useful in determining whether union is delayed or halted, and also contributes to classifying any such non-unions. However, these features may be influenced by the chosen method of treatment. For example, one feature of non-union is a closed medullary cavity (see below) but this will not occur if an intramedullary pin has been used to stabilize the fracture, inadequate though it may have been.

***Radiographic features of delayed union:*** The radiographic features of delayed union include (Figure 5.20):

- Persistent fracture line with evidence of healing
- Open medullary cavity
- Uneven fracture surfaces
- No sclerosis of fracture ends.

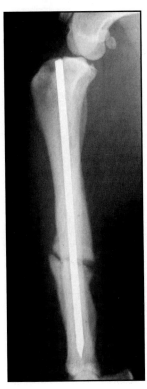

**5.20** ML radiograph of a transverse tibial fracture in a 4-year-old terrier, taken 6 weeks after internal fixation using an intramedullary pin. There was no bridging callus evident radiographically, though the fracture felt stable. This can be termed a delayed union, resulting from some rotational instability. Radiographs taken 12 weeks after treatment showed good bone union.

***Radiographic features of non-union:*** The radiographic features of non-union include (Figure 5.21):

- Gap between fracture ends
- Closed medullary cavity (unless pinned)
- Smooth fracture surfaces
- Sclerosis of fracture ends
- ± Hypertrophy or atrophy of bone ends.

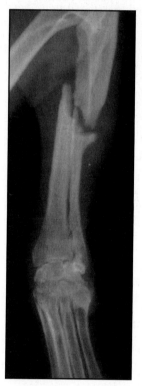

**5.21**
Radiographic appearance of a radial/ulnar fracture in a 3-year-old Labrador Retriever taken 6 weeks after treatment using external coaptation. There is no evidence of bridging callus and the medullary canals have sealed. This appearance constitutes a non-union.

Traditionally, non-unions have been classified according to the Weber–Cech system first described in 1976 (Sumner-Smith and Bishop, 1982). This classification divides non-unions into two broad groups: those that are biologically active (or viable); and those that are biologically inactive (or non-viable). These two groups are then further subdivided according to their cause and radiological appearance (Figures 5.22 and 5.23):

*Biologically active or viable non-unions:* These usually result from instability at the fracture site:

- *Hypertrophic non-union* ('elephant's foot' callus) (Figure 5.22a). There is abundant callus formation but failure to bridge the fracture gap, usually due to rotational instability. This type of non-union is most commonly seen in simple (transverse or short oblique) humeral or femoral fractures treated with an intramedullary pin
- *Slightly hypertrophic non-union* ('horse's foot' callus) (Figure 5.22b). There is some callus formation but without bridging of the fracture gap. The cause is usually rotational or angular instability in simple (transverse or short oblique) radial/ulnar or tibial fractures treated by external coaptation or intramedullary pinning
- *Oligotrophic non-union* (Figure 5.22c). In these cases there is no, or very limited, callus formation. The usual causes are either an avulsion injury treated conservatively, or as above for slightly hypertrophic non-unions in small or toy breed dogs. Additionally, if non-union results from a related systemic disease, e.g. hyperadrenocorticism, then it is this type of non-union that might be expected.

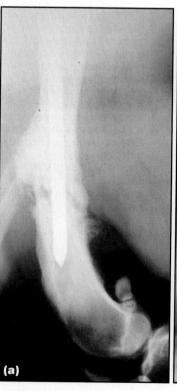 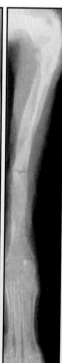 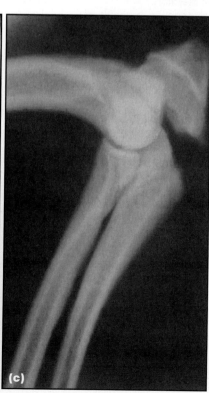

**5.22** Types of biologically active or viable non-unions.
**(a)** Hypertrophic non-union ('elephant's foot' callus). Radiographic appearance of a transverse femoral fracture in a 5-year-old German Shepherd Dog, 4 months after treatment by internal fixation using an intramedullary pin. Note the pin has migrated proximally leaving a radiolucent track in the distal bone segment. **(b)** Slightly hypertrophic non-union ('horse's foot' callus). Radiographic appearance of a radial fracture in a 4-year-old Toy Poodle after 8 weeks of treatment using external coaptation. **(c)** Oligotrophic non-union. Radiographic appearance of an olecranon fracture in a 7-year-old West Highland White Terrier taken 1 month after injury and no specific treatment. There is no evidence of any mineralized callus formation.

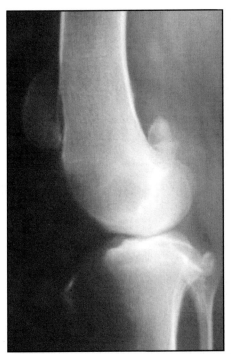

Radiographic appearance of the stifle of a
**5.30** 5-year-old Dobermann, 3 months after hip
luxation. Complications involving infection following
internal stabilization led to excision arthroplasty.
Subsequent to this the dog developed quadriceps
contracture. Note the proximal position of the patella and
over-extended appearance to the femorotibial joint.

### Fracture-associated neoplasia

Although fracture-associated neoplasia is of great interest there are fewer than about 100 cases documented in the literature and the general features of
such cases were reviewed by Stevenson (1991). Most
reports involve dogs, but the condition has been reported in the cat (Fry and Jukes, 1995). Most commonly, clinical signs develop more than 5 years after
primary treatment of the fracture and most of the
fractures involved occurred when the dogs were between 1 and 3 years of age. In some cases the lag
period for the development of a sarcoma is much less
(6–9 months) and it must then be considered that the
fracture might well have been a result of pathology in
the bone rather than a forerunner to its development.
Large breeds of dog are more commonly affected than
the smaller breeds. At the time of sarcoma development the dogs show lameness or a mass that is
gradually increasing in size. Radiographs show changes
typically associated with bone neoplasms, i.e. a mixture of osteolysis, osteoproduction and soft tissue
mineralization (Figure 5.31) (see Chapter 4). They
tend to affect the diaphyses rather than the metaphyses and show a difference in relative incidence between
the various long bones, when compared with primary
bone neoplasms (Stevenson, 1991) (Figure 5.32).

The aetiology of these neoplasms is not understood
and although there are hypotheses regarding factors
which might contribute to their development, none of
these have been proven. The removal of implants after
healing is complete has been hypothesized to reduce
the likelihood of a sarcoma developing. However,

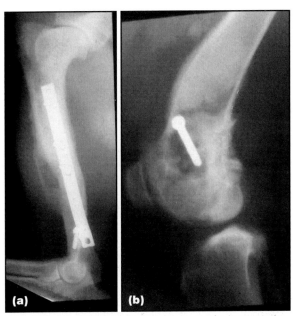

**(a)** Radiographic appearance of a humerus in
**5.31** a 6-year-old Lurcher taken 4 years after treatment
of a humeral non-union fracture. An area of lysis proximal
to the plate is suggestive of neoplasia being the cause of
recent onset lameness. **(b)** Radiographic appearance of a
distal femur in a 9-year-old German Shepherd Dog that
had a distal femoral fracture treated by lag screw fixation
as a puppy. Lysis around the implant and a local
periosteal reaction were associated with pain on
manipulation and palpation of the region. Implant removal
and biopsy confirmed the cause to be osteosarcoma.

| Long bone | Relative incidence (%) | |
|---|---|---|
| | *Primary bone tumour* | *Fracture-associated tumour* |
| Humerus | 20 | 24 |
| Femur | 16 | 49 |
| Radius | 39 | 22 |
| Tibia | 25 | 5 |

**5.32** Relative incidence of sarcoma in the long bones
of dogs; comparison of primary neoplasia with
fracture-associated neoplasia (Stevenson, 1991).

some cases with this problem have not had implants
used at all. Although sarcoma may develop at fracture
sites where healing has been uncomplicated (Fry and
Jukes, 1995), most cases are associated with problematic healing of the original fracture (for example, a
delay in union resulting from instability or infection).

### References and further reading

Braden TD (1991) Posttraumatic osteomyelitis. *Veterinary Clinics of North America: Small Animal Practice* **22**, 781–811
Brinker WO (1978) *Small Animal Fractures*. Michigan State University Press, East Lansing, MI
Brinker WO, Olmstead ML, Sumner-Smith G and Prieur WD (1998) Classification of fractures in small animals. In:*Manual of Internal Fixation in Small Animals, 2nd edn*, pp. 267–270. Springer, Berlin
Butterworth SJ and Innes JF (2001) Incomplete humeral condylar fractures in the dog. *Journal of Small Animal Practice* **42**, 394–398

Caywood DD, Wallace LV and Braden TD (1978) Osteomyelitis in the dog: a review of 67 cases. *Journal of the American Veterinary Medical Association* **172,** 943–946

Fry PD and Jukes HF (1995) Fracture associated sarcoma in a cat. *Journal of Small Animal Practice* **36,** 124–126

Johnson AL (1998) Biomechanics and biology of fracture healing with external skeletal fixation. *Compendium on Continuing Education for the Practicing Veterinarian* **20,** 487–500

Lidbetter DA and Millis DL (2002) Effect of ultrasound stimulation on bone healing in dogs. *Veterinary and Comparative Orthopaedics and Traumatology* **15, No 2** pp. A8. Veterinary Orthopaedic Society Meeting, Spring 2002 [Abstract]

Ness MG, Abercromby RH, May C, Turner BM and Carmichael S (1996) A survey of small animal orthopaedic conditions in small animal veterinary practice in Britain. *Veterinary and Comparative Orthopaedics and Traumatology* **9,** 43–52

Salter RB and Harris WR (1963) Injuries involving the epiphyseal plate. *Journal of Bone and Joint Surgery* **45A,** 587–593

Stevenson S (1991) Fracture-associated sarcomas. *Veterinary Clinics of North America: Small Animal Practice* **21,** 859–872

Sumner-Smith G and Bishop HM (1982) Non-union of fractures. In: *Bone in Clinical Orthopaedics*, ed. G Sumner-Smith, pp. 401–406. WB Saunders, Philadelphia

Wendelberg K, Kaderly R, Dee and Eatone-Wells R (1988) Stress fractures of the acetabulum in 26 racing Greyhounds. *Veterinary Surgery* **17,** 128–134

# 6

# Joints – general

## Graeme Allan and Robert Nicoll

## Indications

Care must be taken to evaluate each joint in isolation from other joints and also from adjacent structures, such as muscles, tendons and ligaments.

- Lameness: most animals with joint problems will be lame, so lameness is the common presenting problem for animals requiring radiography of the joints.
- Pain, restricted range of motion or instability of a joint: while indications of pain or discomfort can assist in localization of lameness to a joint, complete evaluation may be difficult in the conscious patient when pain associated with manipulation prevents adequate assessment for instability or laxity. In such cases sedation and analgesia, or general anaesthesia may be required.
- Swelling or deformity of a joint.
- Muscle atrophy if the condition is chronic.
- Joint trauma: any sign of trauma involving a joint, such as luxation or trauma-induced laxity, is an indication for radiographic examination of a joint. As trauma is a potential trigger for later changes, such as degenerative remodelling and osteoarthrosis in the affected joint, radiographs taken at the time of an injury provide a useful baseline against which to compare later changes.
- Presence of conditions that may have a secondary effect on joints: disorders of growing bones and trauma to long bones may have a secondary effect on the joints adjacent to the affected bone. Asynchronous growth of paired bones, such as the radius and ulna, can lead to incongruity in an adjacent joint. Similarly asymmetrical growth across the physis of a long bone can result in incongruity and/or stress across a joint. Such indirect causes of joint problems may result in secondary osteoarthrosis and need to be considered when giving advice to owners.
- Routine evaluation for inherited conditions: routine phenotypic surveys using radiography are recommended to evaluate dogs for inherited disorders of the skeleton, namely hip and elbow dysplasia (see Chapters 9 and 8).

## Radiography

### Importance of appropriate positioning of each joint

Each joint of the appendicular skeleton is structurally different. Accordingly, while two orthogonal projections are considered a radiographic necessity, the special views required for a full examination of each joint will vary depending on the joint being examined.

### Optimizing radiographic detail

Superior radiographic detail will be obtained when bones and joints of the extremities are radiographed using fine detail receptor systems. This will usually consist of dedicated fine detail intensifying screens, but additional fine detail can be obtained when regular double emulsion film is replaced with single emulsion film and only one intensifying screen is fitted within the cassette. The radiographic benefit of fine detail receptor systems is maximum where structure thickness is less than 8 cm. For high contrast radiography a low kVp technique is recommended. Improved radiographic contrast is aided by tight collimation of the primary X-ray beam. When radiographing joints, image distortion is minimized when the area of interest is centred within the primary X-ray beam and not placed in the periphery of the image, where divergent photons and parallax errors tend to cause image distortion.

### Special views

#### Stress radiography

Due to the fact that ligamentous injury is commonly encountered around joints, special stress techniques have been described to enable fuller appreciation of loss of ligamentous support (Farrow, 1982). This technique may require the application of traction, shearing, wedge or rotational forces during radiography (Figure 6.1). The purpose of stress radiography is to enable palpable laxity to be demonstrated on a radiograph. This technique may also disclose signs of avulsion, chip fractures and luxations that might otherwise be invisible on routine radiographs. Detailed information about stress radiographic techniques is included in the relevant joint chapters.

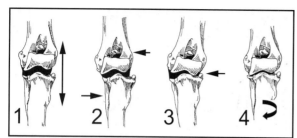

**6.1** Examples of stresses that can be applied to a joint during radiography. (1) Traction. (2) Shearing. (3) Wedge. (4) Rotation. (Courtesy of B Benshoof.)

### Contrast radiography

Both positive and negative contrast studies of joints are performed to highlight intra-articular abnormalities. For positive contrast studies, a water-soluble organic iodinated contrast medium is recommended. For negative contrast a gas such as nitrogen or carbon dioxide is recommended, although room air is frequently used for this purpose. The contrast medium is introduced into the joint following a sterile joint tap. The procedure is most commonly performed in the shoulder joint (see Chapter 7). Double contrast studies have not demonstrated significant benefits.

## Normal radiological anatomy and physiology

Joints of the appendicular skeleton are diarthrodial joints. These are synovial joints, i.e. the capsule is lined by a synovial membrane. The articulating ends of bones comprising each joint are lined with joint cartilage, and synovial fluid is contained within the joint space. Within the stifle joint there are two menisci, fibrocartilaginous plates, that serve to reduce concussion. Menisci are also present in the temporomandibular joints.

### Cartilage and subchondral bone

Subchondral bone is the edge of relatively homogenous epiphyseal bone that forms the apparent margin of the joint surface that is seen on plain film radiographs. The subchondral bone is protected by an intact layer of joint cartilage. The joint cartilage is 'invisible' because it silhouettes with synovial fluid and the opposing cartilage, and thus is only disclosed by arthrography or an alternative imaging technique.

### Soft tissue supporting structures

Synovial joints are surrounded by a fibrous joint capsule. The outer fibrous layer of the joint capsule may be thickened at sites of stress to provide collateral ligaments. In some joints there are intra-articular ligaments, such as the cruciate and meniscal ligaments within the stifles, the round ligaments in the coxofemoral joints, and the complex arrangements of intracarpal and intratarsal supporting ligaments.

### Intra-articular tendons

In some joints tendons of origin of important muscles are located within the joint space, where they are lined with synovium. These include the tendon of the biceps brachii muscle in the shoulder joint and the tendons of the long digital extensor muscle and the popliteal muscle in the stifle joint.

### Synovium

The periarticular blood vessels that supply and drain the epiphyses also provide vascularity to the synovium and the joint capsule. Lymphatic vessels are also present in the synovium as is a network of proprioceptive, pain receptor and sympathetic nerves. Synovial fluid is produced by the synovium and its functions are to:

* Lubricate the contact surfaces of synovial joints
* Transport nutrients to the joint cartilage.

### Sesamoids

Of the 68 sesamoid bones (excluding digit 1 of each foot) that are reported in dogs and cats, 66 may be seen (excluding the iliopubic sesamoid bones) in radiographs of the joints of the appendicular skeleton (Figure 6.2).

| Joint | Sesamoid |
|---|---|
| Shoulder | Clavicle (medial end of tendinous insertion of brachiocephalic muscle) |
| Elbow | Tendon of origin of supinator muscle |
| Carpus | Tendon of abductor pollicis longus muscle |
| Hip | None |
| Stifle | Patella (tendon of insertion of quadriceps femoris muscle) Fabellae (lateral and medial origin of gastrocnemius muscle) Popliteal sesamoid (tendon of popliteus muscle) |
| Tarsus | Lateral plantar tarsometatarsal bone Intra-articular tarsometatarsal bone |
| Metacarpo/ metatarsophalangeal | Paired palmar/plantar sesamoid bones (tendons of insertion of the interosseous muscles) Single dorsal sesamoid (in the extensor tendons) |

**6.2** Sesamoid bones around joints of the appendicular skeleton of dogs and cats.

Sesamoid bones are not always radiographically visible. They represent ossified cartilage within ligaments or tendons, and ossification does not always occur. Their radiological presence varies according to species and sesamoid location. Sesamoid bones are usually homogenous, ovoid osseous structures that are seen in predictable locations. Variation in their usual location, while sometimes normal, has also been interpreted as a sign of associated muscular or tendon injury. Displacement of a sesamoid bone occurs frequently in dogs and cats and may be of traumatic or congenital origin.

## Alternative imaging techniques

### Computed tomography and magnetic resonance imaging

Computed tomography (CT) and magnetic resonance imaging (MRI) are not commonly used to investigate diseases of the joints, although this is mostly a function of access, availability and cost, rather than clinical indication. The increasing availability, combined with demand by owners for more accurate non-invasive assessment of arthropathies, is gradually resulting in greater usage of these imaging modalities, particularly in more complicated or deep joints. CT and MRI provide a significant advantage as a means of evaluating structures that are superimposed upon each other in conventional radiographs and which cannot be adequately imaged with diagnostic ultrasonography. CT and MRI images represent 'slices' of anatomy (tomograms) resulting in cross-sectional views of the structures. Information from these images can be reconstructed in alternative planes or in three dimensions. While CT and MRI both produce tomographic images of a region of interest, they utilize different technologies to produce the image. CT utilizes focussed (pencil thin) beams of X-rays and provides excellent bone and soft tissue information. MRI forms images based upon the distribution of hydrogen ions (protons) within tissues. It provides exquisite differentiation of soft tissues. However, it receives no 'signal' from mineralized tissues and therefore normal subchondral and cortical bone appears as a black region indicative of a signal void.

#### CT *versus* MRI

Both CT and MRI (Figures 6.3 and 6.4) can be utilized when evaluating joints and periarticular tissues. It is unlikely that the veterinary surgeon will have the option of pursuing both imaging modalities within the same patient for the investigation of the same problem. For this reason, the decision as to which technology is likely to be of more use in the investigation of an arthropathy is determined by a number of factors. Each has advantages and disadvantages that need to be considered:

- Availability and access to the modalities
- Suspected underlying disease process: disease processes that involve or arise from bone are best evaluated with CT. However, MRI has superior differentiation of soft tissues, including cartilage. Additionally, newer MRI studies such as MR spectroscopy and diffusion studies may provide information about the metabolic function of tissues in regions of interest. While this is yet to supplant cytological and histological examination of biopsy samples, it has significant application in areas where biopsy is difficult or a higher risk procedure
- Plane of image required: CT acquires data in a plane parallel to the gantry (or in a plane almost parallel to the gantry in helical scanners). MRI can acquire data in any plane required. While it is possible to reconstruct CT images in an alternative plane, image resolution of such reconstructions is lower and inversely proportional to slice thickness of the original data

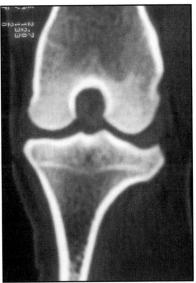

**6.3** CT image of a canine stifle joint made in a dorsal plane with imaging algorithm and windows optimized to assess bone. The cortical and subchondral bone are the most dense structures and are radiopaque. The chondral cartilage, menisci and soft tissues of the joint and adjacent tissues have low contrast and are less well defined. Note that the densely packed bone adjacent to the subchondral surfaces is more opaque than the mixture of cancellous bone and bone marrow within the medullary cavities. The proximal physeal scar of the tibia is a thin radiopaque line parallel to the tibial plateau.

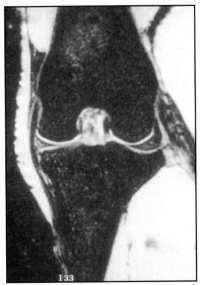

**6.4** MRI of a canine stifle joint in a dorsal plane using an imaging algorithm to optimize the signal from articular cartilage and suppress the signal from fat in the nearby bone marrow and within the fascial planes of adjacent tissues (T2-weighted 3D fat-suppressed Spoiled GRASS sequence). The thin layer of articular cartilage of the femoral condyles and tibial plateau has a hyperintense signal, appearing as a white structure. Mineral and fat in the adjacent bones and bone marrow have little or no signal and appear as dark or black areas; muscle has a hyperintense signal with this algorithm. The medial collateral ligament of the stifle joint appears as a thin hypointense band; the lateral collateral ligament has not been imaged in this plane. The obliquity of the cruciate ligaments in the intercondylar notch provide a mixed signal.

acquisition. (Note: this is not strictly true for helical CT and new multi-slice CT imaging, where data are acquired from a volume of tissue)

- Length of image acquisition process: this is significantly affected by field of view, slice thickness and region of interest. However, it is also influenced by the computing power and age of technology (hardware and software) utilized. Newer technology allows faster image acquisition, reducing the need for prolonged anaesthesia. This has occurred as a consequence of improved hardware (helical multi-slice CT units; highly uniform magnetic fields of more powerful magnets in MR units) combined with faster computing power and new imaging algorithms

- Anaesthesia requirements: general anaesthesia is required for accurate positioning of the patient and maintenance of the position throughout the data acquisition for both CT and MR examinations. MRI units operate in a very strong magnetic field, precluding the use of ferromagnetic materials or equipment in the room. Consequently, conventional anaesthetic machines (including gas bottles) cannot be utilized. Most MR examinations are performed on small animals with either intravenous anaesthesia or with an extended T-piece arrangement running from an anaesthetic machine outside the room. Non-ferromagnetic anaesthetic machines are available but at significant expense

- Cost: there is considerable variation in the cost of CT and MR examinations of veterinary patients. However, when a choice is available, there is usually proportionally little difference in cost between CT and MR examinations relative to the overall cost of undertaking either procedure once anaesthesia and the examination are combined.

### Indications

CT examinations are usually undertaken to evaluate mineralized components of joints. Recent developments in computer software manipulation of CT data allow rapid three dimensional (3D) reconstructions and 'virtual' disarticulation of joints to assist clinicians in diagnosis and therapeutic planning of skeletal disorders.

MRI examinations have greater application for imaging of intra- and periarticular soft tissues, such as ligaments, tendons, menisci and articular cartilage.

### Positioning

For CT examinations it is essential that the patient be symmetrically positioned relative to the plane of the gantry to allow comparative evaluations of the contralateral joint to be made. It is preferable that the long axis of the limb be perpendicular to the plane of the gantry, although in some small dogs and in cats it is often possible to position the patient and limbs parallel with the plane of the gantry.

For MRI examinations symmetry of positioning is essential if the joint of interest is to be compared in the same image. However, joints at the level of or distal to the elbow or stifle should be placed within the smallest

receiving coil available to optimize image signal, and hence quality. Consequently, it may be necessary to image contralateral joints as a separate acquisition sequence.

Folded towels make excellent adjustable supports for the patient and adhesive tape assists in maintaining the position required for imaging throughout the procedure; this is particularly important when sequential pre- and post-contrast studies are made for comparison.

### Field of view and slice thickness

The region of interest selected extends from a level proximal to the origins of the joint capsule and collateral (and other supportive) ligaments, to a level distal to the insertion of these structures on the limb. The slice thickness selected is generally proportional to patient size, so that cats and small dogs will be imaged with thinner slice thicknesses (generally 1–2 mm sequential or overlapped) than larger patients (generally 2–3 mm). In instances where image reconstruction (alternative planes or 3D reconstructions) are required narrow slice thicknesses are preferred.

### Use of contrast agents

As a general rule, if the objective of the examination is to evaluate mineralized structures only, a contrast agent should not be required. However, contrast studies may be preferred when imaging the soft tissues of the joints with CT to assist in the distinction of vascularized tissues from secretions and fluids. In these cases, sterile water-soluble iodinated contrast agents are used.

MRI requires a contrast agent capable of demonstrating its presence by resonating during T1 sequences; generally a compound containing gadolinium is utilized. The differentiation of fluids from soft tissues is more readily apparent in non-contrast MR images than in non-contrast CT images due to its superior differentiation of soft tissues.

Contrast agents are administered as a bolus intravenous injection immediately prior to image acquisition. Contrast CT or MR arthrography can be undertaken by direct injection of the appropriate contrast medium into the joint space.

### 'Windowing' CT and MR images

The display of data acquired in CT and MR examinations in a greyscale image allows post-acquisition manipulation to accentuate certain tissue types. Adjusting the contrast and brightness of the image is achieved by adjusting the window width and window level or centre. This is referred to as 'windowing' the images. In CT examinations it is particular important that regions of interest that contain bone are reviewed in both soft tissue and bone windows. In both CT and MR images, if pre- and post-contrast administration images are compared, it is important the comparison is made using images displayed with the same window width and level.

## Diagnostic ultrasonography

Ultrasonography has limited application in the evaluation of joints due to the strong acoustic shadowing that occurs from mineralized structures. However, diagnostic ultrasonography is useful in the evaluation of intra-articular soft tissues, particularly for those joints which have intra-articular tendons (e.g. biceps tendon in the shoulder (Figure 6.5), extensor tendon in the stifle) or ligaments which are not surrounded by bone (e.g. patellar ligament, Achilles apparatus). It is also used to evaluate periarticular structures, especially when a soft tissue mass or swelling is associated with a joint. Articular ultrasonography has been described for the evaluation of deeper structures, such as the capital epiphysis of young dogs, and the menisci and cruciate ligaments in the stifle, but is not widely practised. Similarly, ultrasonographic evaluation of the elbow for fragmentation of the medial coronoid process and of the shoulder for evidence of osteochondritis dissecans (OCD) have been described, but must be combined with other imaging modalities to determine their full extent. An advantage of ultrasonography is that it permits real-time dynamic study of a structure.

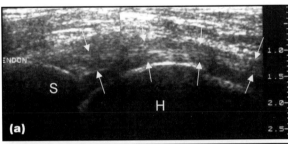
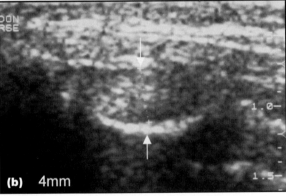

**6.5** Canine biceps tendon ultrasonograms. **(a)** Sagittal plane of composite ultrasound image. The biceps tendon (arrowed) has a linear stippled structure that provides greatest echogenicity when the fibres are under tension and perpendicular to the incident sound waves. Note the hyperechoic margins of the supraglenoid tuberosity (S) and humerus (H), beyond which no useful image is produced due to acoustic shadowing. **(b)** Transverse plane. In cross-section the biceps tendon is an ovoid structure (arrowed). The tendon fibres appear as stippled echoic foci.

## Scintigraphy

Scintigraphy is not commonly utilized for imaging diseases of the joint, but has particular application in the identification of a site of active inflammation and/or increased bone metabolism of patients in which lameness cannot be isolated to a particular region of a limb by either physical examination or radiography. Greater sensitivity can be achieved in localizing an occult lameness to a joint if a three-phase scintigram is performed, so that blood, tissue and bone pools of radioisotope

distribution are assessed. This may be of particular use in early stages of arthroses when only soft tissue inflammation is present, and in animals with active endochondral ossification, when normal bone will show significant uptake of radioisotope (Figure 6.6).

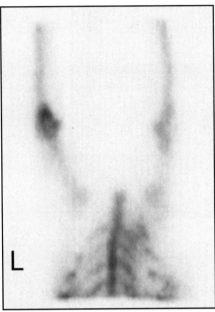

**6.6** Bone phase scintigraphy was used to localize lameness in a 16-month-old Boxer with chronic left forelimb lameness. The aetiology of the lameness could not be identified on physical or radiological examination of the elbows. Scintigraphy demonstrated a greater uptake of radiopharmaceutical in the left elbow than in the right elbow; this asymmetry of uptake localized the lameness to the left elbow. The head was shielded and thus was not visible. (Courtesy of RM Zuber.)

## Abnormal radiological findings

### Radiological signs of joint disease
The following changes may be seen when evaluating a pathological joint (Figure 6.7):

- Soft tissue swelling
- Altered width of a joint space
  - Increased
  - Decreased
- Altered subchondral opacity
  - Irregular margins
  - Decreased opacity
  - Increased opacity
- Osteophyte and enthesophyte formation
  - Intra-articular
  - Periarticular
- Calcification
  - Articular
  - Juxta-articular
- Gas
  - Articular
  - Juxta-articular
- Remodelling the shape of a joint
  - Adaptive remodelling
  - Changed spatial relationships and incongruity.

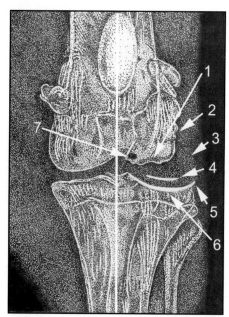

**6.7** The radiological signs of joint disease. The left side is normal and the right side illustrates the pathology. 1 = Uneven subchondral bone surface. 2 = Periarticular new bone formation. 3 = Articular soft tissue swelling. 4 = Intra-articular calcified material. 5 = Osteophyte. 6 = Increase in subchondral bone opacity. 7 = Cyst-like changes within subchondral bone. (Courtesy of B Benshoof.)

## Soft tissue swelling

Soft tissue swelling around and of joints can have many causes. Commonly, synovial effusion is the reason but synovial hypertrophy, joint capsule thickening and inflammation of juxta-articular soft tissues also need to be considered as contributing causes of radiological signs of soft tissue swelling attributed to a joint (Figure 6.8).

*Radiological signs:* Radiological signs of soft tissue swelling include:

- Distortion or displacement of adjacent structures
  - Fatty tissue in fascial planes
  - Articular fat pads
- Visible increase in soft tissue opacity within or around the joint
- Enlarged joint space, sometimes seen as subluxation as in hip dysplasia.

***Causes of articular soft tissue swelling:*** Causes of articular soft tissue swelling include:

- Synovial effusion
- Synovial thickening
- Soft tissue masses.

*Synovial effusion:*

- Inflammation, secondary to trauma of intra-articular structures (such as ligaments or menisci)
- Haemarthrosis (trauma, blood dyscrasias)
- Osteoarthrosis
- Infectious arthritis
- Immune-mediated arthritis.

*Synovial thickening:*

- Chronic synovial inflammation
  - Diffuse
  - Nodular (villonodular)
- Joint capsule fibrosis
- Neoplasia (as in synovial sarcoma).

*Soft tissue masses:*

- Neoplasia, synovial or of other origin
- Villonodular synovitis
- Fluid within articular synovial cysts, associated with osteoarthrosis of affected joint
  - Vertebral articular facets
  - Extension through joint capsule
- Fluid within periarticular synovial cysts arising from tendon sheaths or bursae.

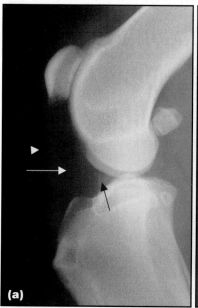

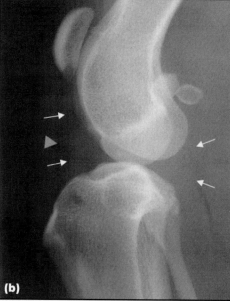

**6.8** ML views of stifle joints. **(a)** Normal stifle. The white arrow identifies the infrapatellar fat pad, which is of a lesser opacity than soft tissue. The white arrowhead points to the cranial surface of the patellar ligament, which is more opaque than adipose tissue. The black arrow points to the meniscus, which has the same opacity as synovial fluid but is more opaque than adipose tissue. **(b)** Abnormal stifle. White arrows point to the cranial and caudal margins of the joint capsule, which is distended by synovial effusion. The white arrowhead points to the caudal border of the patellar ligament. The infrapatellar fat pad and caudal fascial plane have been compressed by the distended joint capsule.

## Altered width of a joint space

Changes in joint space may be difficult to perceive when animals are radiographed in recumbency as the limbs are usually positioned and imaged in a non-weight bearing posture. Incongruity or eccentricity of a joint space may be a consequence of pathology (laxity, malformation or deformation) or asymmetrical stresses applied in positioning of the patient. Some joints (such as the shoulder) are naturally more lax or mobile than others, whereas some (such as the elbow) are not. The joint space that we see on a survey radiograph consists of two opposing layers of joint cartilage separated by a microfilm of synovial fluid ± joint specific articular structures, such as fibrocartilaginous menisci or discs. The cartilage and synovial fluid produce a combined soft tissue opacity between the opacity of the subchondral bone on either side of the joint, creating what we perceive as the radiographic joint space (Figure 6.9). The true joint space can be disclosed by injecting either positive or negative contrast media into the joint space, or by using an advanced imaging study such as MRI.

*Increased width:* Joint spaces may appear wider than normal when there is:

- Stress applied
- Skeletal immaturity
- Synovial effusion
- Joint laxity
  - Ruptured soft tissue supporting structures
  - Inherited laxity (e.g. hip dysplasia)
  - Acquired laxity
- Joint incongruity
- Thickened cartilage.
- Destroyed subchondral bone.

*Reduced width:* Joint spaces may be narrower than normal due to:

- The primary beam not centred properly, i.e. artefactual
- Cartilage attrition
- Muscle contracture.

## Altered appearance of subchondral bone

Subchondral bone is protected by an intact layer of joint cartilage. Its normal radiological appearance is the edge of relatively homogenous epiphyseal bone that forms the apparent margin of the joint surface that we see on survey radiographs.

*Irregularity of margins:* Irregularity of subchondral bone margins is a feature of normal endochondral ossification for several months after birth and is seen particularly in the:

- Greater tubercle of the humerus
- Distal femoral condyle.

Osteochondral fragmentation or destruction may also be seen and can be due to:

- Osteochondrosis/OCD
- Sepsis
- Avascular necrosis
- Immune-mediated joint disease.

*Decreased opacity:* Decreased subchondral bone opacity may indicate:

- Aggressive joint inflammation as in septic arthritis where changes in the constitution of synovial fluid have led to chondrolysis then osteolysis
- Focal lucent subchondral bone lesions, which are a feature of:
  - Osteochondrosis (Figure 6.10)
  - Subchondral osseous cyst-like lesions.

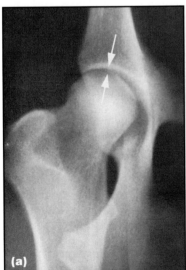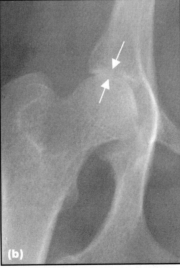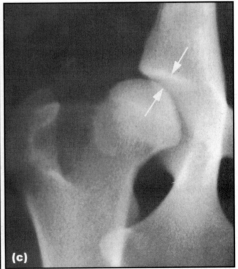

**6.9** VD extended right hip joint views. **(a)** The normal coxofemoral joint space can be seen between the two arrows, which define the radiolucent articular joint space between the femoral head and the cranial acetabular margin. These two joint spaces lie parallel to one another between the cranial effective acetabular edge and the fovea capitalis that represents the insertion of the round ligament. **(b)** Reduced coxofemoral joint space. The arrows point to the absence of a radiolucent space between the femoral head and the cranial acetabular margin. **(c)** The coxofemoral joint space is increased. The arrows define the enlarged lucent, 'V-shaped' coxofemoral joint space. The femoral head is no longer congruent with the acetabulum.

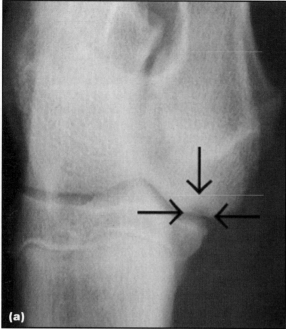

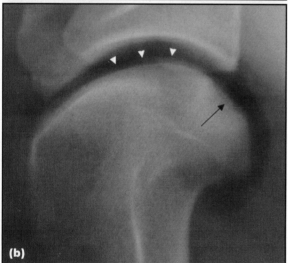

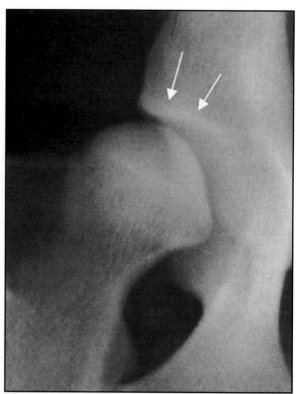

6.11   Extended VD view of a coxofemoral joint. Increased subchondral bone opacity is present in the cranial acetabular margin of this coxofemoral joint (arrowed).

6.10   Changes in subchondral bone.
**(a)** Cr15°LCdMO view of the humero-ulnar articulation. The arrows point to a subchondral lucency surrounded proximally by more opaque bone. This osteolucent change is an example of medial humeral condylar OCD. **(b)** ML view of shoulder joint. On the caudal border of the head of the humerus there is an osteochondral lesion in which poorly defined mineralized material is located. The cavity is surrounded distally by a crescent of increased bone opacity. The black arrow points to the cavitated lesion. The white arrowheads define the surface of the joint cartilage covering the humeral head, which has been defined by the addition of gas to the joint space (pneumoarthrogram).

*Increased opacity:* Increased subchondral bone opacity (Figure 6.11) may indicate:

- Cartilage attrition, with or without exposure of the subchondral bone surface
- Inflammation, in situations where cartilage fragmentation has exposed the subchondral bone
- Stress or trauma-induced remodelling, in situations where eccentric stress occurs across a joint.

## Osteophytes and enthesophytes

*Osteophytes:* An osteophyte can be defined as an outgrowth of bone at the margin of the articular surface of a synovial joint. Most commonly osteophytes are seen as smoothly marginated and homogenous osseous proliferations, as either undulating or nodular bone outgrowths from bone surfaces, sometimes adjacent to the articular surfaces of a joint. The initiating change is neochondrogenesis, which leads to ossification of new tissue to produce osteophytes. The presence of periarticular osteophyte formation is one of the defining features of osteoarthrosis in animals.

*Enthesophytes:* An enthesophyte is a focal proliferation of new bone to form a bony spur at an enthesis (Rogers *et al.,* 1997). An enthesis is the site of attachment of a ligament, tendon or fibrous capsule to a bone. Enthesophytes form when the enthesis is disturbed. The underlying disturbance may be due to either trauma or inflammation. The result is fibrocartilaginous development at the enthesis, which subsequently becomes mineralized.

In specific locations these new bone proliferations may also arise from an intra-articular structure, such as the origin or insertion of an intra-articular tendon or ligament (e.g. extensor fossa of the distal femur or intercondylar origin of the cruciate ligaments). They may also occur at the site of fibrous joint capsular attachment to bone (Figure 6.12) or from the reflection of the synovium.

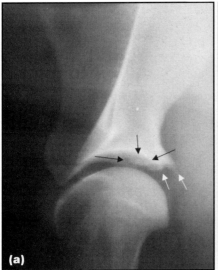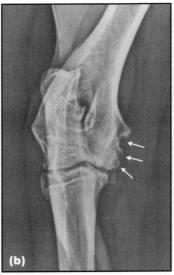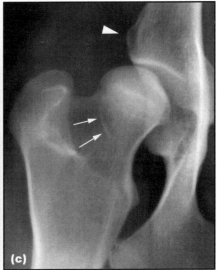

**6.12** **(a)** ML view of shoulder joint. Periosteal new bone proliferation is noted on the medial edge and the caudal margin of the glenoid. The white arrows point to a focal spur of new bone proliferation; these changes represent enthesophytes. The black arrows point to calcified material that was located within the scapulohumeral joint. It was an osteochondral fragment from an OCD lesion located in the glenoid. **(b)** CrCd elbow view. Roughened periosteal new bone formation is present on the medial epicondyle (arrowed). A small lucent cavity is present in the subchondral bony surface of the medial humeral condyle. These changes were caused by humeral OCD and secondary arthrosis of the elbow. **(c)** Extended VD view of coxofemoral joint. The arrows point to enthesophyte lining the axial surface of trochanteric fossa. The arrowhead points to enthesophytes on the craniodorsal margin of the acetabulum.

## Calcification

Intra-articular new bone formation may be seen as enthesophytes at specific locations, or as seemingly free fragments of bone or calcified soft tissue. Such calcifications are not usually 'floating' within the synovium but are attached to or incorporated into a structure, which most commonly is the synovium. In the stifle, meniscal calcification may also occur. True 'joint mice', or floating calcific bodies, usually arise as osteochondral fragments from diseased cartilage. It may be difficult to distinguish free intra-articular calcific bodies from fixed articular or extra-articular calcific bodies (Figure 6.13).

***Intra-articular calcification:*** Calcification within the confines of a joint may be due to:

- 'Joint mouse'
  - Loose fragments of calcified soft tissue
  - Free osteochondral fragments
- Not all 'joint mice' are opaque, and thus may require special studies such as MRI or arthrography to disclose them
- Fixed foci of calcification or ossification
  - Calcified menisci
  - Calcification within the synovium (e.g. synovial osteochondroma)
- It may be difficult to distinguish loose from fixed calcified particles (Figures 6.14 and 6.15).

***Juxta-articular calcification:*** Calcification in the juxta-articular soft tissues may be due to:

- Tendinopathies
- Synovial sheaths
- Changes in normal extra-articular ossified structures such as sesamoid fragmentation.

**Articular and periarticular**

Accessory centre of ossification
- Caudal glenoid rim
- Distal acromion

Osteochondral fragmentation
- Osteochondritis dissecans
- Fragmented medial coronoid process of the ulna
- Septic arthritis
- Avascular necrosis of the femoral head
- Trauma

Osteoarthrosis

Articular fractures

Avulsed or ununited centres of ossification
- Ununited anconeal process

Avulsion of ligaments
- Origin of cranial cruciate ligament
- Origin of long digital extensor tendon
- Medial humeral epicondyle

Sesamoid bone anomalies
- Bi-partite sesamoid
- Fractured sesamoid
- Fragmented sesamoid

Soft tissue calcification
- Synovial osteochondromatosis
- Meniscal calcification

Intra-articular calcifying tendinopathies
- Biceps tendon

Patella cubiti **(a)**

**6.13** **(a)** Articular and periarticular calcified bodies in the dog and cat. (Adapted from Mahoney and Lamb (1996).) (continues) ▶

**Juxta-articular**

Sesamoid bones
• Clavicle
• Fabellae

Calcinosis circumscripta (tumoral calcinosis)

Myositis ossificans

Calcifying tendinopathies [a]
• Thoracic limb
    Infraspinatus muscle insertion
    Supraspinatus muscle insertion [a]
    Coracobrachialis muscle insertion
    Flexor carpi ulnaris muscle origin
    Flexor carpi radialis muscle origin
    Superficial and deep flexor tendons
• Pelvic limb
    Gluteus muscle insertion [a]
    Iliopsoas muscle insertion
    Biceps femoris
    Quadriceps femoris
    Gastrocnemius muscle origin
    Common calcaneal tendon [a]          **(b)**

**6.13** (continued) **(b)** Juxta-articular calcified bodies in the dog and cat. [a] Commonly observed calcifying tendinopathies. (Adapted from Mahoney and Lamb (1996).)

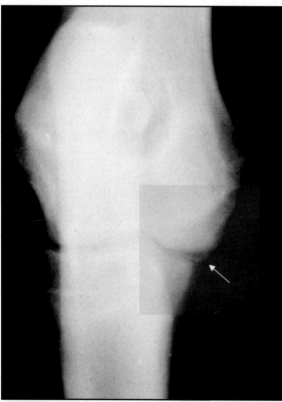

**6.14** CrCd view of elbow. The arrow points to a fragment of bone adjacent to the medial humeral condyle. This bony fragment represents either an osteochondral fragment from the humeral condylar surface or fragmentation of the medial coronoid process of the ulna.

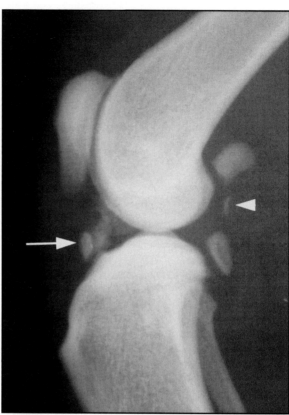

**6.15** ML view of a feline stifle. Ossified fragments of tissue are present within this cat's stifle. The arrow points to a cranially located mineralization, which may represent either a synovial osteochondroma or calcification of the meniscus. The arrowhead points to caudally located calcified material, which is probably within or attached to the synovium.

**Gas**

Causes of gas in joints include the following:

• Iatrogenic
    – Procedural, as the result of an investigative procedure
        – arthrotomy
        – arthrography
        – arthrocentesis
    – Excessive tension on a joint or disc space
        – Vacuum phenomenon (distraction radiography of the coxofemoral joint; distraction of the vertebral column)
• Spontaneous vacuum phenomenon
    – Intervertebral disc disease
    – OCD of the shoulder
• Trauma and infection
    – Penetrating injury
    – Gas-forming organisms.

The prevailing theory of the vacuum phenomenon is that naturally occurring intra-articular gas migration represents diffusion of nitrogen from extracellular fluid into an adjacent joint space when there is negative pressure in the joint. This may occur naturally or be induced by applying traction to a joint. Intra-articular gas slowly diffuses out of the joint, a process that takes several hours, after normal intra-articular pressure is re-established (Figure 6.16).

*Radiological features of severe sprains:* Radiological features of severe sprains include:

- Periarticular soft tissue swelling
- Avulsion fractures at points of attachments of ligaments, tendons and capsules to bones
- Joint instability or subluxation
- Spatial derangement of the osseous components of a joint.

Tendon and ligament injuries can be examined using an imaging technique that provides more optimal structural detail of soft tissues, such as MRI or ultrasonography.

### Congenital and developmental conditions

*Inherited disorders:* Joint disorders with established genetic transmission occur in both dogs and cats (Figure 6.17).

| Disorder | Mode of inheritance |
|---|---|
| Elbow dysplasia | Polygenic |
| Hip dysplasia | Polygenic |
| Osteochondrosis | Polygenic |
| Mucopolysaccharidosis | Autosomal recessive |
| Osteochondrodystrophy of Scottish Fold cats | Autosomal dominant |
| Alaskan Malamute chondrodysplasia | Recessive |
| Avascular necrosis of the femoral head | Autosomal recessive |
| Incomplete ossification of the humeral condyle | Recessive |

**6.17** Inherited skeletal disorders affecting the joints of dogs and cats.

*Canine hip and elbow dysplasia:* Canine hip and elbow dysplasia are inherited disorders that result in incongruent hip and elbow joints. Their underlying aetiopathogenesis is complex but it is generally accepted that their cause is polygenic and their phenotypic expression can be influenced by environmental factors such as nutrition, rate of growth and exercise (Hedhammar *et al.*, 1974). They are the subject of specific control schemes based on radiography in most countries.

*Osteochondrosis:* Dogs are genetically predisposed to osteochondrosis in its various manifestations. It affects many joints and is also one component of the elbow dysplasia group of disorders, although it also commonly occurs in other joints such as the shoulder, stifle and tarsus in dogs (see relevant chapters). Local ischaemia is thought to be the key initiating factor for osteochondrosis. Failure of the joint cartilage to mineralize leads to thickened and weakened articular cartilage that is prone to rupture and so exposes the underlying subchondral bone to synovial fluid. The sequence of cartilage fragmentation and subchondral bone lysis produces joint pain and lameness. This phase of the disorder is called osteochondritis dissecans. The incidence of osteochondrosis is exacerbated by over consumption and over supplementation of food.

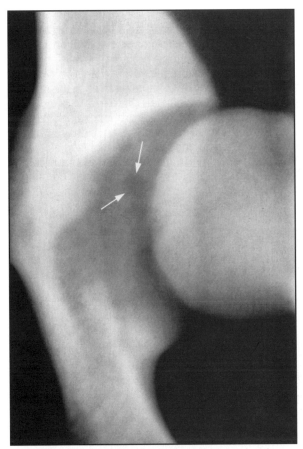

**6.16** VD flexed view of the right hip joint using the Penn-HIP® technique in the distracted position. The arrows point to small gas bubbles within the synovial fluid typical of the vacuum phenomenon.

### Changes in shape or spatial relationships
Joint laxity or instability is a common precursor to osteoarthrosis. The principle of laxity as a precursor to osteoarthrosis can apply to any joint. Signs of joint laxity (such as subluxation) can be detected by palpation and special radiographic techniques. Changes in shape represent remodelling of joint components to accommodate joint laxity or incongruity. A typical example is the shallow acetabulum and flattened femoral head in hip dysplasia. Changes in relative position of joint components are commonly seen and include coxofemoral subluxation, altered angle of the proximal tibial plateau and elbow incongruity.

### Joint disorders

#### Trauma
Radiography is used to identify fractures that enter a joint and to verify postoperatively that surgical repair has adequately restored joint congruity. Physeal injuries of any type may result in joint incongruity and subsequent eccentric load transfer through a joint, causing osteoarthrosis. Care must be taken when evaluating bone fractures to determine whether they enter a joint.

Trauma that produces sprains, joint instability or subluxation/luxation can be evaluated radiographically. Some form of stress radiography is recommended when evaluating joint instability in order that the extent of soft tissue trauma can be more adequately assessed.

*Mucopolysaccharidoses:* These are a group of genetic lysosomal storage disorders characterized by abnormal cartilage formation, and subsequent bone and joint malformation. Several subtypes of the disorder exist, the best studied being MPS VI which occurs in cats of Siamese ancestry. There are two underlying genotypes and three phenotypic modes of expression of MPS VI, which range from minimal bone and joint malformation to bizarre remodelling of the vertebrae (see Chapter 16) and severe osteoarthrosis (Crawley *et al.*, 1998). Other forms of MPS reported in dogs and cats include MPS I, II, III, IV and VII. These share characteristics of bone malformation and osteoarthrosis.

*Scottish Fold osteochondrodysplasia:* This is an inherited disorder causing defective cartilage formation of all cartilaginous structures, affecting both bone growth and the architecture of joints. Radiological changes manifest in the joints, being most easily recognized in the extremities of the appendicular skeleton (see Chapter 11). Ankylosing arthropathy of the carpi and tarsi gradually develops and the metacarpi, metatarsi and phalanges may be misshapen and of variable length. Soft tissue mineralization at entheses may produce large enthesophytes. The caudal vertebral elements are often malformed with the tail being shorter and wider than normal. Affected animals are lame and often cannot run or jump.

*Joint luxation and subluxation:* Congenital joint luxation, which occurs more commonly in the shoulder and elbow than in other joints, can lead to extensive degenerative remodelling of joint surfaces (Figure 6.18). In specific instances, occult (unidentified) trauma to the neonate may result in a joint luxation that becomes evident as the animal grows. In such cases, differentiation of congenital malformation from traumatic deformation can be difficult; and salvage surgery may be the only option by the time these malformations are identified. Patellar luxation, which may be of traumatic or congenital origin, occurs in dogs and cats (see Chapter 10).

Developmental subluxation of the coxofemoral joint, the consequence of joint laxity, is an underlying cause of hip dysplasia in dogs and cats. Signs of joint laxity may be camouflaged during routine radiography of the hips and usually requires specific stress radiography to disclose it (Smith *et al.*, 1990; Farese *et al.*, 1998; Fluckiger *et al.*, 1999) (Figure 6.19).

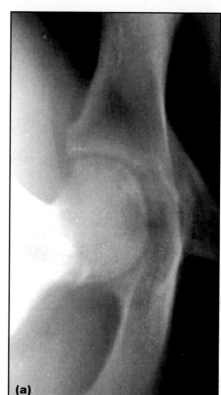

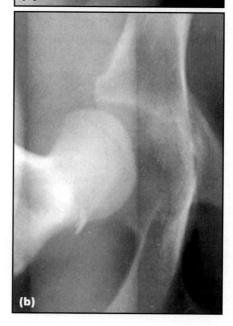

**6.19** VD view of the right hip joint using the Penn-HIP® technique. **(a)** The compressed position demonstrating excellent coxofemoral joint congruency. **(b)** The distracted position demonstrating increased joint volume, indicating excessive joint laxity and poor joint congruency.

**6.18** **(a)** CdCr view. Congenital luxation of the shoulder of a dog. The humeral head has luxated proximally and medially. The glenoid has remodelled as a consequence of chronic malarticulation. **(b)** CrCd view. Congenital luxation of the elbow. The radial head is luxated proximally and laterally with respect to the humeral condyle.

## Nutritional and metabolic conditions

As described above, the effects of food consumption and growth rate influence the phenotypic expression of osteochondrosis, canine hip and elbow dysplasia. More specific nutritional disorders that affect bones and joints include the following:

- Hypervitaminosis A
- Nutritional secondary hyperparathyroidism
- Rickets.

**Hypervitaminosis A:** Hypervitaminosis A reduces proliferation and differentiation of cartilage cells, leading to a crippling polyarthropathy in cats of any age. This clinical syndrome can be identified after feeding a vitamin A laden diet to cats for a few months. Radiological changes become evident after 10 weeks of such a diet and consist of ankylosing spondylopathy and periarticular enthesopathy, which may result in ankylosis of affected joints. The changes are most pronounced in the cervical vertebral column and the shoulder and elbow joints (Figure 6.20).

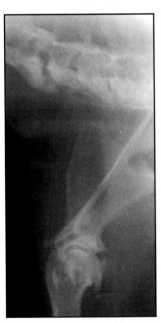

**6.20** ML view of the shoulder and part view of the cervical vertebral column showing signs of hypervitaminosis A in a cat. There is an extensive ankylosing spondylopathy involving the bodies of the cervical vertebral column and signs of arthrosis involving the scapulohumeral joint.

**Nutritional secondary hyperparathyroidism:** Of the various manifestations of hyperparathyroidism, the nutritional form of the disease is the most common. Radiological signs of generalized skeletal osteopenia are seen in both the appendicular and axial skeleton, where cortical thinning and relative radiolucency of bones are the predominant findings. The common cause is a diet low in calcium but rich in phosphorus, which leads to low serum calcium and so stimulates the parathyroid glands to produce parathyroid hormone. Subsequent bone resorption leads to generalized osteopenia (see Chapter 3).

**Rickets:** This disorder is generally regarded as being the result of a dietary deficiency of vitamin D or its precursors. Histological manifestations of rickets are seen in physeal cartilage where there is decreased calcification of the matrix in the zone of hypertrophied

cartilage cells. This, in combination with other changes leads to physeal thickening, which is one of the defining radiological features of rachitic animals. Consequential changes such as wide metaphyses, unbalanced growth of paired bones and bowing of long bones may also occur.

## Osteoarthrosis

Primary osteoarthrosis is a common age-related disorder of joints of the appendicular skeleton of dogs and cats. Radiological and necropsy surveys of cat and dog populations that have no history of lameness, or of an inciting cause of osteoarthrosis, demonstrate typical radiological and necropsy signs of osteoarthrosis with a high prevalence in the shoulder and elbow joints. Radiological signs of osteoarthrosis generally correlate poorly with clinical signs of osteoarthrosis.

The chronological sequence of radiological changes in osteoathrosis has been reported as:

- Increased subchondral opacity
- Bony remodelling of normal joint contours
- Formation of osteophytes and enthesophytes
- Calcification in and around the joints.

Contributing (secondary) causes of osteoarthrosis include:

- Joint instability/laxity
- Cartilage disorders
  - Osteochondrosis
  - Fragmented medial coronoid process
- Disorders that cause joint inflammation
  - Septic arthritis
  - Haemarthrosis
  - Immune-mediated polyarthropathies
  - Avascular necrosis of the femoral head
- Environmental factors
  - Food intake
  - Growth rate
  - Body size.

## Infection

Infectious arthritides may be caused by any infectious agent, be it bacterial, viral, protozoal or fungal. Entry of pathogens into the joint may be by direct penetration (trauma, surgery) or via haematogenous dissemination. The distribution of joint involvement may be mono- or polyarticular.

In the early stages of the infectious process articular soft tissue swelling is the predominant sign, but as the infection becomes established subchondral bone erosion may occur. There may also be signs of variation in width of joint spaces but these changes are always difficult to interpret in non-weight bearing radiographs. Later changes of periosteal proliferation, possibly reflecting synovial and capsular inflammation, will be observed in some cases. Subchondral bone erosion is the first stage of secondary osteomyelitis, which can become extensive as infections spread from the joint into adjacent bone (Figure 6.21).

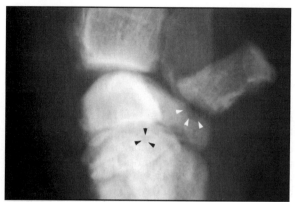

**6.21**  ML view of a canine carpus. Subchondral bone lucency (a sign of erosive bone disease) can be seen in many locations in the bones of this carpus. The white and black arrowheads point to two of these lucent bone changes. This radiograph is an example of an erosive arthropathy, in this case caused by septic arthritis.

### Immune-mediated polyarthropathies

Joint disorders that are immune-mediated are classified as erosive or non-erosive. Typically multiple joints are involved so they are by definition polyarthropathies. Whenever there is multiple joint swelling it should be regarded as a potential sign of haematogenously disseminated septic arthritis or an immune-mediated joint disease. Non-erosive immune-mediated polyarthropathies present signs of increased articular soft tissue swelling without evidence of erosion.

Bone erosion is only seen in the more advanced stages of immune-mediated joint disease and may affect subchondral and periarticular bone. It is more likely to be seen in canine rather than feline rheumatoid arthritis. Rheumatoid arthritis in dogs and cats is a rare condition. In dogs it mainly affects the distal joints of the extremities of small or toy breeds. Dogs with rheumatoid arthritis eventually lose much bone to erosion of affected joints. Joint laxity secondary to ligamentous destruction eventually also becomes a problem. In the feline form of rheumatoid arthritis periosteal proliferation and mineralization are the predominant radiological changes and occur exclusively in young male cats. An erosive arthropathy form of the disease has also been reported. The most reliable test for immune-mediated joint disease is synovial biopsy of affected joints.

### Neoplasia

Neoplasms that arise from or invade joints and periarticular tissues may be of several types. They can originate from any tissue of the joint (fibrous tissue, vasculature, fat, cartilage or synovium) or periarticular tissues even though the most commonly considered primary joint neoplasm is the synovial cell sarcoma. From both a radiological and histological perspective this neoplasm can be mimicked by several neoplasms that are not specific for joints. Joint neoplasms are characterized as invading bone on either side of a joint, behaviour that other neoplasms do not usually exhibit.

***Synovial cell sarcoma:*** Synovial cell sarcoma is a slowly growing soft tissue neoplasm that arises from the synovium, which may be located either inside or outside a joint. These neoplasms are much more common in dogs than in cats. Initially they present as a soft tissue swelling but eventually invade adjacent bone. When bone changes ultimately develop they consist of both cortical erosion and multiple lucent cyst-like changes in underlying cancellous bone. Synovial cell sarcomas grow slowly and eventually metastasize in about 50% of cases. Approximately 20% of cases have distant metastasis (lymph nodes, spleen and lungs) at the time of initial diagnosis and therefore wider examination is required so that the neoplastic process can be properly staged. Median disease-free intervals of greater than 36 months have been reported in cases where amputation was undertaken. Local resection is not recommended (Vail *et al.*, 1994).

***Miscellaneous joint neoplasms:*** A range of neoplasms that are not of synovial origin have been reported invading the joints of dogs. These include fibrosarcoma, rhabdomyosarcoma, fibromyxosarcoma, malignant fibrous histiocytoma, liposarcoma, undifferentiated sarcoma and lipoma.

### Miscellaneous

***Epiphyseal and physeal changes:*** Signs of epiphyseal disease are more generally associated with bone diseases but there are specific epiphyseal and physeal abnormalities that also relate to the joints (see Chapters 3, 5, 8 and 9).

*Physeal separation:*

* Capital femoral physeal separation – separation of the capital physis, whether or not of traumatic origin, is an intra-articular disorder.
* Eccentric stress, secondary to eccentric growth from a damaged physis – asymmetrical growth following a physeal injury can subject a joint to eccentric load bearing, resulting in osteoarthrosis.

*Epiphyseal fractures:* Complete Salter–Harris types III and IV fractures involve the articular surface.

*Avascular necrosis of the epiphysis:*

* Femoral capital epiphysis – this is seen mainly in toy and terrier breeds. Secondary osteoarthrosis of the coxofemoral joint results.
* Feline capital physeal dysplasia syndrome – this is a form of epiphysiolysis, radiologically similar to traumatic femoral capital physeal separation that appears to occur spontaneously, suggesting an underlying physeal weakness.

*Ossification centres that fail to unite:*

* Ununited anconeal process – the physis of the anconeal process communicates with the humero-ulnar joint and provides a large 'joint mouse' when the anconeal process fails to unite (see Chapter 8).

- Incomplete ossification of the humeral condyle – this is a congenital problem reported in spaniels, predisposing affected dogs to sagittal articular fractures of the humeral condyle. The medial and lateral condyle ossification centres fail to unite, leaving an intercondylar cleavage is confluent with the elbow joint (Figure 6.22; see Chapter 8).

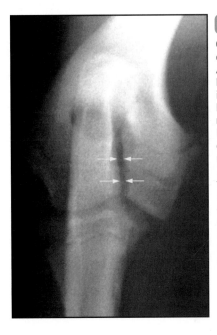

**6.22**

CrCd view of canine elbow. A radiolucent line (arrowed) is present between the medial and lateral humeral condyles. This represents incomplete fusion of the humeral condyle, a condition that has been reported in spaniels.

### Disorders of the synovium:

*Synovial cysts:* Fluctuant soft tissue swelling(s) adjacent to a joint may represent a synovial cyst. These thin walled, fluid-filled cysts may arise from the synovium of a joint, or a tendon sheath or bursa. Although benign, synovial cysts can attain large proportions. Their extent can be determined by injecting an organic iodine-based contrast medium into the cyst lumen, followed by radiography (positive contrast cystography).

*Synovial osteochondromatosis:* Calcified tissue adjacent to a joint may represent mineralization of metaplastic cartilage that has developed within the synovium of a joint, or tendon sheath and bursa. These synovial osteochondromatoses are benign lesions that are generally not regarded as a source of joint pain or lameness. Reported in both cats and dogs they can be confused with meniscal calcification when present in the stifle. They may be multiple and tend to be rounded.

*Villonodular synovitis:* A condition better reported in horses than in dogs, villonodular synovitis produces a fibrous mass that arises from the synovium. The presence of the mass may result in adjacent bone destruction, in which case the condition can be confused radiologically with an invasive neoplasm.

*Haemarthrosis:* A haemorrhagic arthropathy that may arise from trauma or an underlying disorder of haemostasis. Trauma, anti-coagulant (rodenticide) toxicosis, haemophilia, von Willebrand's disease, factor VII, X and XI deficiency and liver disease are potential causes of haemarthrosis. Chronic or recurrent haemarthrosis can lead to subchondral erosion once cartilage destruction, mediated by the release of chondrolysins in haemorrhagic synovial fluid, has developed.

*Hypertrophic osteopathy:* Hypertrophic osteopathy is not really a joint disorder but at one time was called hypertrophic osteoarthropathy because of bone proliferation on or around joints in affected animals. A change in nomenclature has occurred due to the significantly greater prevalence of this condition to involve the diaphyses of bones rather than periarticular structures in affected patients (see Chapter 4).

*Calcinosis circumscripta:* Foci of ectopic calcification of soft tissues, often in periarticular locations, is a condition that is over represented in young dogs of large breeds, particularly German Shepherd Dogs. Sometimes called tumoral calcinosis, it has been identified in a variety of locations but most commonly near joints of the appendicular skeleton. It typically has a multiple punctate mineralized appearance (see Chapter 1).

### References and further reading

Crawley AC, Yogalingam G, Muller VJ and Hopwood JJ (1998) Two mutations within a feline mucopolysaccharidosis type VI colony cause three different phenotypes. *Journal of Clinical Investigation* **101**, 109–119

Farese JP, Todhunter RJ, Lust G, Williams AJ and Dykes NL (1998) Dorsolateral subluxation of hip joints in dogs measured in a weight-bearing position with radiography and computed tomography. *Veterinary Surgery* **27**, 393–405

Farrow CS (1982) Stress radiography: applications in small animal practice. *Journal of the American Veterinary Medical Association* **181**, 177–184

Fluckiger MA, Friedrich GA and Binder H (1999) A radiographic stress technique for evaluation of coxofemoral joint laxity in dogs. *Veterinary Surgery* **28**, 1–9

Hedhammar A, Wu F-M and Krook L (1974) Overnutrition and skeletal disease. *Cornell Veterinarian* **64**, Suppl 5, 83–114

Mahoney PN and Lamb CR (1996) Articular, periarticular and juxta-articular calcified bodies in the dog and cat: a radiographic review. *Veterinary Radiology and Ultrasound* **37**, 3–19

Pedersen NC, Pool RR and O'Brien T (1980) Feline chronic progressive polyarthritis. *American Journal of Veterinary Research* **41**, 522–535

Rogers J, Shepstone L and Dieppe P (1997) Bone formers: osteophyte and enthesophyte formation are positively associated. *Annals of Rheumatic Disease* **56**, 85–90

Smith GK, Biery DN and Gregor TP (1990) New concepts of coxofemoral joint stability and the development of a clinical stress-radiographic method for quantitating hip joint laxity in the dog. *Journal of the American Veterinary Medical Association* **196**, 59–70

Vail DM, Powers BE, Getzy DM, Morrison WB, McEntee MC, O'Keefe DA, Norris AM and Withrow SJ (1994) Evaluation of prognostic factors for dogs with synovial sarcoma: 36 cases (1986–1991) *Journal of the American Veterinary Medical Association* **205**, 1300–1307

van Bree H (1992) Vacuum phenomenon associated with osteochondrosis of the scapulohumeral joint in dogs: 100 cases (1985–1991) *Journal of the American Veterinary Medical Association* **201**, 1916–1917

# 7

# The shoulder joint and scapula

## Henri van Bree and Ingrid Gielen

## Indications

Shoulder lameness, although a common condition in the dog, can be difficult to localize. Even when the lameness has been localized to the shoulder, identifying the precise cause can be unrewarding and frustrating. Occasionally it will be difficult to determine whether a specific structure is normal or abnormal. Numerous anatomical variants of the skeletal system exist that can easily be diagnosed erroneously as disease. In such cases, it is often helpful to take a radiograph of the contralateral shoulder for comparison or consult radiographs of other animals of similar age and breed.

Frequently there is a poor correlation between the radiological findings and clinical signs. There may be extensive changes present, such as osteoarthrosis, with no lameness. When a radiological finding is equivocal, additional follow-up radiographs may be helpful; bone is metabolically active and lesions, such as a bone neoplasm, sometimes change in appearance in a relatively short period of time. It is also very important to remember that the musculoskeletal system may appear normal even in the presence of disease. For example, more than 50% of the bone mineral content may be removed before a bone is radiologically more radiolucent than normal.

The radiological assessment of the shoulder joint should include evaluation of alignment, subchondral bone, joint space and adjacent periarticular soft tissues. Many of the joint tissues, such as cartilage, synovial membrane, fibrous capsule and collagenous structures, are not visible on plain film radiographs and therefore can only be evaluated indirectly. Arthrography and ultrasonography can be helpful in visualizing some of these structures.

The following are some of the indications for radiography of the shoulder joint:

- Any lameness associated with a shoulder problem, i.e. pain on manipulation of the joint itself or any structures in the shoulder area
- Swelling or deformity of the shoulder region
- Atrophy of the adjacent shoulder muscles.

## Radiography and normal anatomy

Technically excellent radiographs must be made. Failure to perceive a lesion is often related to poor radiographs as a result of underexposure, overexposure, improper positioning or as a result of an insufficient number of radiographic views. It should be remembered that since a radiograph is only a two-dimensional image, a minimum of two views, preferably perpendicular to each other, are usually necessary. This is especially true in traumatic lesions.

For radiographic examination of the shoulder joint it is necessary to heavily sedate or even anaesthetize the animal because manipulation of the affected leg usually is painful, and for radiation safety reasons. Optimal detail is obtained by using a grid, especially in larger dogs.

## Standard views

### Scapula

#### Mediolateral views:

- Scapula positioned dorsal to the vertebral column.

For this mediolateral (ML) view the patient is placed in lateral recumbency with the affected leg on the cassette and pushed dorsally to displace the scapula dorsal to the vertebral column. Usually the proximal part of the scapula will be slightly overexposed (Figure 7.1a).

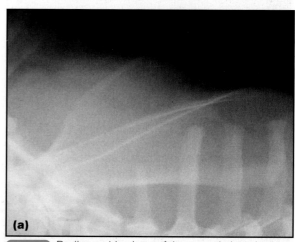

**7.1** Radiographic views of the scapula in a dog. **(a)** ML view with scapula positioned dorsal to the vertebral column. (continues) ▶

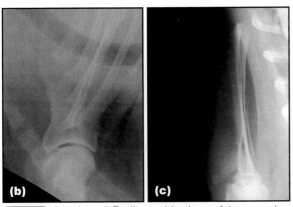

7.1 (continued) Radiographic views of the scapula in a dog. **(b)** ML view with scapula superimposed over the cranial lung field. **(c)** CdCr view.

- Scapula superimposed over the cranial lung field.

For this ML view the patient is placed in lateral recumbency with the affected leg on the cassette and pulled caudally and ventrally. The neck and body of the scapula can be evaluated although superimposition of the rib structures is present (Figure 7.1b).

*Caudocranial view:* For a caudocranial (CdCr) view the patient is placed in dorsal recumbency with the front legs extended cranially as far as possible. The patient's thorax should be rotated 10–15 degrees away from the scapula under examination in order to avoid superimposition of the rib cage. The scapular spine should be parallel to the cassette. The beam should be centred on the scapula. The scapular spine will usually be slightly overexposed (Figure 7.1c).

### Shoulder joint

*Mediolateral view:* The patient is placed in lateral recumbency with the affected leg on the cassette. The affected limb should be extended cranially and ventrally and the unaffected limb should be drawn caudally to separate the limbs. The neck should be extended dorsally to alleviate superimposition of the neck muscles and trachea (Figure 7.2).

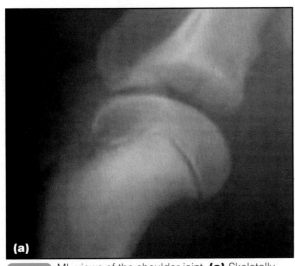

7.2  ML views of the shoulder joint. **(a)** Skeletally immature dog. (continues) ▶

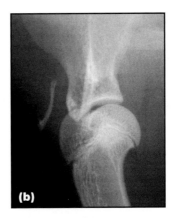

7.2  (continued) ML views of the shoulder joint. **(b)** Skeletally immature cat. Note the presence of the clavicle.

*Caudocranial view:* The positioning is similar to the corresponding view of the scapula except that the beam is centred on the shoulder joint (Figure 7.3).

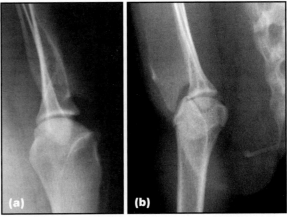

7.3  CdCr views of the shoulder joint. **(a)** Dog. **(b)** Cat. Note the presence of the clavicle.

### Special views

#### Intertubercular groove
Sometimes it can be advantageous to take a *tangential view* of the intertubercular groove (i.e. flexed cranio-proximal-craniodistal oblique view (CrPr-CrDiO)) (Figure 7.4). This view can demonstrate new bone formation in the groove and identify calcification in the biceps and supraspinatus tendons. This view is technically difficult to take and, if available, CT will provide more information.

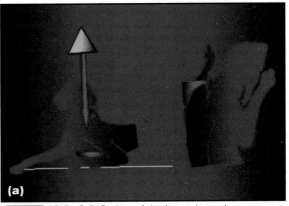

7.4  CrPr-CrDiO view of the intertubercular groove. **(a)** Sketch of positioning. (continues) ▶

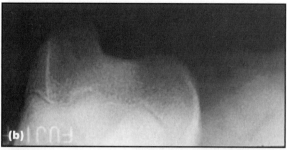

**7.4** (continued) CrPr-CrDiO view of the intertubercular groove. **(b)** Radiograph of skeletally immature dog.

## Normal anatomy

In the dog the scapula is a large, flat bone composed of a body with a longitudinal flat spine, a neck and the articular surface or glenoid. In the cat it is a shorter bone and a metacromion process extends caudally from the spine and acromion process. The coracoid process of the supraglenoid tubercle is a significant bony process extending from the medial side of the supraglenoid tubercle. In the dog, the coracoid process is insignificant.

The scapula is formed by multiple separate centres of ossification in immature animals. Of great importance is the supraglenoid tubercle because its physis may be mistaken for a fracture line (Figures 7.5 and 7.6). In doubtful cases a comparison with the contralateral limb is useful.

The major difference between the dog and cat is the presence of clavicles in cats (see Figures 7.2b and 7.3b). In large dogs the clavicles can be seen as rudimentary, poorly mineralized structures, which are sometimes visible bilaterally (Figures 7.7 and 7.8).

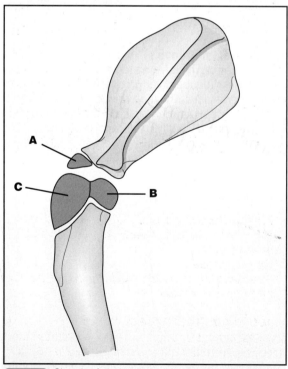

**7.5** Sketch of skeletally immature shoulder region, illustrating centres of ossification in an immature dog. A = Supraglenoid tubercle; B = Humeral head; C = Greater tubercle.

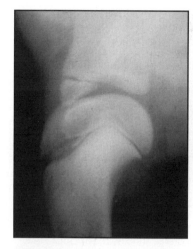

**7.6** ML view of a shoulder joint of a skeletally immature dog. Note the physeal line of the supraglenoid tubercle, which should not be mistaken for a fracture line.

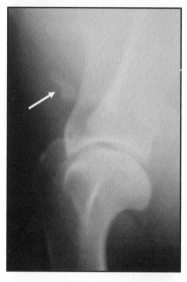

**7.7** ML view of a shoulder joint of a large dog. Note the rudimentary clavicle (arrowed).

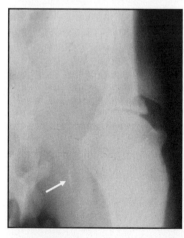

**7.8** CdCr view of a shoulder joint of a large dog. Note the rudimentary clavicle, which is just visible as a mineralized structure medial to the humerus (arrowed).

Calcified opacities around or within the shoulder joint are common findings and the majority of them are usually incidental findings. To associate them with pathology their origin should be identified, which is not always an easy task, and they should be correlated with clinical findings (Figure 7.9). Pathological calcified opacities are described later.

When viewing the shoulder joint, the joint space should be of equal width throughout. The head of the humerus should be smooth and rounded with no flattened areas. The spine of the scapula in the CdCr view

| Normal articular or periarticular shoulder joint mineralized opacities |
| --- |
| Clavicles in the cat (see Figures 7.2b and 7.3b) |
| Rudimentary clavicles in some dogs (see Figures 7.7 and 7.8) |
| Centres of ossification in young animals (supraglenoid tuberosity) (see Figures 7.5 and 7.6) |
| Separate ossification centre of the caudal rim of the glenoid (see Figure 7.42) |

**7.9** Normal articular or periarticular shoulder joint mineralized opacities.

should be checked for fractures. The so-called 'accessory ossification centre' of the caudal aspect of the glenoid in dogs should not be confused with osteochondritis dissecans (OCD), which occurs on the caudal aspect of the head of the humerus. The entire radiograph should be examined, including the cervical vertebrae and soft tissues, ribs, trachea and cranial lung fields.

## Physeal closure times

For information on physeal closure times see Chapter 3.

## Contrast studies

Arthrography of the shoulder joint is the most common arthrographic procedure used in small animal orthopaedics. It is an interesting and simple technique for imaging some shoulder problems in the dog.

### Positive contrast arthrography

A non-ionic, low osmolar contrast medium (preferably) is injected (1–4 ml) intra-articularly. The contrast medium should be diluted to 100 mg I/ml otherwise it can be too opaque and mask lesions. Exposures have to be made within 5 minutes post-injection because of the rapid absorption of the contrast medium by the synovial membrane. Several bursae are present around the scapulohumeral joint (Figure 7.10). The bicipital tendon sheath and subscapular recess are always visible whereas the infraspinatous bursa is only occasionally seen (Figure 7.11).

Technical pitfalls and artefacts encountered in arthrography include:

- Contrast medium injected or leaking into the periarticular tissues
- Insufficient or excessive contrast medium
- Contrast medium too opaque
- Air bubbles mimicking small joint mice. Air bubbles always have a round and smooth appearance.

Arthrography can outline the:

- Articular cartilage
- Synovial membrane

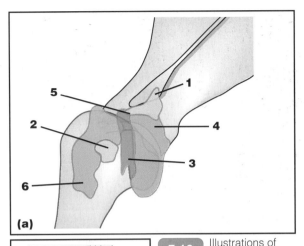

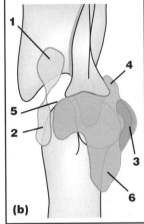

**7.10** Illustrations of the different bursae and pouches around the shoulder joint. **(a)** ML view. **(b)** CdCr view. 1 = Acromial bursa of infraspinatus muscle; 2 = Subtendinous bursa of infraspinatus muscle; 3 = Synovial tendon sheath of coracobrachialis muscle; 4 = Subscapular recess; 5 = Supraspinous recess; 6 = Intertubercular synovial tendon sheath.

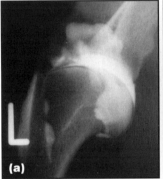
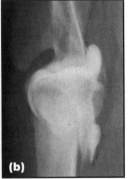

**7.11** Normal positive contrast arthrogram in the dog. **(a)** ML view. **(b)** CdCr view.

- Biceps tendon and associated synovial sheath (but cannot identify smaller lesions within the biceps tendon)
- Various bursae
- A cartilage flap in shoulder osteochondrosis (OC)
- Radiolucent joint mice.

### Negative contrast arthrography

Room air can be used as a negative contrast medium. The articular cartilage can be visualized but a distinction between a loose flap or thickened cartilage is usually not possible (Figure 7.12). Such a contrast study has the same effect as the vacuum phenomenon.

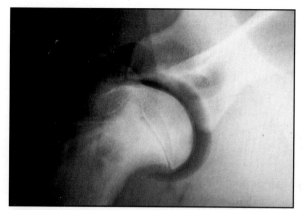

**7.12** ML view of a negative contrast arthrogram of a humeral OC lesion. The articular cartilage can be visualized but a distinction between a loose flap or thickened cartilage is not possible.

## Double contrast arthrography

Double contrast arthrography is a combination of the injection of a positive contrast medium and some air, and can provide good images (Figure 7.13). Unfortunately, because the shoulder joint space is rather small, bubble formation may hinder accurate interpretation.

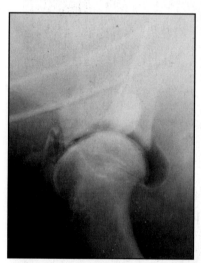

**7.13** ML view of a double contrast arthrogram of a humeral OCD lesion. The detached flap is clearly visible.

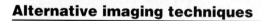

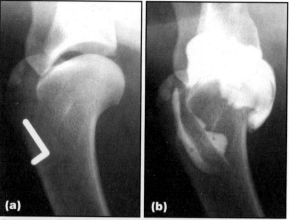

**(a)** **(b)**

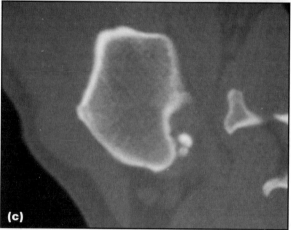

**(c)**

**7.14** Mineralization of the supraspinatus tendon of insertion. **(a)** Plain radiograph. **(b)** Positive contrast arthrogram. **(c)** CT image. Two mineral-like opacities within the supraspinatus tendon are visible. The arthrogram is helpful in localizing the opacities to outside the intertubercular groove. On the transverse CT image the locality and shape of these opacities is clearly defined.

## Alternative imaging techniques

Besides routine and more advanced imaging techniques, arthroscopy is a very useful imaging modality to directly visualize shoulder pathology with the advantage that treatment can be performed at the same time.

## Computed tomography

In some conditions the use of computed tomography (CT) can be justified, especially in situations where the superimposition of bony structures needs to be avoided, when evaluating the extent of pathology, or to determine the source of calcifications or fragments seen on plain film radiographs (Figure 7.14). New bone formation in the bicipital groove can be easily seen (Figure 7.15). CT may also be useful in cases with suspect demineralization as this technique can detect loss of bone content at an earlier stage (Figure 7.16) than conventional radiography.

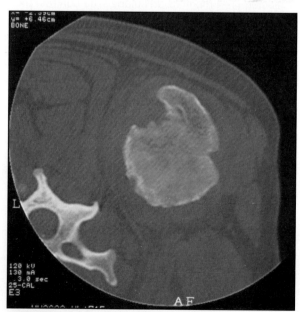

**7.15** Transverse CT image of new bone formation in the bicipital groove due to bicipital tenosynovitis.

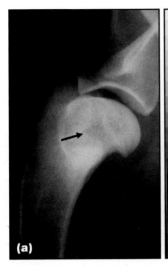

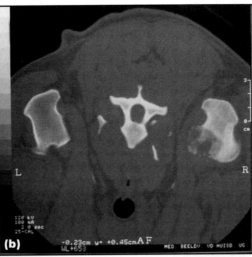

**7.16** Early proximal humeral primary bone neoplasm. **(a)** ML view showing an area of bony lysis surrounded by sclerosis (arrowed). **(b)** Transverse CT image in which the extent and exact localization of the lesion is better appreciated in the medial aspect of the humerus.

## Magnetic resonance imaging

Magnetic resonance imaging (MRI) has been evaluated for detecting OC lesions in the canine humeral head and was found to be useful in assessing the extent and severity of subchondral bone lesions (van Bree *et al.*, 1993). Although articular cartilage discontinuity can be detected, loose flaps are not always demonstrated (Figure 7.17).

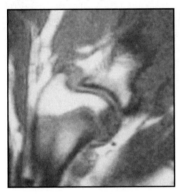

**7.17** T1-weighted MRI image of an OCD lesion. The extent and severity of subchondral bone involvement can clearly be appreciated. Although discontinuity in the delineation of the caudal humeral head can be detected, the detached flap cannot be demonstrated.

## Ultrasonography

Ultrasonography can be used in the shoulder joint for the diagnosis of muscle and tendon injury, and the evaluation of OC lesions. For this examination a high frequency linear transducer is used and the dog may have to be anaesthetized if joint manipulation is painful. The dog is placed in lateral recumbency with the shoulder to be examined uppermost. To visualize the humeral head, the acromion of the scapula is palpated and used as a landmark. Just distal to the acromion, the transducer is positioned in a craniocaudal direction and maintained in this position while the joint is adducted and maximally endorotated to obtain an adequate window of the caudal aspect of the humeral head. The humeral head is visible as a hyperechoic convex curvilinear line with a strong acoustic shadow and the cartilage as an anechoic layer (Figure 7.18a) covered by the joint capsule, the tendons of the infraspinatus and teres minor muscle and the acromial part of the deltoid muscle. For evaluation of the bicipital tendon sheath cross-sectional images at the level of the bicipital groove (Figure 7.18b) and longitudinal images at the level of the attachment on the supraglenoid tubercle should be taken (Figure 7.18c).

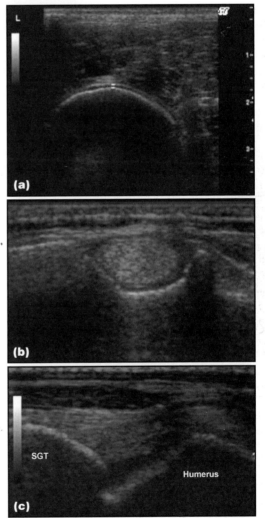

**7.18** Ultrasonographic images of a normal canine shoulder joint. **(a)** The humeral head is visible as a hyperechoic convex curvilinear line with a strong acoustic shadow and the cartilage as an anechoic layer covered by the joint capsule and superficial muscles. The thickness of the articular cartilage is 0.6 mm. **(b)** For the evaluation of the bicipital tendon sheath cross-sectional images at the level of the bicipital groove and **(c)** longitudinal images at the level of the attachment on the supraglenoid tubercle (SGT) are taken. Note the homogenous structure of the normal biceps tendon.

## Scintigraphy

Scintigraphy can be used to localize lameness originating in the shoulder region and to evaluate the significance of equivocal radiological findings.

## Abnormal radiological findings

Shoulder conditions can be classified as originating from the bony parts or soft tissues.

## Trauma

### Fractures

Radiography will assist in confirming the presence and extent of fractures. Two views are necessary to evaluate the degree of displacement (Figure 7.19). Scapular fractures may occur in the area of the scapular spine, body, neck, acromion and supraglenoid tuberosity. In the immature animal it is important that the fracture line not be confused with a growth plate (see Figures 7.6 and 7.20). Glenoid fractures are intra-articular fractures and result in complete limb dysfunction or severe lameness.

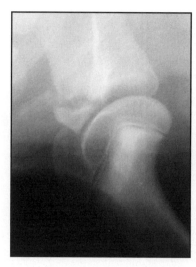

**7.20**

ML view of the shoulder joint of an immature animal showing an avulsion fracture of the supraglenoid tubercle. This fracture line should not be confused with the normal physis (see Figure 7.6).

Fractures of the proximal part of the humerus are uncommon because this is the thickest part of the bone. Fractures of the head of the humerus are usually seen in young animals with open, growing physes. A Salter–Harris type I fracture of the proximal physis of the humerus is occasionally seen (Figure 7.21). In addition, because of the close proximity of the scapula and shoulder joint to the thorax, fractures are commonly associated with various types and degrees of thoracic trauma, and a complete thoracic radiographic examination should be routinely performed.

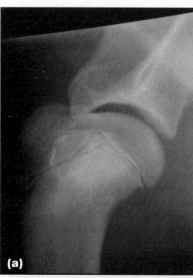

**7.19**

Multiple intra-articular fracture of the shoulder joint. **(a)** ML view. **(b)** CdCr view. Both views are necessary to evaluate the degree of displacement and the extent of the fractures.

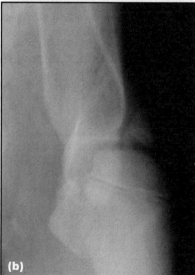

**(a)**

**(b)**

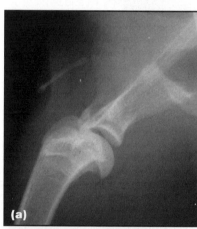

**7.21**

Salter–Harris type I fracture of the proximal physis of the humerus in a cat. **(a)** ML view. **(b)** CdCr view. The two views are necessary to evaluate the full extent of the fracture.

**(a)**

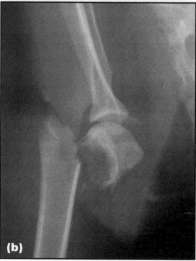

**(b)**

## Luxations and subluxations

Luxations of the scapulohumeral joint can be congenital (see later) or acquired and can occur in any direction (cranial, caudal, medial and lateral). Medial luxations occur most often in toy breeds and are usually congenital. Lateral luxations occur infrequently and are seen primarily in large-breed dogs as a result of trauma. Cranial and caudal luxations are very rare.

Traumatic luxation is usually due to automobile trauma but may also be due to falls from a height or by twisting injuries to the shoulder. Since trauma is the basic injury, there is no breed, age or sex predilection. Luxation is usually unilateral but may also occur bilaterally. Traumatic subluxation results from trauma that is sufficient to create joint instability but not enough to result in total luxation. Subluxation often leads to chronic instability, osteoarthrosis and progressive disuse of the limb.

Standard radiographic views will demonstrate the position of the humeral head relative to the glenoid cavity. Two views are necessary, since a lateral view with complete shoulder extension may reduce the shoulder or allow for positioning that appears to be reduced. Typically the lateral view will demonstrate superimposition of the humeral head over the glenoid with no joint space visible. Care should be taken to look for fractures of the medial glenoid rim, which will probably preclude closed reduction (Figure 7.22).

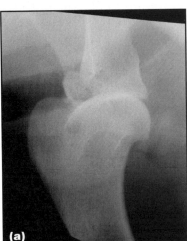
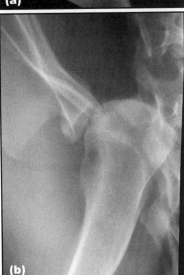

**7.22** Traumatic medial shoulder luxation. **(a)** ML view. **(b)** CdCr view. Note the fracture fragment of the medial glenoid rim, which will probably preclude closed reduction.

## Biceps tendon rupture

Traumatic rupture of the tendon of the biceps brachii muscle can occur but is rare. In the growing dog (4 to 8 months) there is generally an avulsion of the supraglenoid tuberosity, which can be seen radiologically. In the mature dog, the rupture of the tendon occurs near its origin. The diagnosis can be difficult and usually there are no signs on plain film radiographs. The diagnosis can be confirmed by positive contrast arthrography, which reveals leakage of contrast media from the tendon sheath, or by loss of the normal tendon filling defect (Figure 7.23). This condition can be easily visualized with ultrasonography (Figure 7.24).

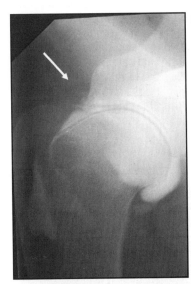

**7.23** ML view of a positive contrast arthrogram of a traumatic rupture of the biceps tendon. The arthrogram reveals leakage of contrast medium from the tendon sheath (arrowed) and loss of the normal tendon filling defect. Effusion in the area of the caudal pouch can also be appreciated.

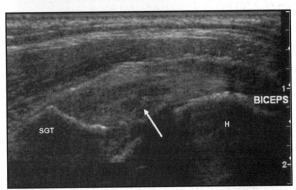

**7.24** Longitudinal ultrasonographic view of a traumatic partial rupture of a biceps tendon. H = Humerus; SGT = Supraglenoid tubercle. Note the inhomogenous and hypoechoic areas within the tendon (arrowed) in comparison with Figure 7.18c.

## Congenital and developmental conditions

### Congenital luxation

Congenital shoulder luxation occurs predominantly in miniature dog breeds. The luxation may be uni- or bilateral; in all reported cases luxation has been medial. Congenital shoulder luxation usually manifests itself as shoulder lameness and is first apparent to owners from three to eight months of age, although some animals may be older. In addition, although the luxation may not occur until well after the dog has reached skeletal maturity, these luxations are considered congenital because of the anatomical predisposition to luxation. Some dogs with chronic luxations become weight bearing on the affected limb(s), but varying degrees of muscle atrophy and bony crepitus may develop. Radiography will prove the position of the luxation and may demonstrate a flattened or convex glenoid cavity (Figure 7.25). Congenital subluxation, characterized by joint laxity, flattened humeral head and shallow glenoid has also been described.

### Shoulder osteochondrosis

In dogs one of the most common predilection sites for OC is the caudal humeral head. OC is an abnormality of endochondral ossification in which the cartilage of the epiphysis fails to form subchondral bone. This results in thickened abnormal cartilage, which is susceptible to injury. OCD is the form of OC in which the articular cartilage is fissured and forms a cartilage flap. In most dogs, this flap will remain within its subchondral bed, hindering the ingrowth of granulation tissue. In some dogs, this cartilage flap eventually dislodges and may then be resorbed, remain a free body (joint mouse) or grow in size, nourished by synovial fluid, to eventually ossify. A joint mouse may cause lameness by intermittently becoming interposed between articulating surfaces or, when small enough, it can enter the biceps tendon sheath to lodge here. Most of the time, the free flap will migrate towards the caudal pouch of the shoulder joint. Often these flaps become overgrown by synovium, which can be observed arthroscopically. Joint mice may be seen within the bicipital tendon sheath (Figure 7.26), the caudal pouch (Figure 7.27) and, rarely, within the bursa subscapularis (Figure 7.28). The final result of shoulder OCD may be secondary osteoarthrosis, even when treated correctly. Despite apparent lameness in only one limb, both shoulders should be radiographed because often there may be bilateral lesions. It is also advisable to evaluate the hip joints for signs of hip dysplasia as, in the authors' experience, this is often seen concurrently with shoulder OC.

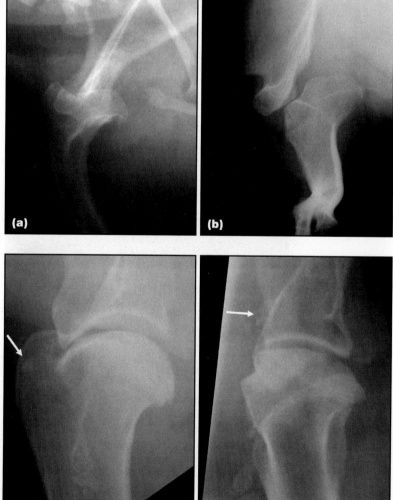

**7.25** Congenital medial shoulder luxation. **(a)** ML view. **(b)** CdCr view. Note the flattened abnormal form of the glenoid cavity.

**7.26** Joint mice in the distal bicipital tendon sheath. **(a)** ML view. **(b)** CdCr view. Mineralized opacities within the supraspinatus muscle are also visible (arrowed).

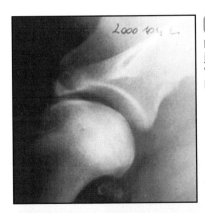

**7.27** ML view of a joint mouse within the caudal pouch.

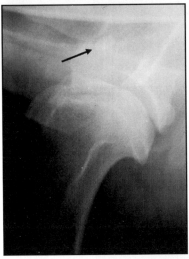

**7.28** ML view of a joint mouse within the bursa subscapularis (arrowed), which is an uncommon finding.

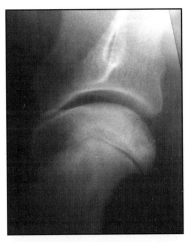

**7.30** ML view of a classical shoulder OC lesion, a flattening and an irregular radiolucent subchondral defect involving the caudal aspect of the humeral head can be seen.

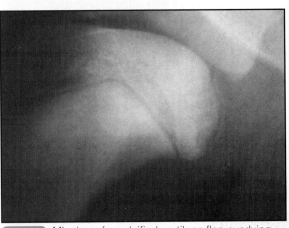

**7.31** ML view of a calcified cartilage flap overlying the subchondral defect.

The most common radiological finding of shoulder OC lesions is a flattening or an irregular, radiolucent subchondral defect of variable size, involving the caudal aspect of the humeral head (Figures 7.29 and 7.30). This is caused by thickening of the articular cartilage in that area. If there is calcification of a cartilage flap, it is usually seen overlying the subchondral defect (Figure 7.31), although it may be seen elsewhere if detached (see Figure 7.27). Additional findings may include subchondral sclerosis surrounding the defect (Figures 7.29 and 7.30) and osteoarthrosis in chronic cases (Figures 7.28 and 7.32). In 20% of cases a vacuum phenomenon can be seen (Figure 7.32) (see also Chapter 6).

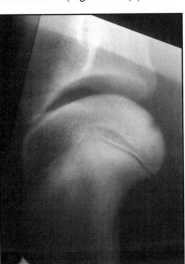

**7.29** ML view of a small OC lesion involving the caudal aspect of the humeral head.

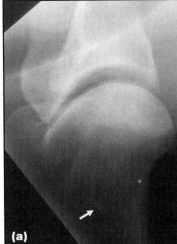

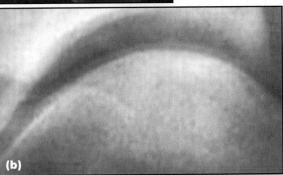

**7.32** (a) ML view of an osteochondrotic shoulder joint with a vacuum phenomenon; the articular cartilage is seen as a grey line superimposed on the subchondral bone. A joint mouse within the bicipital tendon sheath is visible (arrowed) as well as arthrotic changes. (b) Close-up view.

Although a correlation has been demonstrated between the size of the subchondral defect, the presence of a vacuum phenomenon, and the status of the overlying articular cartilage and the associated clinical signs, plain film radiographs cannot be used to assess the status of the articular cartilage or the presence of radiolucent joint mice. Positive contrast arthrography helps to assess whether a non-mineralized cartilage flap is present with an accuracy of 80%, and this finding helps to determine whether a dog should be treated conservatively or surgically. Using positive contrast arthrography, the status of the articular cartilage covering the subchondral defect can be evaluated and classified to determine treatment options:

- Contrast medium going underneath the cartilage usually correlates with signs of pain and lameness (Figure 7.33) and the joint should be surgically or arthroscopically treated
- The detection of thick cartilage covering the subchondral defect (Figure 7.34) or a detached cartilage flap lodged in the caudal pouch of the joint capsule (Figure 7.35) is associated in most cases with lack of clinical signs and such a lesion can usually be left untreated
- In some dogs with acute severe lameness, a detached cartilage flap migrating towards the caudal pouch can be detected (Figure 7.36).

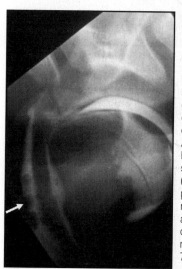

**7.33**

ML view of a positive contrast arthrogram of a clinical OCD lesion. Contrast medium is seen underneath the cartilage, which correlates with signs of pain and lameness. Artefactual air bubbles, mimicking small joint mice (arrowed), are also present. They have a round and smooth appearance in contrast to real joint mice (see Figures 7.37 and 7.38).

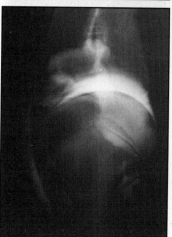

**7.34**

ML view of a positive contrast arthrogram of a non-clinical OCD lesion. Thick cartilage is covering the subchondral defect with no contrast medium visible underneath the cartilage.

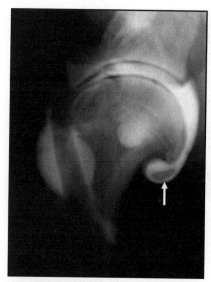

**7.35**

ML view of a positive contrast arthrogram showing a detached cartilage flap lodged in the caudal pouch of the joint capsule (arrowed). In most cases, such a finding is associated with no clinical signs and the lesion can be left untreated.

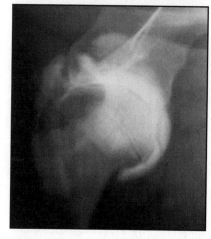

**7.36**

ML view of a positive contrast arthrogram showing a detached cartilage flap migrating towards the caudal pouch. Notice also the joint effusion. Such dogs are presented with an acute severe lameness.

Detached flaps in the caudal pouch may migrate cranially to interfere with joint function or enter the bicipital tendon sheath. About 10% of joint mice are located here. Not all these joint mice are calcified and are thus not always visible on plain film radiographs. Arthrography can be used to visualize joint mice in the bicipital tendon sheath and helps in deciding whether they should be removed (Figure 7.37). The bicipital tendon sheath may have large pouches and when a joint mouse is detected within such a pouch, it can usually be left untreated (Figure 7.38). On the other hand, if a joint mouse is hindering the mechanical action of the biceps tendon it should be removed.

Results of a recent study (Vandevelde *et al.*, 2005) comparing ultrasonography with radiography, arthrography and arthroscopy, suggest that all radiologically diagnosed subchondral lesions in the humeral head can be visualized, with the use of ultrasonography, as a concave deviation of the hyperechoic subchondral bone line with a variable length according to the extent of the lesion. The results also suggest that the presence of a second hyperechoic line at the bottom of the subchondral defect, seen on ultrasound examination, is a pathognomonic sign for the presence of a flap (Figure 7.39). It was suggested that ultrasonography might present an alternative to positive contrast arthrography.

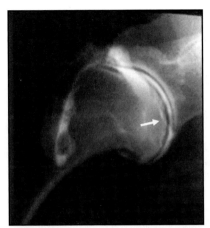

**7.37** ML view of a positive contrast arthrogram showing a joint mouse in the bicipital tendon sheath. This large joint mouse hinders the mechanical action of the biceps tendon and should be removed. Notice also that the cartilage flap looks fragmented (arrowed) meaning that smaller cartilage fragments may break off and form joint mice.

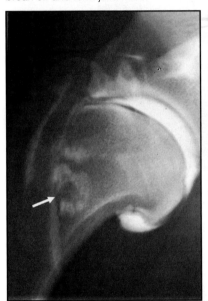

**7.38** ML view of a positive contrast arthrogram showing a joint mouse in the bicipital tendon sheath within a larger pouch (arrowed). This mouse is not hindering the biceps tendon and can be left untreated.

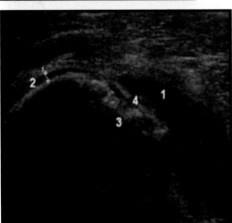

**7.39** Longitudinal ultrasound image of a clinical OCD lesion. Note the presence of a second hyperechoic line at the bottom of the subchondral defect, which is a pathognomonic sign for the presence of a flap. 1 = Joint effusion; 2 = Normal articular cartilage cranial to the lesion; 3 = Subchondral bed of the OCD lesion; 4 = Hyperechoic line representing the detached flap.

## Shoulder dysplasia

Shoulder dysplasia is a rare and confusing condition, and the clinical symptoms are not clear. It has been reported in the Dachshund and other breeds. Butterworth (1994) believes it is a condition similar to hip dysplasia, whilst others (Morgan *et al.*, 2000) consider it a different pathological condition, believing it to be part of the congenital shoulder luxation complex encountered in small-size breeds. Morgan *et al.* (2000) consider shoulder dysplasia to be a faulty development of the caudal portion of the ossification centre of the humeral head. In some dogs this fails to form, resulting in a collapse of the caudal portion of the humeral head. The glenoid cavity (because of the lack of support from the convex humeral head) also fails to form and develops into a convex surface, poorly congruent with the flattened humeral head (Figure 7.40). The condition has been associated with lameness but it is important to rule out other possible diagnoses before concluding that shoulder dysplasia is the cause of the problem. Nevertheless, like some congenital shoulder luxations, a surprising amount of functional compensation is possible and the condition is sometimes incidentally discovered in sound adult dogs.

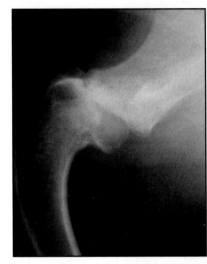

**7.40** ML view of a shoulder with shoulder dysplasia. The glenoid cavity, because of the lack of support by a convex humeral head, has failed to form and has therefore developed into a convex surface, which is incongruent with the flattened humerus.

## Separate ossification centre of the caudal rim of the glenoid

The presence of a separate ossification centre of the caudal rim of the glenoid is described in the dog, although there is no proof in the literature that such an ossification centre actually exists. It appears radiologically as a small radiopaque projection located just caudal to the glenoid (Figure 7.41). In some cases it may have the appearance of a fracture (Figure 7.42) but in most instances it is an incidental finding. Lameness occurs when the fragment is loosely embedded in the joint capsule. Such an unstable fragment can act as a free body in the joint and can cause synovitis and pain. With the use of positive arthrography, impingement of the joint capsule can be demonstrated and the fragment is visible as a filling defect (Figure 7.43). Arthroscopic removal of these fragments alleviates the clinical symptoms. The use of CT can be very helpful to delineate the position and structure of the fragment. Lameness can be attributed to this condition only after other causes of forelimb lameness have been excluded.

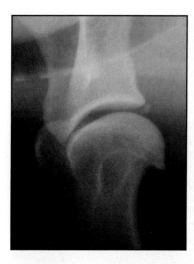

**7.41**

ML view of a separate ossification centre of the caudal rim of the glenoid. It appears radiologically as a small radiopaque projection located just caudal to the glenoid. Note also the presence of an arthrotic spur at the caudal end of the humeral head, probably an incidental finding.

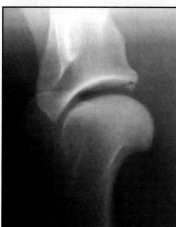

**7.42**

ML view of an ossification centre of the caudal rim of the glenoid with the appearance of a fracture. This dog was presented with clinical shoulder lameness.

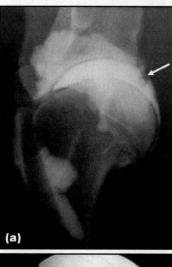

(a)

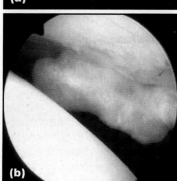

(b)

**7.43**

**(a)** ML view of a positive contrast arthrogram of the dog in Figure 7.42, demonstrating impingement of the joint capsule. Lameness occurred when the fragment became loosely embedded in the joint capsule. The fragment is visible as a filling defect (arrowed). **(b)** The corresponding arthroscopic view shows an unstable fragment acting as a free body in the joint and causing synovitis and pain.

## Degenerative conditions

### Omarthrosis

Shoulder osteoarthrosis may be primary, as a result of ageing (often clinically insignificant), or more often secondary, as a consequence of a shoulder problem such as OCD. It is characterized by osteophytes on the caudal glenoid rim and caudal articular margin of the humeral head (Figure 7.44). In more advanced cases capsular enthesophytes may be seen in the intertubercular groove region and superimposed on the humeral head.

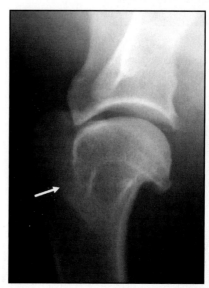

**7.44**

ML view of a shoulder joint with osteoarthrosis. It is characterized by osteophytes on the caudal glenoid rim and caudal articular margin of the humeral head. Osteophytes in the intertubercular groove region (arrowed) and superimposed on the humeral head can also be appreciated.

### Tenosynovitis and partial rupture of the biceps tendon

Bicipital tenosynovitis is a common cause of forelimb lameness in the dog and may be difficult to diagnose. Many breeds can be affected but it is more common in large mature dogs, although immature animals can be affected as well. Lameness is usually chronic and progressive and may be uni- or bilateral. The cause of the disease remains controversial. Inflammation plays a role in most instances. It has been suggested that the pathology may be a result of a degenerative process (Gilley *et al.*, 2002) whilst other authors (Rivers *et al.*, 1992) mention chronic repetitive trauma as a possible aetiology. The mechanism of injury can be direct, indirect, overuse or migration of joint mice from humeral OCD lesions. The association of biceps tendon lesions with shoulder instability has been reported but is still controversial. These lesions can eventually result in tears and partial ruptures or, rarely, a complete rupture of the biceps tendon.

The diagnosis may be confirmed by radiography of the shoulder, although often radiographs show no changes, especially in the acute phase. The most sensitive radiological indicator of bicipital tenosynovitis is sclerosis along the bicipital groove (Figure 7.45). Other radiological signs include dystrophic calcification of the tendon, avulsion fractures of the attachment of the tendon, demineralization of the supraglenoid tubercle, osteophytes in the intertubercular groove or mineralized fragments within the tendon sheath (Figures 7.46 and 7.47). Positive contrast arthrography may demonstrate changes in the contour of the bicipital groove and tendon, incomplete filling of the synovial sheath, filling defects and irregularities (Figure 7.48). Ultrasonography is very useful in diagnosing this condition (Figure 7.49). Diagnosis can also be performed by arthroscopic examination of the tendon and associated sheath (Figure 7.50). Arthroscopic tenotomy of the attachment of the biceps tendon from the supraglenoid tuberosity immediately alleviates symptoms of pain and lameness.

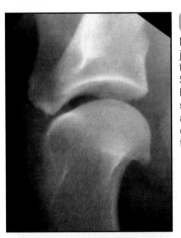

**7.45**
ML view of a shoulder joint with bicipital tenosynovitis. Sclerosis along the bicipital groove and supraglenoid tubercle as well as irregular delineation of the tubercle is visible.

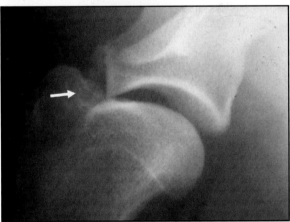

**7.46** ML view of a shoulder joint with biceps tendon pathology. Radiological signs include dystrophic calcification of the tendon (arrowed) and new bone formation in the area of its attachment.

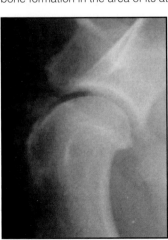

**7.47**
ML view of a shoulder joint showing an avulsion fracture of the attachment of the biceps tendon. Demineralization of the supraglenoid tubercle, osteophytes in the intertubercular groove and signs of osteoarthrosis are also visible.

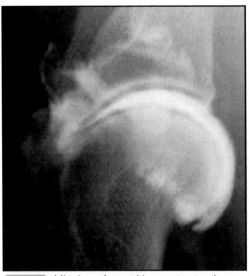

**7.48** ML view of a positive contrast arthrogram demonstrating incomplete filling of the synovial sheath, filling defects and absence of delineation of the bicipital attachment due to partial avulsion of the biceps tendon. Effusion can also be appreciated.

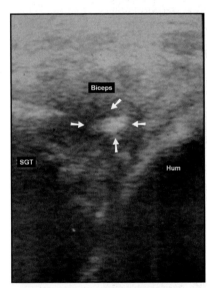

**7.49**
The corresponding longitudinal ultrasonographic view of the shoulder of the patient in Figure 7.48, demonstrating the fragment (arrowed) within the avulsed biceps tendon. Hum = Humerus; SGT = Supraglenoid tubercle.

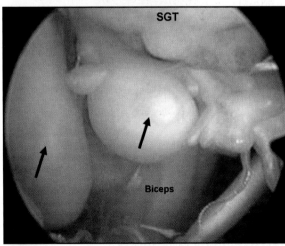

**7.50** Arthroscopic view of a partially ruptured biceps tendon. Fibres and hypertrophied stumps (arrowed) of the biceps are visible. SGT = Supraglenoid tubercle.

## Neoplasia

### Synovial sarcoma

Synovial sarcoma is an uncommon neoplasm in the dog and represents about 2% of all primary and secondary bone neoplasms. It is of mesenchymal origin, occurring mainly in the vicinity of a joint. Subsequent invasion of the joint and adjacent bones may occur. Synovial sarcoma usually affects male, middle-aged, large-breed dogs. The rate of growth can vary from very slow to very rapid. The neoplasm is usually poorly defined and infiltrates the deeper structures. The initial radiological change is a soft tissue mass in the area of the joint. In the later stages punctate lytic areas, involving either the diaphysis and the adjacent epiphyseal-metaphyseal area or the epiphyseal-metaphyseal area alone, are seen. Bones on either side of the joint may be affected.

### Bone neoplasms

The proximal humerus is a predilection site for primary malignant bone neoplasia in the dog. In most cases, radiography is all that is needed to make the diagnosis but sometimes there are ambiguities. Different radiological signs are possible, varying from very lytic to productive changes. Most of the time there is a mixed pattern. In the early stages infectious and degenerative lesions may be possible differential diagnoses (see Figures 7.16a and 7.51) (see also Chapter 4).

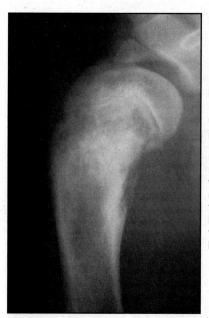

**7.51**

ML view of a proximal humerus with osteomyelitis. An osteolytic area surrounded by osteosclerosis and a proliferative periosteal reaction are visible. The radiological features should be differentiated from a primary bone neoplasm.

### Infection

Infection of the shoulder joint is rarely seen and then usually in young dogs. Initially there will be no radiological changes, but as the condition advances, a mixture of subchondral bone lysis and active periarticular bone formation develops (see also Chapter 6).

### Miscellaneous conditions

Pathological calcified opacities in or around a joint are often seen (Figure 7.52) and must be distinguished from normal structures (see Figure 7.9).

| **Abnormal articular or periarticular shoulder joint mineralized opacities** |
|---|
| Osteochondrosis:<br>• Mineralized cartilage flaps (see Figure 7.31)<br>• Osteochondral fragments (joint mice) in: caudal pouch (usual) (see Figure 7.27); bicipital tendon sheath (10%) (see Figure 7.26); bursa subscapularis (rare) (see Figure 7.28)<br>Avulsion fracture of the supraglenoid tubercle (see Figure 7.20)<br>Avulsion fracture of the biceps tendon attachment (see Figure 7.47)<br>Calcifying tendinopathy of the biceps tendon (see Figure 7.46)<br>Calcifying tendinopathy of the supraspinatus tendon (see Figure 7.14)<br>Synovial osteochondromatosis (see Figure 7.53)<br>Calcinosis circumscripta (see Figure 7.56)<br>Hypervitaminosis A in the cat (see Figure 7.55)<br>Avulsion fractures of the infraspinatus tendon (can mimic mineralization in the bicipital groove).<br>Fragment adjacent to the caudal rim of the glenoid (see Figure 7.43)<br><br>(For normal mineralized opacities see Figure 7.9.) |

**7.52** Abnormal articular or periarticular shoulder joint mineralized opacities.

### Synovial osteochondromatosis

Shoulder synovial osteochondromatosis (chondrometaplasia) is an uncommon condition. The synovial membrane of the shoulder joint or the bicipital tendon sheath undergoes a nodular cartilaginous metaplasia, and sometimes the cartilage becomes replaced by cancellous bone. Synovial osteochondromatosis can be either primary (idiopathic) or secondary (a response to chronic irritation). The nodules may stay adherent to the synovium, or break free and form joint mice. Although, theoretically benign, these joint mice can cause cartilage trauma or bicipital tenosynovitis if they migrate into the bicipital tendon sheath. Radiologically, multiple mineralized nodules are seen within the joint capsule and its recesses. On positive contrast arthrography, radiolucent nodules appear as filling defects (Figure 7.53). Concurrent omarthrosis is frequently observed.

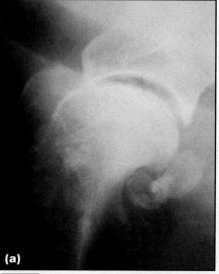

(a)

**7.53** ML views of a shoulder joint with synovial osteochondromatosis. **(a)** Plain film radiograph shows multiple mineralized nodules within the joint capsule and its recesses. (continues) ▶

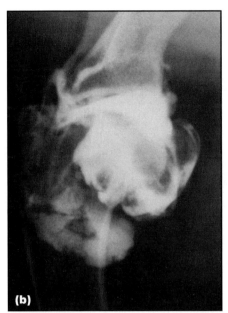

**7.53** (continued) ML views of a shoulder joint with synovial osteochondromatosis. **(b)** Positive contrast arthrogram. Radiolucent nodules appear as filling defects within the joint.

### Infraspinatus muscle contracture

Infraspinatus contracture is a uni- or bilateral fibrotic myopathy of the infraspinatus muscle, which is usually secondary to trauma in hunting or working dogs. Clinical signs include an acute lameness, pain and swelling in the shoulder region. The lameness subsides, but a gait abnormality develops 2–4 weeks after injury as progressive muscle fibrosis and contracture occur. Clinical signs include a characteristic adduction of the elbow, abduction of the foreleg, and external rotation of the carpus and paw. The limb is circumducted with each stride of the leg. Palpation of the shoulders reveals outward rotation of the humerus as the elbow is flexed. Radiological examination may reveal narrowing of the lateral scapulohumeral joint space on the CdCr view (Figure 7.54). Treatment consists of resection of the

fibrous musculotendinous portion of the muscle, including tenotomy of the tendon of insertion. Limb and joint functions are immediately improved and prognosis for full recovery is excellent.

### Mineralization of the supraspinatus muscle

Mineral-like opacities within the supraspinatus tendon of insertion are a common radiological finding and are due to dystrophic mineralization. Their clinical significance is unclear but in the authors' experience they are seldom a primary cause of lameness. Any age or breed of dog can be affected, but this condition is more common in large breeds, particularly Rottweilers. A presumptive diagnosis of the clinical significance of these mineral-like opacities can be made only by excluding other cases of thoracic limb lameness. They appear on ML views as irregular linear or more oval opacities in different locations. Mineralization of the biceps tendon may be indistinguishable from that of the supraspinatus tendon if only a ML radiograph is taken. To delineate the location of dystrophic calcification a flexed CrPr-CrDi oblique view of the intertubercular groove can be helpful. Arthrography is also helpful in localizing the source of mineralization outside the intertubercular groove (see Figure 7.14b). CT is also very useful to define the localization and the structures of these densities (see Figure 7.14c).

### Hypervitaminosis A

Hypervitaminosis A is diagnosed, mostly in cats older than three years, due to vitamin A intoxication. These animals may present with forelimb lameness due to proliferative new bone formation at tendon and ligament insertion or origins around the shoulder joint (Figure 7.55) and other joints. Radiological changes are also characteristically seen in the spine (see also Chapter 15).

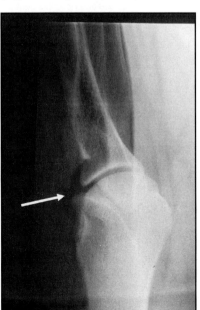

**7.54** CdCr view of a shoulder joint with infraspinatus muscle contracture revealing narrowing of the lateral scapulohumeral joint space (arrowed).

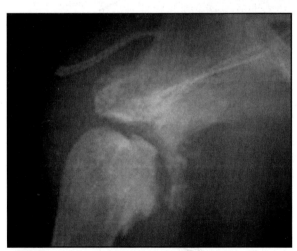

**7.55** ML view of the shoulder joint of a cat suffering from hypervitaminosis A, revealing proliferative new bone formation around the shoulder joint.

### Calcinosis circumscripta

Calcinosis circumscripta is an ectopic mineralization characterized by deposition of calcium salts (calcium phosphate crystals, including hydroxyapatite crystals) in soft tissues. It occurs most commonly in young, large-breed dogs with a higher incidence seen in German Shepherd Dogs. The lesions are generally solitary and occur in specific anatomical locations, such as the lateral metatarsus and digits, the elbow, the shoulder (Figure 7.56), the spine, the hip, the tongue and the foot pads.

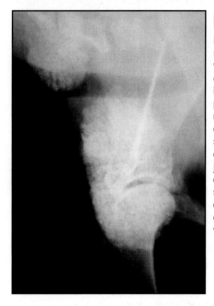

**7.56**

ML view of a shoulder joint with calcinosis circumscripta. Note the punctate mineralized opacities superimposed on the shoulder joint. The same opacities are seen in the area of the caudal cervical vertebrae.

## References and further reading

Bardet JF (1999) Lesions of the biceps tendon: diagnosis and classification. *Veterinary and Comparative Orthopaedics and Traumatology* **12,** 188–195

Barthez P and Morgan J (1993) Bicipital tenosynovitis in the dog, evaluation with positive contrast arthrography. *Veterinary Radiology* **34**, 325–330

Begon D, Mialot JP and Guérin C (1988) Aspects radiographiques de l'épaule du chien en croissance. *Le point vétérinaire* **19**, 683–690

Butterworth S (1994) The shoulder. In: *BSAVA Manual of Small Animal Arthrology*, ed. JEF Houlton and RW Collinson, pp. 149–174. BSAVA Publications, Cheltenham

Cook JL, Cook CR, Tomlinson JL, Millis DL, Starost M, Albrecht MA and Payne JT (1997) Scapular fractures in dogs: epidemiology, classification and concurrent injuries in 105 cases (1988–1994). *Journal of the American Animal Hospital Association* **33**, 528–532

Dennis R, Kirberger RM, Wrigley RH and Barr FJ (2001) Appendicular skeleton. In: *Handbook of Small Animal Radiological Differential Diagnosis*. pp.31–41. WB Saunders, London

Flo GL and Midleton D (1990) Mineralization of the supraspinatus tendon in dogs. *Journal of the American Veterinary Medical Association* **197**, 95–97

Gilley RS, Wallace LJ and Hayden DW (2002) Clinical and pathologic analyses of bicipital tenosynovitis in dogs. *American Journal of Veterinary Research* **63**, 402–407

Kramer M, Gerwing M, Hach V and Schimke E (1997) Sonography of the musculoskeletal system in dogs and cats. *Veterinary Radiology and Ultrasound* **38**,139–149

Kramer M, Gerwing M, Shepperd C and Schimke E (2000) Ultrasonography for the diagnosis of diseases of the tendon and tendon sheath of the biceps brachii muscle. *Veterinary Surgery* **30**, 64–71

Kriegleder H (1995) Mineralization of the supraspinatus tendon: clinical observations in seven dogs. *Veterinary and Comparative Orthopaedics and Traumatology* **8**, 91–97

Laitinen OM and Flo GL (2000) Mineralization of the supraspinatus tendon in dogs: a long-term follow-up. *Journal of the American Animal Hospital Association* **36**, 262–267

Long CD and Nyland TG (1999) Ultrasonographic evaluation of the canine shoulder. *Veterinary Radiology and Ultrasound* **40**, 372–379

Mayerhofer E (1987) Rontgenologische Untersuchungen zur Peritendinitis calcarea im Schultergelenksbereich des Hundes. *Journal of Veterinary Medicine A* **34**, 501–507

Morgan JP, Wind A and Davidson AP (2000) In: *Hereditary Bone and Joint Diseases in the Dog.* pp 21–40. Schlütersche, Hannover

Olivieri M, Piras A, Marcellin-Litle DJ, Borghetti P and Vezzoni A (2004) Accessory caudal glenoid ossification centre as possible cause of lameness in nine dogs. *Veterinary and Comparative Orthopaedics and Traumatology* **3**, 131–135

Rivers B, Wallace L and Johnston GR (1992) Biceps tenosynovitis in the dog: radiographic and sonographic findings. *Veterinary and Comparative Orthopaedics and Traumatology* **5**, 51–57

Schawalder P, Prieur WD and Koch H (1998) Dysplasien und Wachstumsstörungen. In: *Kleintierkrankheiten Band 3: Orthopädische Chirurgie und Traumatologie*, ed. KH Bonath and D Prieur, pp. 356–413. UTB-Reihe, Ulmer

van Bree H (1990) Evaluation of the prognostic value of positive-contrast shoulder arthrography for bilateral osteochondrosis lesions in dogs. *American Journal of Veterinary Research* **7**, 1121–1125

van Bree H (1992) Vacuum phenomenon associated with osteochondrosis of the scapulohumeral joint in dogs: 100 cases (1985–1991). *Journal of the American Veterinary Medical Association* **201**, 1916–1917

van Bree H (1993) Comparison of diagnostic accuracy of positive-contrast arthrography and arthrotomy in evaluation of osteochondrosis lesions in scapulohumeral joints in dogs. *Journal of the American Veterinary Medical Association* **203**, 84–88

van Bree H (1994) Evaluation of subchondral lesion size in osteochondrosis of the scapulohumeral joint in dogs. *Journal of the American Veterinary Medical Association* **204**, 1472–1474

van Bree H, Degryse H, Van Ryssen B, Ramon F and Desmidt M (1993) Pathologic correlations with magnetic resonance images of osteochondrosis lesions in canine shoulders. *Journal of the American Veterinary Medical Association* **202**, 1099–1105

van Bree H and Van Ryssen B (1998) Diagnostic and surgical arthroscopy in osteochondrosis lesions. *The Veterinary Clinics of North America: Small Animal Practice* **28**, 161–189

van Bree H, Van Ryssen B and Desmidt M (1992) Osteochondrosis lesions of the canine shoulder: correlation of positive contrast arthrography and arthroscopy. *Veterinary Radiology and Ultrasound* **33**, 342–347

Vandevelde B, Saunders J, Kramer M, Van Ryssen B and van Bree H (in press) Ultrasonographic evaluation of osteochondrosis lesions in the canine shoulder: comparison with radiography, arthrography and arthroscopy. *Veterinary Radiology and Ultrasound*

# 8

# The elbow joint

## Robert M. Kirberger

## Indications

The following are some of the indications for radiography of the elbow joint:

- Pain on manipulation of the joint
- Joint instability
- Swelling or deformity of the joint
- Atrophy of the adjacent muscles
- Evaluation of inherited conditions
- Elbow dysplasia grading
- Abnormal long bone growth.

## Radiography and normal anatomy

The elbow is a composite joint consisting of three bones, resulting in a structurally complex joint with superimposition of several clinically significant structures. Several views may be needed to identify the various components. Radiographs are usually taken in lateral or sternal recumbency. They may also be made in dorsal recumbency or with horizontal beam radiography but these are not described here.

### Standard views

#### Mediolateral extended

For a mediolateral extended (ML extended) view the patient is positioned in lateral recumbency lying on the affected limb. The upper limb is retracted caudally and the head and neck are slightly extended. The angle between the humerus and radius and ulna is 120 degrees. The beam is centred on the medial epicondyle (Figures 8.1–8.4). This view optimizes the following:

- Evaluation of elbow incongruity
- Osteophytes on the cranial aspect of the joint and lateral epicondylar crest
- Medial coronoid process is superimposed on the radial head.

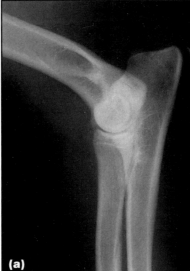

**8.2**
**(a)** ML extended view of the elbow of a 5-year-old Dobermann.
**(b)** Diagrammatic representation of the structures seen in (a).

(a)

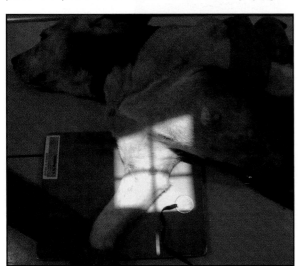

**8.1** Positioning for the ML extended view of the elbow.

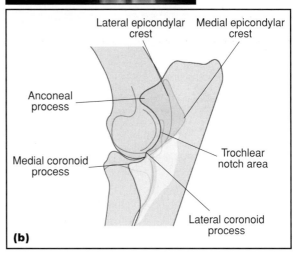

Lateral epicondylar crest
Medial epicondylar crest
Anconeal process
Medial coronoid process
Trochlear notch area
Lateral coronoid process
**(b)**

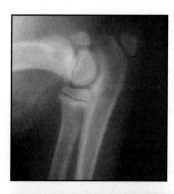

**8.3** Incompletely extended ML view of the elbow in an 8-week-old Spaniel. Note the separate ossification centres for the olecranon and medial epicondyle.

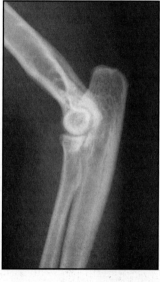

**8.4** ML extended view of the elbow in an adult cat.

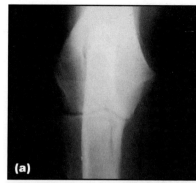

**8.6** (a) CrCd view of the elbow in a 5-year-old Dobermann. (b) Diagrammatic representation of the structures seen in (a).

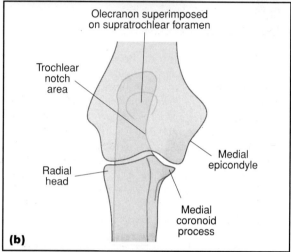

(a)

(b)

Olecranon superimposed on supratrochlear foramen

Trochlear notch area

Radial head

Medial epicondyle

Medial coronoid process

### Craniocaudal

For a craniocaudal (CrCd) view the patient is positioned in sternal recumbency ensuring the humerus, radius and ulna are in a straight line. The head is elevated and retracted away from the affected limb. A thin foam pad under the elbow may prevent rotation. The beam is centred on the joint space just distal to the prominent medial epicondyle (Figures 8.5–8.9). This view optimizes the following:

- Visibility of medial humeral condyle osteochondral defects
- Osteophytes on the medial humeral epicondyle
- Humeral condylar fractures.

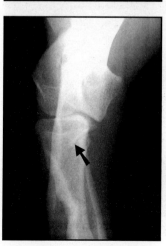

**8.7** CrCd view of the elbow of an 8-week-old Spaniel. Note incompletely fused humeral condyles.

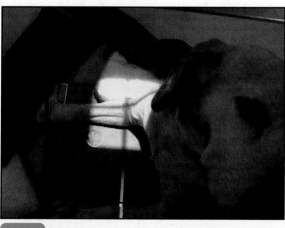

**8.5** Positioning for the CrCd view of the elbow.

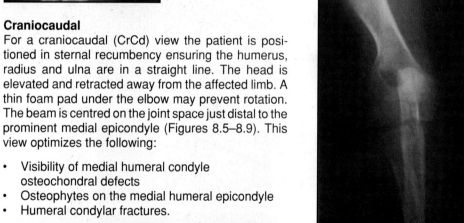

**8.8** CrCd view of the elbow in a 7-month-old Basset Hound. There is also an incomplete fracture of the proximal ulna (arrowed).

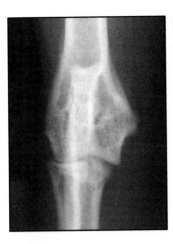

8.9   CrCd view of the elbow of an adult cat.

## Special views

### Mediolateral maximally flexed

For a mediolateral maximally flexed (ML flexed) view the patient is positioned in lateral recumbency lying on the affected limb. The upper limb is retracted. The distal antebrachium is pulled towards the neck so that the angle between the humerus and radius and ulna is <45 degrees. The carpus should not be elevated to maintain the elbow in a true lateral position. The beam is centred on the medial epicondyle (Figures 8.10–8.12). This view optimizes the following:

• Evaluation of osteophytes on the anconeal process
• Diagnosis of ununited anconeal process.

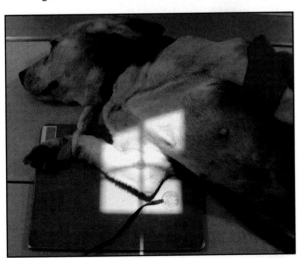

8.10   Positioning for the ML flexed view of the elbow.

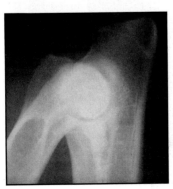

8.11   ML flexed view of the elbow in a 5-year-old Dobermann.

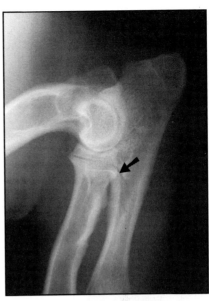

8.12   ML flexed view of the elbow in a 7-month-old Basset Hound. There is also an incomplete fracture of the proximal ulna just caudal to the radial head (arrowed).

### Extended supinated mediolateral

For an extended supinated mediolateral (Cd75°MCrLO) view the patient is positioned in lateral recumbency lying on the affected limb. The upper limb is retracted. The joint is maximally extended and the limb supinated about 15 degrees. The beam is centred on the medial epicondyle. This view optimizes the cranial border of the medial coronoid process (Figure 8.13).

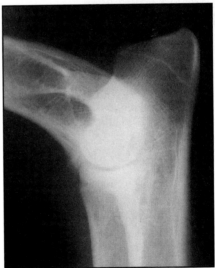

8.13   Cd75°MCrLO view of the elbow in a 5-year-old Dobermann.

### Craniolateral-caudomedial oblique

For a craniolateral-caudomedial oblique (Cr15°LCdMO) view the patient is positioned in sternal recumbency ensuring the humerus, radius and ulna are in a straight line and the limb is pronated 15 degrees (15–50 degrees is the range in the literature). The beam is centred on the joint (Figures 8.14 and 8.15). This view optimizes the following:

• Visibility of medial humeral condyle osteochondral defects
• The medial coronoid process as it is isolated from other structures, improving visibility of fragments.

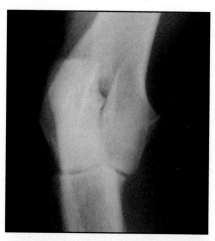

**8.14**
Cr15°LCdMO view of the elbow in a 5-year-old Dobermann.

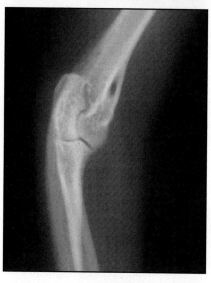

**8.15**
Cr15°LCdMO view of the elbow in a cat. Note the normal supracondylar foramen on the distomedial aspect of the humerus.

### Craniomedial-caudolateral oblique

For a craniomedial-caudolateral oblique (Cr45°MCdLO) view the patient is positioned in sternal recumbency ensuring the humerus, radius and ulna are in a straight line and the limb is supinated 45–50 degrees. The beam is centred on the joint (Figure 8.16). This view optimizes the following:

- Visibility of the lateral humeral condyle
- Incomplete ossification of the humeral condyle; best seen on 15 degree supination.

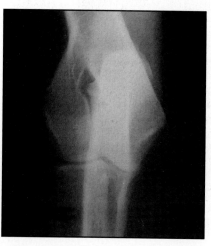

**8.16**
Cr45°MCdLO view of the elbow in a 5-year-old Dobermann.

### Distomedial-proximolateral oblique

Distomedial-proximolateral oblique (Di35°MPrLO) view is also known as the medlap view. The patient is positioned in lateral recumbency lying on the affected limb. The upper limb is retracted. The joint is flexed to 90 degrees, the antebrachium elevated 35 degrees and the extremity supinated 40 degrees. A foam wedge may be used for this. The beam is centred on the medial epicondyle (Figure 8.17). This view optimizes the medial coronoid process, which is now seen proximal to the humero-radial joint.

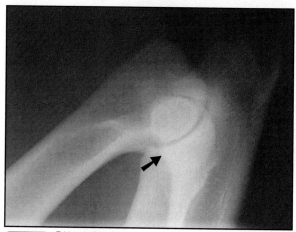

**8.17**
Di35°MPrLO view of the elbow in a Rhodesian Ridgeback. Arrow indicates the medial coronoid process.

### Physeal closure times

For information on physeal closure times see Chapter 3.

### Incidental findings

In larger breed dogs a sesamoid may be seen in the origin of the supinator muscle on CrCd or Cr45°MCdLO views. The sesamoid is located laterally or craniolaterally to the radial head and may have a distinct articulation with the radius (Figure 8.18). It should not be confused with joint mice, chip fractures or a medial coronoid process fragment which lies medially.

The supratrochlear foramen may be absent in small chondrodystrophic breeds.

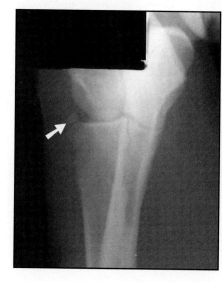

**8.18**
Cr45°MCdLO view of the elbow of an adult large-breed dog showing the supinator longus sesamoid on the craniolateral aspect of the joint (arrowed).

In cats the supinator muscle sesamoid is rarely seen, and then usually on ML views where it may be located just craniodorsal to the radial head or superimposed upon it. The latter may mimic a fractured medial coronoid process (Figure 8.19). On CrCd views of the distal feline humerus the supracondylar foramen may appear as a cortical defect depending on the angle of the view. The cat has no supratrochlear foramen.

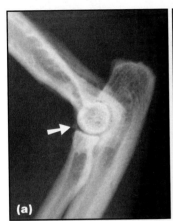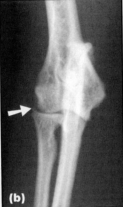

**8.19** **(a)** ML extended view of the elbow of a 9-year-old cat showing the 1 mm wide supinator longus sesamoid just cranioproximally to the radial head (arrowed). **(b)** Cr45°MCdLO view of the elbow of the same cat with the supinator longus sesamoid seen craniolaterally to the radial head (arrowed).

## Contrast studies

Positive contrast arthrography has been described in the elbow but is rarely used.

## Alternative imaging techniques

Due to the difficulty in visualizing incomplete humeral condyle ossification, joint incongruity and medial coronoid process pathology with routine radiography, multiplanar imaging techniques are ideal for these problems, particularly in those cases with no significant findings on plain film radiography.

### Computed tomography

The excellent contrast resolution, good bony detail and the ability to evaluate the elbow in sagittal or transverse planes markedly increases the diagnostic accuracy of computed tomography (CT) over plain films. Pathology, such as irregularity or cyst-like lesions of the radial notch of the ulna or humeral condyle, may be seen that is not visible on plain films.

### Magnetic resonance imaging

Magnetic resonance imaging (MRI) has the same advantages as CT and additionally can evaluate cartilage more accurately. As such it is more beneficial for determining cartilaginous defects of the medial coronoid process.

## Scintigraphy

This is rarely used in the elbow but may be used to localize pathology to the elbow joint in cases of lameness of unknown origin. Some authors have found it useful in the diagnosis of fragmented medial coronoid process but the active physes in the growing dog may hamper interpretation.

## Abnormal radiological findings

### Trauma

#### Fractures

*Condylar fractures:* Humeral condylar fractures may be associated with minimal trauma secondary to incomplete ossification of the humeral condyle, especially in spaniels (see developmental disorders).

- Lateral condylar fractures are the most common, as this condyle bears the most weight via the radial head and its weak attachment to the humeral diaphysis. The fracture line runs from the articular surface between the medial and lateral condyles into the supratrochlear foramen and then into the lateral humeral cortex. On ML views the proximal radial articular surface superimposes on the medial humeral condyle. On CrCd views the lateral condyle usually remains *in situ* on the radial head and both are displaced proximally.
- 'Y' or 'T' condylar fracture. Incomplete ossification between the medial and lateral humeral condyles may predispose to this fracture, particularly in spaniels. The fracture line runs from the articular surface between the medial and lateral condyles into the supratrochlear foramen and then into both the lateral and medial humeral cortices (Figure 8.20).
- Medial condylar fractures are rare (Figure 8.21) (see avulsion fractures below).

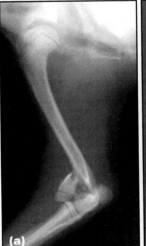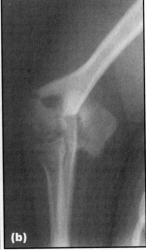

**8.20** **(a)** ML extended view of the elbow of a skeletally immature miniature Dobermann with a 'Y' condylar fracture. **(b)** CdCr view of the elbow of the same dog.

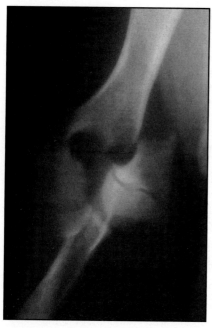

**8.21**
CrCd view of the elbow of a skeletally immature dog with a medial condylar fracture.

*Monteggia fracture:* This is a proximal ulnar fracture (articular or non-articular) accompanied by cranial luxation of the proximal radius and distal ulnar fragment (Figure 8.22).

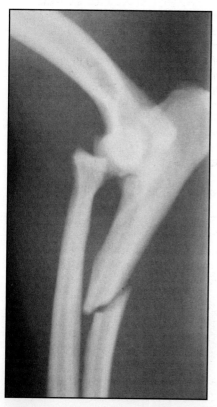

**8.22**
ML extended view of the elbow of a skeletally mature dog with a Monteggia fracture.

*Olecranon avulsion fracture:* Fractures may occur through the olecranon physis in immature animals, or occur more distally and involve the semilunar notch in skeletally mature animals. The fragment is distracted proximally by the triceps muscle. These avulsion fractures need to be differentiated from patella cubiti (see below).

*Medial epicondyle avulsion fracture:* Usually associated with a traumatic incident, resulting in varying sized fragments seen medially or mediodistally to the medial epicondyle on CrCd or Cr15°LCdMO views (Figure 8.23). This condition needs to be differentiated from the rare ununited medial humeral epicondyle (see below).

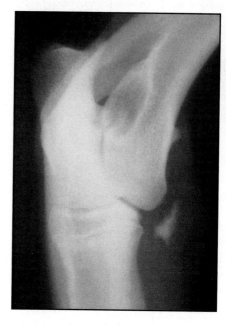

**8.23**
Cr15°LCdMO view of the elbow in a skeletally immature dog with an avulsion fracture of part of the medial epicondyle.

*Physeal fractures:* For information on physeal fractures see Chapter 5.

**Luxations and subluxations**

*Primary as a result of elbow trauma:* Primary luxations (Figure 8.24) and subluxations (Figure 8.25) are uncommon as the elbow is a complex joint with strong ligaments, and therefore fractures of the adjacent bones are more likely to occur. They may be caused by a dog being suspended by its limb from a fence. The ML views may appear relatively normal but humeral and radial/ulnar joint surfaces will overlap. On CrCd views the radius and/or ulna are usually luxated laterally. Periarticular chip fragments of various sizes or avulsion fractures are often present. In chronic cases secondary osteoarthrosis will be present.

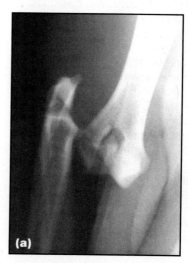

**8.24** **(a)** CdCr view of the elbow of a skeletally mature Staffordshire Bull Terrier with complete elbow luxation. Specks of avulsion fragment were seen on the original film. (continues) ▶

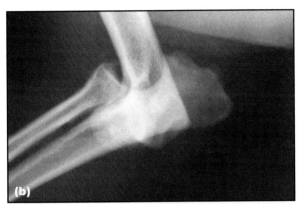

8.24 (continued) **(b)** ML extended view of the elbow of the same dog.

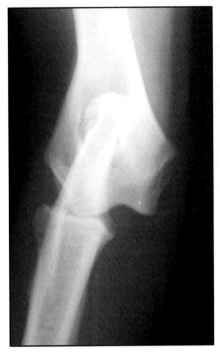

8.25 CrCd view of the elbow of a skeletally mature dog with elbow subluxation. An avulsion fragment speck was seen adjacent to the medial epicondyle on the original films.

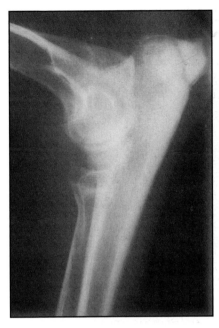

8.26 Dog with premature closure of the distal radial physis with secondary widening of the humero-radial joint space.

- Chondrodystrophic breeds display retarded ulnar growth with secondary humero-ulnar subluxation. Development of lameness or osteoarthrosis is variable.
- Retained endochondral cartilage cores in the distal ulnar physes may have a similar effect to premature closure of the distal ulnar physis. However, these cases will be bilateral.
- Fractures of the radius and ulna in the growing dog or cat may result in synostosis of the bones during the healing phase, which may result in ulnar subluxation at the elbow.

*Congenital:* See below.

## Congenital and developmental

### Congenital radial and/or ulnar luxation

*Primary:* These dogs usually present from one month of age onwards. Lesions may be uni- or bilateral and both elbows should always be radiographed, even if one appears clinically normal. In puppies changes may be difficult to interpret due to the wide joint cartilage and physes. Secondary osteoarthritic changes develop with time. Congenital elbow luxation may also occur concomitantly with ectrodactyly (cleft hand deformity) (see Chapter 3).

Three types of luxation are recognized:

- Proximal ulnar luxation is the most common form and presents with marked limb dysfunction. It is seen mainly in small breeds such as the Yorkshire Terrier and Boston Terrier as well as the Cocker Spaniel, English Bulldog and Staffordshire Bull Terrier. The ulna usually luxates laterally. The anconeal process may be underdeveloped and the ulna rotated 90 degrees resulting in a lateral projection of the ulna on a CrCd radiograph (Figure 8.27)

*Secondary to distal antebrachium pathology:* Premature closure or retarded growth of the distal ulnar or proximal or distal radial physes during the active growth phase results in secondary elbow joint subluxation. Ununited anconeal processes may also develop with ulnar growth disturbance in breeds with a separate ossification centre in the anconeal process (i.e. not part of the elbow dysplasia complex; see below). The practitioner should also look for additional radiological signs of these conditions affecting the elbow joint (see Chapter 3).

- Traumatic premature closure of the distal ulnar physis results in distal subluxation of the trochlear notch relative to the humeral condyles and radial head.
- Traumatic premature closure of the proximal or distal (more severe) radial physis results in proximal subluxation of the trochlear notch relative to the humeral condyles and radial head. The humero-radial joint space will be widened (Figure 8.26).

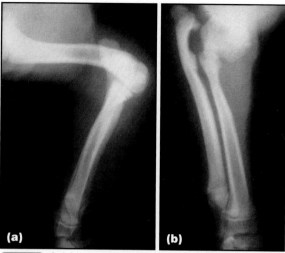

**8.27** **(a)** ML semi-extended view of the elbow of a skeletally immature dog with congenital ulnar luxation. **(b)** CrCd view of the elbow of the same dog.

- Proximal radial luxation or subluxation usually occurs in larger breeds such as Shetland Sheepdogs and Bulldogs. Clinically there may only be mild deformity or lameness. The radius usually luxates caudolaterally. The radial head is often underdeveloped and rounded (Figure 8.28)
- Both the radius and ulna can also luxate, usually laterally, and are rotated 90 degrees.

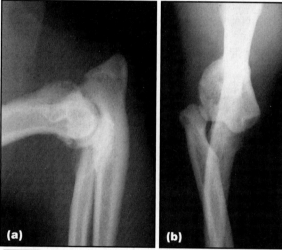

**8.28** **(a)** ML flexed view of the elbow of a 9-year-old Staffordshire Bull Terrier with congenital radial luxation. **(b)** CrCd view of the elbow of the same dog. Note the marked osteophytic reaction on the lateral supracondylar crest and rounded radial head.

**Secondary:** Elbow malformation and radial head luxation has been described secondary to congenital radio-ulnar synostosis in a cat (Rossi *et al.*, 2003).

### Elbow dysplasia

Elbow dysplasia is the abnormal development of the elbow joint. The term dysplasia is derived from the Greek words *dys* meaning abnormal and *plassein* meaning to form. Elbow dysplasia is an all-encompassing term comprehensible to the dog-breeding fraternity and has gained popular recognition, particularly in communicating scientific information to the public.

Developmental elbow abnormalities included in the term elbow dysplasia are:

- Fragmented medial coronoid process (FMCP)
- Ununited anconeal process (UAP)
- Osteochondritis dissecans (OCD) of the medial humeral condyle
- Elbow incongruity.

More than one condition may be present in the same elbow and both elbows may be affected, although pathology may differ between elbows. These conditions, singly or in combination, result in irreversible elbow osteoarthrosis with resultant pain and lameness. Osteochondrosis is the most likely underlying cause for all the conditions included in elbow dysplasia (Olsson, 1993). Underdevelopment of the trochlear notch with secondary incongruity is postulated by others to be the primary cause (Morgan *et al.*, 2000). In the elbow joint articular cartilage involvement results in OCD, whilst non-articular cartilage alterations are assumed to result in FMCP, UAP and elbow incongruity, probably as a result of small growth abnormalities of the long bones making up the elbow joint. The cartilaginous growth disturbance is likely to have genetic and environmental causes. The latter are mainly nutritional or minor trauma. The most important nutritional factors are an excessively energy-rich diet and over-supplementation with calcium. Trauma is usually minimal and associated with hyperactivity or excessive bodyweight. Figure 8.29 illustrates these interrelationships. As the condition is often bilateral both elbows should be radiographed even if only one shows clinical signs. This is particularly the case in predisposed breeds, working and breeding dogs. In affected dogs a skeletal survey should be considered to rule out hip dysplasia and other potential OCD lesions.

***Fragmented medial coronoid process:*** Fragmentation of the medial coronoid process is the most common clinical entity causing elbow osteoarthrosis. The cartilaginous medial coronoid process has no separate ossification centre and ossifies from its base to the tip, with ossification complete at 20–22 weeks. In affected dogs there is increased pressure on the cartilaginous medial coronoid as a result of disparate growth between the radius and ulna or alternatively by an incongruent trochlear notch. Osteochondrosis results in the inability of the deeper chondrocytes in the thick layer of cartilage to survive, and they undergo chondromalacia with eventual fissuring of the cartilage and subsequent fragmentation. The fragments may remain cartilaginous, or may ossify at the normal time or at a later stage as a result of receiving a blood supply through its fibrous connection with the annular ligament or joint capsule. The fragments may remain in place or displace slightly and may increase in size over time. Fragments are often poorly visualized radiologically, especially on lateral views, for the following reasons:

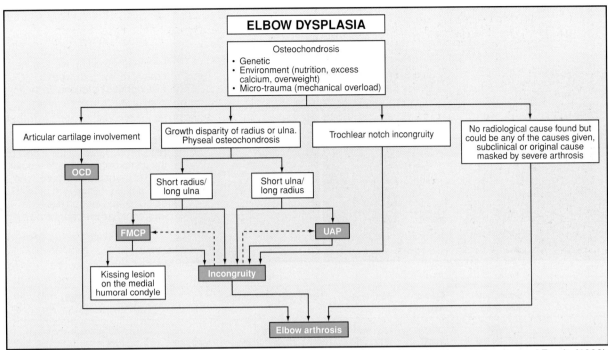

**8.29** Interrelationship between elbow dysplasia and elbow osteoarthrosis. (Adapted from Kirberger and Fourie (1998) with permission from the *Journal of the South African Veterinary Association*.)

- The fragment remains cartilaginous
- Minimal or no fragment displacement
- The fragment is fissured and not separated
- The separation line is often in a sagittal plane, which is perpendicular to the primary beam in ML views and is thus not seen
- The fragment is most often located laterally on the coronoid process and is thus hidden between the body of the coronoid process and the radial head.

The diagnosis is confirmed by seeing the fragment (Figures 8.30 and 8.31) but this is often impossible. The radiological diagnosis is then made based on the presence of secondary arthritic changes, or if the medial coronoid process cannot be defined clearly or has a convex, flattened or irregular outline (Figures 8.32 and 8.33). Clinical presentation, age and breed predisposition also need to be taken into consideration when radiological changes are equivocal (Figure 8.34).

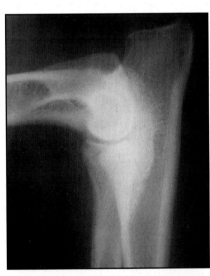

**8.31** ML semi-extended view of the elbow of a 1-year-old Rottweiler with a rounded medial coronoid process.

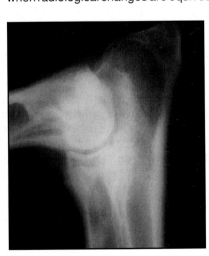

**8.30** ML semi-extended view of the elbow of an 8-month-old German Shepherd Dog with a triangular medial coronoid fragment.

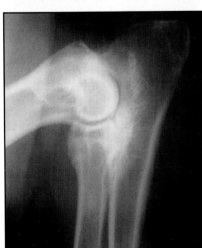

**8.32** ML flexed view of the elbow of a skeletally mature dog with an absent or flattened medial coronoid process. Note early osteophyte formation on the anconeal process.

111

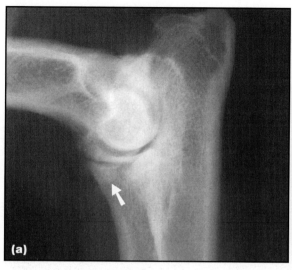
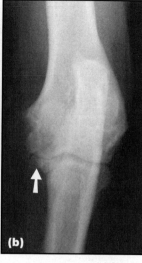

**8.33** **(a)** ML extended view of the elbow of a 4-year-old Rottweiler with a large separate medial coronoid fragment superimposed on the cranial radius (arrowed). Osteophytic reactions on the cranial margins of the joint and on the anconeal process, and sclerosis of the trochlear notch area are present. **(b)** Cr15°LCdMO of the elbow of the same dog with the triangular medial coronoid fragment seen with adjacent ulnar and medial epicondylar osteophytes. The fragment has probably grown over time.

| Condition | Breeds most susceptible | Age first seen from | Best views | Primary radiological changes | Interpretation pitfalls |
|---|---|---|---|---|---|
| Fragmented medial coronoid process | Rottweiler, Labrador and Golden Retrievers, Bernese Mountain Dog, Newfoundland, German Shepherd Dog | 7 months or older | Cd75°MCrLO Cr15°LCdMO Di35°MPrLO ML extended | Separate fragment(s) Blunted, irregular, osteopenic or absent medial coronoid process Distal trochlear notch sclerosis Joint incongruity may be present (see below) Often only diagnosed based on secondary arthritic changes | Laterally located sesamoid in the supinator muscle Medial coronoid osteophytes mimicking a fragment especially on the Cd75°MCrLO view |
| Ununited anconeal process | German Shepherd Dog, Great Dane, Irish Wolfhound, St. Bernard, Chow Chow, Basset Hound, Bullmastiff, Boerboel | 5 months | ML flexed | Irregular vertical radiolucent line through caudal anconeal process Joint incongruity may be present (see below) | Open physis of anconeal process <22 weeks of age On ML extended views the separate physis of the medial epicondyle mimics the pathology (closed by 5 months) |
| Osteochondritis dissecans | Labrador and Golden Retrievers, Rottweiler | 4–5 months | CrCd Cr15°LCdMO ML extended ML flexed | Radiolucent area on medial humeral condyle with possible sclerotic rim Subchondral saucer defect Mineralized flap (rare) Flattening of the cranioventral aspect of the medial condyle | May have minimal secondary osteoarthrosis |
| Joint incongruity | Bernese and Swiss Mountain Dogs | 4 months or older | ML extended | Step formation between lateral coronoid process and adjacent radial head Medial coronoid process located more proximally Asymmetrical widening of humeroulnar joint Widened humeroradial joint Indistinct outline of trochlear notch Cranial displacement of the humerus towards the cranial radial head margin | Poorly positioned and centred views |

**8.34**   Breed incidence, best radiographic views and primary radiological signs of elbow dysplasia.

***Ununited anconeal process:*** Ununited anconeal processes typically occur in larger breeds, which often have a separate anconeal process ossification centre. This ossification centre appears at 11–14 weeks and is united with the olecranon at 20–22 weeks (e.g. Greyhounds 14–15 weeks, German Shepherd Dogs 16–20 weeks). If ossification fails it is seen as an UAP, which may be completely separated or joined to the ulna by fibrous or fibrocartilaginous tissue (Figure 8.35). Overgrowth of the radius with a relatively shorter ulna is postulated to be the cause (Olsson, 1993). The radius forces the humeral trochlea in a proximal direction and the floor of the olecranon fossa exerts more pressure than normal on the anconeal process, damaging the anconeal process ossification centre. If osteochondrosis is present, the entire structure is less resistant to trauma and a tear in the weakened cartilage prevents osseous bridging of the gap. Morgan *et al.* (2000), on the other hand, proposed a hypothesis of a primary incongruent joint, with an abnormally developed slightly elliptical trochlear notch, which, if present before anconeal process ossification is complete, results in similar pressures on the anconeal process.

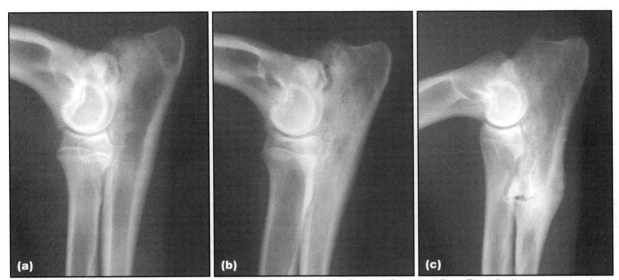

**8.35** **(a)** ML extended view of the right elbow of a 6-month-old German Shepherd Dog. The left elbow was normal. Note the irregularly wide vertical radiolucent line in the anconeal process. The humero-anconeal joint space is slightly widened, indicating minor displacement of the anconeal process. **(b)** Same dog at 7.5 months of age. **(c)** Same dog 9 months after ulna osteotomy with fusion of the ununited anconeal process.

An ununited anconeal process is occasionally seen together with FMCP (Figure 8.36), which is important to diagnose as the surgical approaches to treatment are different.

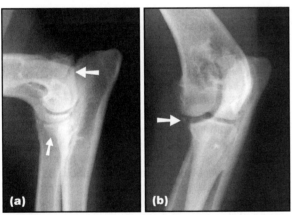

**8.36** **(a)** ML semi-extended view of the elbow of a 2-year-old Boerboel with an united anconeal process (large arrow), a fragmented medial coronoid process (small arrow) and extensive osteoarthrosis. **(b)** Cr15°LCdMO of the elbow of the same dog to illustrate the separate medial coronoid fragment (arrowed) accompanied by osteophytic reactions on the remaining medial coronoid process.

**Osteochondritis dissecans:** The OCD lesion involves the medial humeral condyle (Figures 8.37 to 8.39). The pathophysiology is very similar to that described for FMCP. Osteochondritis dissecans without concomitant FMCP is very rare. The cartilage flap rarely mineralizes *in situ*. The cartilage flap may separate and form a joint mouse, which may be located within the radial fossa (hidden radiologically) or lie medial to the joint where it may become attached to the joint capsule and ossify. Osteochondritis dissecans should not be confused with kissing lesions on the medial humeral condyle (see below). The radiological changes are described in Figure 8.34.

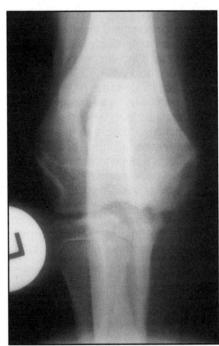

**8.37** CrCd view of the elbow of a 7-month-old dog with an OCD semicircular defect in the medial humeral condyle.

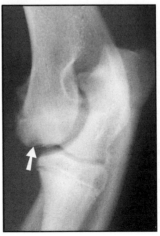

**8.38** Cr15°LCdMO view of the elbow of an 8-month-old Boerboel with an OCD lesion on the medial humeral condyle. Note the break in the continuity of the subchondral bone, faint mineralized cartilage flap (arrowed) and triangular radiolucency extending proximally. There was also a fragmented medial coronoid process not visible on this view.

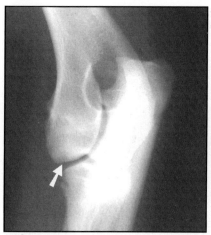

**8.39**
Cr15°LCdMO view of the elbow of a 7-month-old Rottweiler with a similar but less severe OCD lesion as in Figure 8.38. Only the triangular radiolucency (arrowed) with some adjacent sclerosis is seen.

*Joint incongruity:* The incongruity may involve the humero-ulnar, humero-radial and radio-ulnar joints separately or together (see Figures 8.29 and 8.40). According to Morgan *et al.* (2000) the incongruity is due to the trochlear notch developing in a slightly elliptic shape with the articular curvature of the trochlear notch being too small to fully encompass the humeral trochlea. If the incongruity occurs after 6 months it may be present on its own, with only elbow osteoarthrosis resulting. If present before 6 months, incongruity may also predispose the dog to FMCP, OCD and UAP owing to increased mechanical forces on these structures, and incongruity may thus be seen together with these conditions. Intermediate and heavy-set breeds have a longer proximal ulna relative to the adjacent radius than in other breeds. Morgan *et al.* (2000) postulate that this reflects a need to accommodate a trochlear notch of sufficient size to encompass a heavier and larger humeral trochlea. Insufficient development of the trochlear notch with resultant incongruity is thus most likely in these larger dogs. Incongruity may not always be evident at the time of the radiographic examination due to compensatory adjustments during

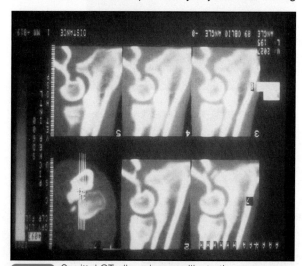

**8.40**  Sagittal CT elbow images illustrating severe humero-ulnar incongruity and step formation between the lateral coronoid process and the adjacent radial head. (Reproduced from Kirberger and Fourie (1998) with permission from the *Journal of the South African Veterinary Association.*)

growth. According to Olsson (1993) the incongruity is caused by asynchronous growth as discussed under FMCP. The incongruity may decrease in more mature animals due to compensatory growth adjustments.

*Kissing lesions:* Kissing lesions on the opposing humeral condylar surface often accompany a fragmented medial coronoid process but are not visible radiologically and are abrasions of the condylar cartilage caused by the more proximally located ossified medial coronoid fragment. The kissing lesion is usually located more laterally than OCD lesions and it is believed that they develop later than OCD lesions.

*Heritability:* The frequency of osteoarthrosis caused by elbow dysplasia in the dog population varies from 30% to 50%, with males generally more frequently and severely affected. Elbow dysplasia is inherited as a multifactorial polygenic threshold trait and the sire and dam affect the prevalence of the pathology. Thus, it requires more than one gene to express the phenotype in an individual and the product of the genes must build up to a certain threshold before it affects the development of the trait. Osteochondritis dissecans and FMCP appear to be inherited independently from each other as polygenic traits. Elbow joints should be radiographed in susceptible breeds at the same time as hip dysplasia examinations to save costs. The two conditions may also occur at the same time. Breeding animals, particularly of susceptible breeds, should be selected by their phenotypic status and by information on the elbow status of parents, grandparents, litter mates and offspring already born.

*Control programmes:* Screening programmes to grade elbow osteoarthrosis have been established in various countries to determine the degree of elbow involvement and to limit breeding with severely affected dogs. Elbow screening is also important in the large percentage of dogs that have elbow dysplasia but show no clinical signs. Elbow grading does not, however, predict the type of lesion present and thus does not correlate with the degree of lameness that may be evident.

The International Elbow Working Group (IEWG) was established in 1989 to lower the incidence and promote a greater worldwide understanding of elbow dysplasia. The group consists of veterinary surgeons, veterinary radiologists, geneticists and dog breeders, and meets annually in different parts of the world to discuss current knowledge and promote elbow screening schemes. More information on the IEWG can be obtained from their website http://www.iewg-vet.org. The IEWG has established guidelines for elbow screening and these have been adopted by the Fédération Internationale Cynologique and World Small Animal Veterinary Association as the official standard. Control programmes in different countries are encouraged to utilize the IEWG criteria when initiating screening programmes. The current IEWG elbow screening protocol includes submission of at least flexed ML radiographs of both elbows from 12 months onwards for osteophyte evaluation. The films must be permanently identified and of good quality. Additional views may be required in certain countries.

The flexed ML view has been proven to be a sensitive predictor of elbow osteoarthrosis, resulting from elbow dysplasia even though the inciting cause is not always evident. Grading is as follows:

| Location | Best view in descending order | Graphic representation |
|---|---|---|
| Dorsally on anconeal process | ML flexed<br>ML extended | |
| Cranial aspect of joint | ML extended | |
| Lateral epicondylar crest | ML flexed<br>ML extended | |
| Medial epicondyle | Cr15°LCdMO<br>CrCd | |
| Medial coronoid process | CrCd<br>Cr15°LCdMO | |
| Along trochlear notch particularly more distally | ML extended<br>ML flexed | |

**8.41** Location of osteophytic reactions on various views.

**Grade 1** (mild osteoarthrosis) – osteophytes <2 mm anywhere in the elbow but particularly at one or more of the following sites (Figures 8.41 and 8.42a):

- On the dorsal border of the anconeal process
- On the cranioproximal edge of the radius
- On the proximal edge of the medial coronoid process
- On the proximal edge of the lateral epicondylar crest
- Sclerosis in the area caudal to the distal end of the ulnar trochlear notch and the proximal radius.

**Grade 2** (moderate osteoarthrosis) – osteophytes 2–5 mm high at one or more locations as described for Grade 1.

**Grade 3** (severe osteoarthrosis) – osteophytes > 5 mm high at one or more locations as described for Grade 1 (Figure 8.42b).

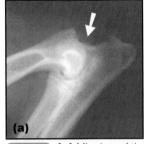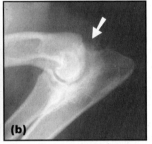

**8.42** **(a)** ML view of the elbow illustrating Grade 1 osteophyte formation on the anconeal process (arrowed). **(b)** ML view of the elbow illustrating Grade 3 osteophyte formation on the anconeal process (arrowed) and additional osteophytic reactions on the lateral supracondylar crest and cranial aspect of the joint.

Osteophytes may also be evaluated on a CrCd radiograph at the following locations:

- Distal aspect of medial humeral condyle
- Medial aspect of medial coronoid process.

In addition, if the primary pathology is evident it should be noted. Screening should be performed at a standard and narrow age interval, i.e. as close to 12 months as possible, as increasing age has a significant influence on the prevalence and severity of elbow osteoarthrosis. Dogs with clinical signs of elbow pathology, or offspring bred with a high risk of developing elbow osteoarthrosis, are radiographed at an earlier age so that affected dogs may be submitted for surgery before osteoarthrosis changes develop.

*British Veterinary Association/Kennel Club Elbow Dysplasia Scheme:* The requirements for submission of films for elbow dysplasia grading in the United Kingdom are outlined below. Dogs may be radiographed from one year onwards and radiographs may be made at the same time as hip dysplasia radiographs. The Kennel Club Registration Certificate of the dog and any related transfer or change of name documents are required. The owner signs an Owner's Declaration verifying the details of the dog and the veterinary surgeon signs the Submitting Veterinary Surgeon's Certificate verifying the microchip or tattoo number and patient details.

The BVA scheme requires a flexed and extended ML view of each elbow. The Kennel Club Registration Number, or other appropriate identification if not registered, the date of the radiographs and left and right markers must be imprinted in the film emulsion. Optimal image quality is essential. If any of the above criteria are not strictly adhered to the films will be returned to the submitting veterinary surgeon. The clinician should send the films and forms to the British Veterinary Association, 7 Mansfield Street, London W1M 0AT.

The radiographs are evaluated by two official BVA scrutineers and the radiographs and result certificates are usually posted back to the submitting veterinary surgeon within three weeks. Dogs that are registered with the Kennel Club have their results published in their relevant documents. Owners are advised only to select breeding stock with overall elbow grades of 0 or 1.

More details on the BVA Elbow Scheme as well as procedure and information notes are available on the BVA web site at http://www.bva.co.uk.

### Ununited medial humeral epicondyle
This is a rare condition of unknown aetiology occurring mainly in young Labradors and German Shepherd Dogs. It has also been associated with elbow dysplasia but is not currently recognized to be part of this syndrome. Single or multiple mineralized fragments of varying size and shape are located adjacent to the medial epicondyle on CrCd views. The condition may be accompanied by adjacent bone defects.

### Medial epicondylar spur
This is believed to be a traumatic enthesopathy of the flexor tendon origins and may result in lameness. It is seen mainly in larger dogs and rarely in the cat. It has also been associated with elbow dysplasia but is not currently recognized to be part of this syndrome. The changes are best seen on the ML flexed view. A variably sized distally projecting enthesophyte (spur) arises from the most caudodistal aspect of the medial epicondyle (Figure 8.43). A separate linear focus of mineralization may also be seen adjacent to the medial epicondyle, tending to have a somewhat curved appearance and is often superimposed on the anconeal process (Figures 8.44 and 8.45). The changes are not readily seen on CrCd views. Additional osteoarthrosis changes may be present in the joint but it is uncertain if these are directly related to the spur formation or are just part of concomitant elbow dysplasia.

### Incomplete ossification of the humeral condyle
The condition is caused by disturbed ossification of the humeral condyles, resulting in a mechanically weak midline. This is due to persistence of the thin cartilaginous plate separating the ossification centres of the capitulum and trochlea. These ossification centres should normally fuse at 2–3 months. Affected dogs may be clinically normal, be lame, particularly if there are secondary changes, or the area may be predisposed to fractures, which often occur with normal activity. Bilateral fractures may also occur. If a dog is presented with a unilateral humeral condylar fracture the opposite limb must also be radiographed. There tends to be a high failure rate

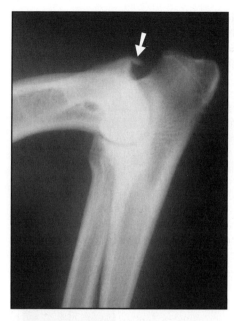

**8.43** Medial epicondylar spur (arrowed).

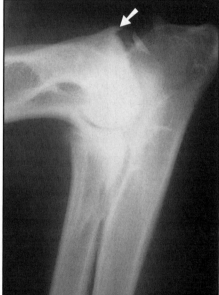

**8.44** Early medial epicondylar spur (arrowed) and mineralization of an adjacent flexor tendon in a dog.

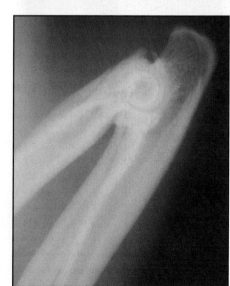

**8.45** Early medial epicondylar spur and mineralization of an adjacent flexor tendon in a cat.

with surgical repair and if incomplete ossification is diagnosed in the normal limb, a prophylactic transcondylar screw must be considered. The condition is seen most commonly in middle-aged male spaniels where a genetic basis with a recessive mode of inheritance is suspected. It is also being seen more often in other breeds, including Labrador Retrievers.

On CrCd, or preferably Cr15°MCdLO, views a vertical radiolucent line up to 1 mm diameter, extending proximally from the trochlear articular surface to the physeal scar or supratrochlear foramen is seen (Figure 8.46). A solid periosteal proliferation may be seen on the lateral epicondylar crest in cases with a complete vertical radiolucent line. The condition is more readily diagnosed with CT (Figure 8.47). A fragmented medial coronoid process and secondary osteoarthrosis may also be seen.

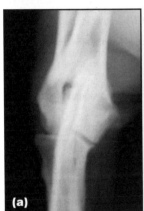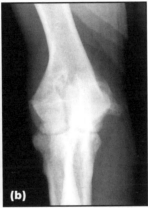

**8.46** **(a)** 8-year-old Springer Spaniel presented with a long oblique fracture of the right humerus. There is incidental incomplete ossification of the humeral condyles. **(b)** Left elbow of the same dog with a prominent radiolucent line of incomplete ossification of humeral condyles. Extensive osteoarthrosis present is not related to the incomplete ossification.

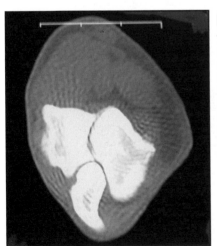

**8.47** Transverse CT image of the elbow of a 3-year-old Springer Spaniel with incomplete ossification of the humeral condyles.

### Distractio cubiti/dysostosis enchondralis
The condition results from asynchronous growth of the radius and ulna in chondrodystrophic breeds, resulting in elbow incongruity and pain starting at skeletal maturity. Distal subluxation of the trochlear notch relative to the humeral condyles and radial head is the end result. It is seen commonly in Basset Hounds (Figure 8.48).

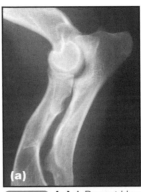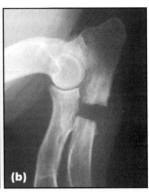

**8.48** **(a)** A Basset Hound with marked elbow incongruity. **(b)** The same dog after ulnar ostectomy.

### Patella cubiti
Patella cubiti is a very rare fusion effect through the trochlear notch with proximal distraction of the olecranon and proximal ulnar metaphysis by the triceps muscle. The avulsed fragment has the shape of a patella.

## Metabolic disorders

### Hypervitaminosis A
Seen in older cats that often present with forelimb gait abnormalities and abnormal neck movement due to cervical ankylosis. The lameness is due to proliferative new bone formation at tendon and ligament insertion or origins, typically at the triceps insertion on the olecranon (Figure 8.49; see Chapter 16 for cervical changes).

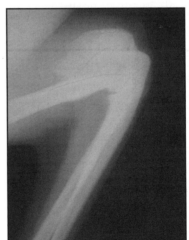

**8.49** ML view of the elbow of a cat with proliferative new bone formation at the triceps tendon insertion due to hypervitaminosis A.

## Osteoarthrosis
The osteophytic changes typically seen in osteoarthrosis have been described (see Figure 8.41). In larger breeds with elbow osteoarthrosis, particularly if bilateral, elbow dysplasia will be the most likely aetiology. Where the primary cause cannot be determined it will be impossible to distinguish elbow osteoarthrosis caused by elbow dysplasia from traumatic or chronic inflammatory changes, especially in unilateral osteoarthrosis. Often middle-aged or older dogs present with acute lameness. On radiographs these dogs may show extensive osteoarthrosis of undetermined origin, which in predisposed breeds is likely to have been elbow dysplasia, and the owners may not have been aware of the

joint changes occurring in their dog. Minor traumatic injuries to such compromised joints may set up acute inflammatory reactions, resulting in the sudden lameness. It is advisable in these cases to aspirate synovial fluid from the joint to rule out concomitant early infectious arthritis.

## Infection

For information on infection see Chapter 6.

## Neoplasia

For information on neoplasia see Chapter 6.

## Miscellaneous

### Synovial cysts

These cysts have been described in older cats and cause mild lameness. Radiologically there is periarticular soft tissue swelling, more extensive medially. If a water-soluble iodine-based contrast medium is injected into the cyst it communicates with the joint. Mild signs of osteoarthrosis may be present. (For further information see Chapter 6.)

## References and further reading

Carpenter LG, Schwarz PD, Lowry JE, Park RD and Steyn PF (1993) Comparison of radiologic imaging techniques for diagnosis of fragmented medial coronoid process of the cubital joint in dogs. *Journal of the American Veterinary Medical Association* **203**, 78–83

Culvenor JA and Howelett CR (1982) Avulsion of the medial epicondyle of the humerus in the dog. *Journal of Small Animal Practice* **23**, 83–89

Dennis R, Kirberger RM, Wrigley RH and Barr FJ (2001) Appendicular skeleton. In: *Handbook of Small Animal Radiological Differential Diagnosis*. pp.42–45. WB Saunders, London

Haudiquet PR, Marcellin-Little DJ and Stebbins ME (2002) Use of the distomedial-proximolateral oblique radiographic view of the elbow joint for examination of the medial coronoid process in dogs. *American Journal of Veterinary Research* **63**, 1000–1005

Hornof WJ, Wind AP, Wallack ST and Schulz KS (2000) Canine elbow dysplasia. The early radiographic detection of fragmentation of the coronoid process. *Veterinary Clinics of North America: Small Animal Practice* **30**, 257–266

Kirberger RM and Fourie SL (1998) Elbow dysplasia in the dog: pathophysiology, diagnosis and control. *Journal of the South African Veterinary Association* **69**, 43–54

Marcellin-Little DJ, DeYoung DJ, Ferris KK and Berry CM (1994) Incomplete ossification of the humeral condyle in Spaniels. *Veterinary Surgery* **23**, 475–487

May C and Bennett D (1988) Medial epicondylar spur associated with lameness in dogs. *Journal of Small Animal Practice* **29**, 797–803

Milton JL and Montgomery RD (1987) Congenital elbow luxations. *Veterinary Clinics of North America: Small Animal Practice* **17**, 873–888

Morgan JP, Wind A and Davidson AP (2000) Elbow dysplasia. In: *Hereditary Bone and Joint Diseases in the Dog*. pp 41–91. Schlütersche, Hannover

Olsson SE (1993) Pathophysiology, morphology, and clinical signs of osteochondrosis in the dog. In: *Disease Mechanisms in Small Animal Surgery*. 2nd edn, ed. MS Bojrab *et al.*, pp.777–796. Lea & Febiger, Philadelphia

Ravesti GL, Biasibetti M, Schumacher A and Fabiani M (2002) The use of computed tomography in the diagnostic protocol of the elbow in the dog: 24 joints. *Veterinary Comparative Orthopaedics and Traumatology* **15**, 35–43

Reichle JK, Park RD and Bahr AM (2000) Computed tomographic findings in dogs with cubital lameness. *Veterinary Radiology and Ultrasound* **41**, 125–130

Rossi F, Vignoli M, Terragni R, Pozzi L, Impallomeni C and Magnani M (2003) Bilateral elbow malformation in a cat caused by radioulnar synostosis. *Veterinary Radiology and Ultrasound* **44**, 283–286

Snaps FR, Balligrand MH, Saunders JH, Park RD and Dondelinger RF (1997) Comparison of radiography, magnetic resonance imaging, and surgical findings in dogs with elbow dysplasia. *American Journal of Veterinary Research* **58**, 1367–1370

Wosar MA, Lewis DD, Neuwirth L, Parker RB, Spencer CP, Kubilis PS, Stubbs WP, Murphy ST, Shiroma JT, Stallings JT and Bertrand SG (1999) *Journal of the American Veterinary Medical Association* **214**, 52–58

# The hip joint and pelvis

## Darryl N. Biery

## Indications

The following are some of the indications for radiography of the pelvis and hip joints:

- Pelvic limb lameness
- Trauma with suspected fracture of pelvis
- Pain or instability on manipulation of the hip joint or pelvis
- Hip dysplasia control programmes for breeding status.

## Radiography and normal anatomy

The pelvis is composed of the ilium, ischium, pubis and acetabular bones (Figures 9.1 to 9.4). These bones fuse at approximately 12–16 weeks of age to form each of the two hemipelves. The acetabulum, a cotyloid or cup-shaped lunate cavity, is formed by the fusion of four bones (ilium, ischium, acetabulum and pubis) for the pelvic component of each hip joint. The femoral head fits into the acetabulum and together they form the hip joint. The closure of the centre of ossification on the dorsal aspect of the ilial wings is highly variable in the dog and may remain completely unossified throughout life. On a lateral or lateral oblique view it is important not to mistake this variation of normal for a fracture (Figure 9.5). Similarly, the normal unossified caudal ischial ossification centres and triangular centre at the pelvic symphysis should also not be mistaken as a fracture or other lesion in a skeletally immature dog.

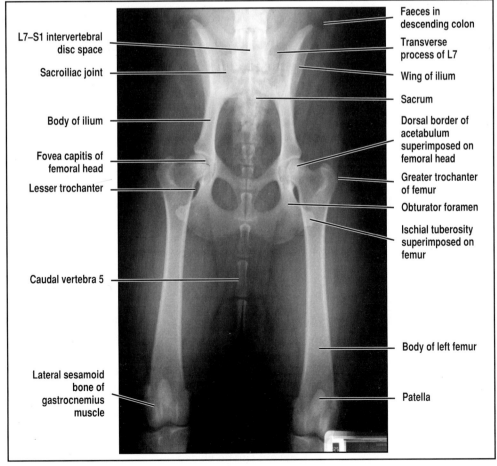

**9.1** VD extended hip view of a normal skeletally mature dog.

L7–S1 intervertebral disc space

Sacroiliac joint

Body of ilium

Fovea capitis of femoral head

Lesser trochanter

Caudal vertebra 5

Lateral sesamoid bone of gastrocnemius muscle

Faeces in descending colon

Transverse process of L7

Wing of ilium

Sacrum

Dorsal border of acetabulum superimposed on femoral head

Greater trochanter of femur

Obturator foramen

Ischial tuberosity superimposed on femur

Body of left femur

Patella

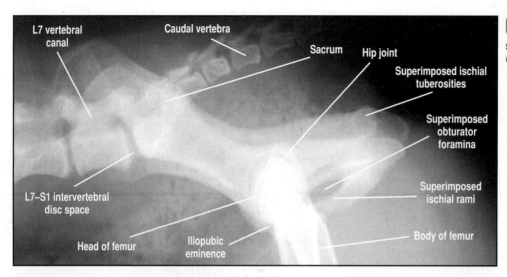

L7 vertebral canal

Caudal vertebra

Sacrum

Hip joint

Superimposed ischial tuberosities

Superimposed obturator foramina

Superimposed ischial rami

L7–S1 intervertebral disc space

Head of femur

Iliopubic eminence

Body of femur

**9.2** Lateral view of a normal skeletally mature dog's pelvis.

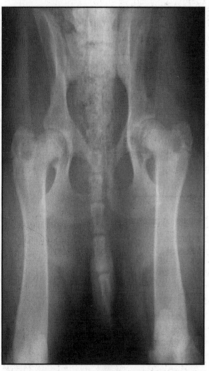

**9.3** VD extended hip view of a normal skeletally immature dog.

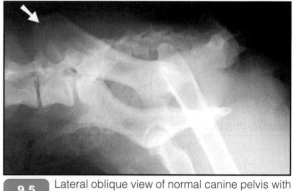

**9.5** Lateral oblique view of normal canine pelvis with incomplete ossification of the ilial wing (arrowed).

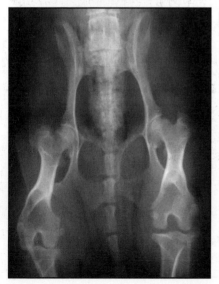

**9.4** VD extended hip view of pelvis and hips of a normal Dachshund.

## Standard views

### Pelvis

Diseases of the pelvis are most commonly diagnosed on a lateral recumbent (right-left or left-right) radiographic view and an orthogonal ventrodorsal view. Occasionally, a lateral oblique view of the pelvis is necessary to visualize some lesions that might be obscured by superimposition of the opposite hemipelvis and hip.

*Ventrodorsal view:* For a ventrodorsal (VD pelvis) view (Figure 9.6) the patient is positioned in dorsal recumbency with the pelvis and pelvic limbs positioned symmetrically and the X-ray beam centred over the hips. It is not essential to fully extend the pelvic limbs as it is for a hip dysplasia study. If the patient experiences pain when placed in the VD position, a dorsoventral (DV) view of the pelvis can be taken.

*Lateral view:* For a lateral view (Figure 9.7) the patient is positioned in either right or left lateral recumbency with the X-ray beam centred on the hip joints. The affected side is usually placed down next to the table top to minimize distortion and maximize sharpness, but if painful, the affected side of the patient can be placed up.

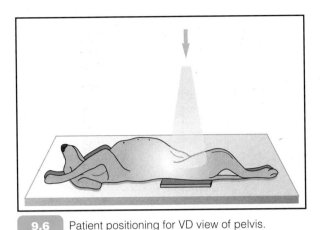

9.6   Patient positioning for VD view of pelvis.

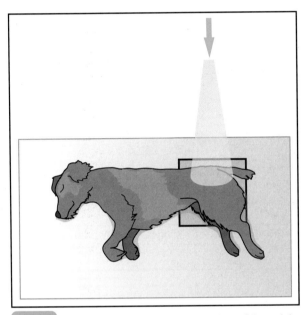

9.7   Patient positioning for a lateral view of the pelvis.

## Hip joint

***Ventrodorsal view:*** For a VD (extended hip) view (Figure 9.8) the patient should be positioned symmetrically in dorsal recumbency with the femurs fully

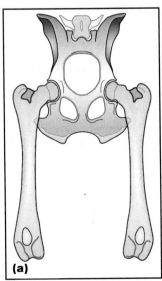

9.8   VD hip extended view. **(a)** Illustration of proper radiographic positioning of pelvis, hips and femurs. (continues) ▶

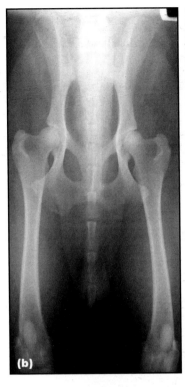

9.8   (continued) VD hip extended view. **(b)** Radiograph of normal hips with proper positioning of pelvis and femurs. Note the pelvic symmetry and position of patellas over centre of distal femurs.

extended and parallel, and the stifles rotated slightly inward so that the patellas are superimposed over the centre of the distal femurs. The X-ray beam should be centred over the middle of the hips and the radiograph should include the entire pelvis and femurs. This is the standard hip dysplasia evaluation view. However, as this view is commonly an insensitive method for detecting femoral head subluxation (laxity), accurate patient positioning and radiographic quality are extremely important (Figure 9.9). Chemical restraint, preferably general anaesthesia, is recommended to obtain proper patient positioning and for radiation safety of personnel.

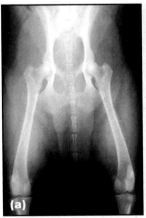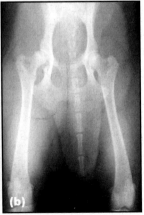

9.9   VD extended hip view of canine pelvis for hip evaluation. **(a)** No abnormality is seen but there is improper positioning with slight asymmetry of the pelvis, the femurs are not parallel to each other and the patellas are not superimposed upon the middle of the distal femurs. **(b)** Repeat radiograph of same dog. Now the right femoral head appears subluxated with better positioning of the femurs and patellas but the pelvis is still slightly tilted.

## Special views

### Pelvis and hip joint: ventrodorsal flexed view

The VD flexed (hip) view (Figure 9.10) is also known as the frog-leg view and is particularly useful for articular fractures that are equivocal on VD extended hip views. The patient is placed in dorsal recumbency with the pelvic limbs spread in a symmetrical flexed and abducted position. The X-ray beam is centred in the middle of the pelvis at the level of the hips.

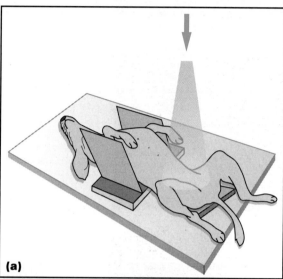

**(a)**

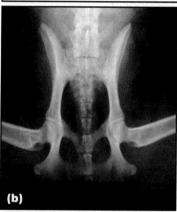

**(b)**

**9.10** VD flexed frog-leg view of pelvis and hips. **(a)** Patient positioning. **(b)** Radiograph of normal pelvis and hips.

### Pelvis: inlet and outlet views

The inlet view is also known as the ventrocranial-dorsocaudal (V20°Cr-DCd) view and the outlet view is also termed the ventrocaudal-dorsocranial (V20°Cd-DCr) view. The patient is placed in dorsal recumbency with the pelvis and rear legs positioned symmetrically and the X-ray tube tilted 20 degrees cranially or caudally (Figure 9.11). These views have been proposed as being helpful when the standard lateral and ventrodorsal views are inconclusive.

### Hip joint: lateral view

The lateral view (Figure 9.12) is particularly useful for hip and pelvic lesions poorly visible on the standard views. The patient is positioned in lateral recumbency on the affected side and the unaffected leg is abducted to be out of the radiographic field.

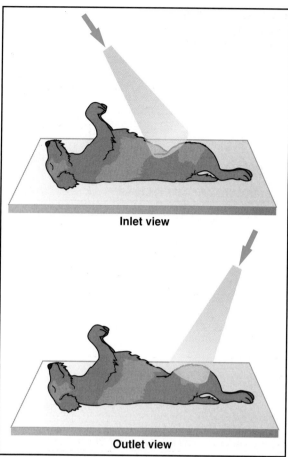

**Inlet view**

**Outlet view**

**9.11** Patient positioning for the inlet (V20°Cr-DCd ) and outlet (V20°Cd-DCr) views of the pelvis.

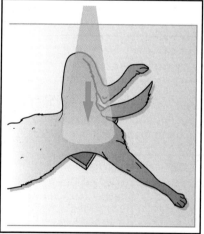

**9.12** Patient positioning for a lateral view of the hip.

### Hip dysplasia additional views

Additional views for hip dysplasia evaluation (e.g. compression, distraction and dorsal acetabular rim) are described later (see Hip dysplasia).

### Physeal closure times

Ossification centre closure times in the dog are as follows:

- Acetabulum 4–6 months
- Ischial tuberosities 8–10 months
- Iliac crest 1–2 years, or may remain open permanently.

## Incidental findings

One or more accessory ossification centres may be present as variants of normal and be visible radiographically. For example, an ossicle on the dorsal acetabular rim (Figure 9.13), which when present, is usually seen on the VD view in medium to large-breed dogs.

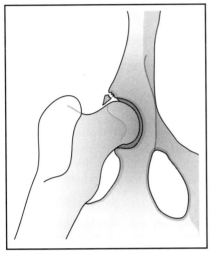

**9.13**

Illustration of ossicle on dorsal acetabular rim of canine pelvis.

## Contrast studies
Contrast studies are not commonly used.

## Alternative imaging techniques

### Computed tomography
Computed tomography (CT) is being used more frequently as a more sensitive imaging modality for the pelvis and hips, especially for soft tissue lesions adjacent to the pelvis and hips, surgical planning of fracture repair and staging of neoplastic disease.

### Diagnostic ultrasonography
Ultrasonography has not been found to be helpful in assessment of the bony structures of the pelvis and the hips. Dynamic ultrasonographic images can be made during movement of the hip, but determination of laxity varies with age and has not been as reliable as other methods.

### Magnetic resonance imaging
Magnetic resonance imaging (MRI) is not in common use.

## Abnormal radiological findings

### Trauma

#### Fractures
Fractures of the pelvis due to blunt trauma are common in dogs and cats. On radiographic examination, many of the fractures have minimal displacement whilst others are more serious with concurrent sacroiliac joint or soft tissue injuries of the urinary bladder, urethra and abdominal wall. Sometimes more than the standard VD and lateral radiographic views (such as a lateral oblique view) are needed to adequately visualize intra-articular

acetabular fractures, reduction in the pelvic canal size, grossly displaced fragments and 'free floating' fragments of the ilium, ischium and pubic bones. Most fractures usually involve more than one bone of the pelvis (Figure 9.14). If only one bone is fractured, a concurrent sacroiliac luxation or subluxation is usually present. The majority of complications relate to malunion and soft tissue injuries in the region of the pelvic fractures (Figure 9.15) or to other body regions. With severe trauma, concurrent pneumothorax or pulmonary contusion is not uncommon. Many pelvic fractures heal with a fibrous union, rather than a bony callus as is common with other bones.

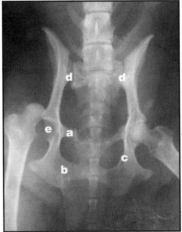

**9.14**

Multiple pelvic fractures.
a = Cranial ramus of the right pubic bone;
b = Right ischium;
c = Left ischium;
d = Bilateral sacroiliac subluxations;
e = Right coxofemoral luxation.

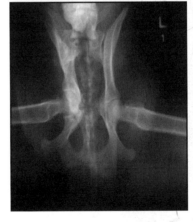

**9.15**

Old right sacroiliac subluxation and pelvic fractures, resulting in malunion of the right hemipelvis with narrowing of the pelvic canal and chronic constipation.

All fractures involving the acetabulum represent intra-articular fractures and are usually categorized according to two-part or three-part fractures that involve the cranial, dorsal, caudal or central portion of the acetabulum. The more severe acetabular fractures involve the dorsal weight bearing surface for the femoral head and central fractures that impinge upon the pelvic canal structures (Figure 9.16).

All physeal fractures of the femoral head are intra-articular and most occur in immature dogs and cats. In mature animals, similar trauma usually results in hip luxation rather than a fracture. If not adequately reduced with internal fixation, many physeal fractures will progress to a fibrous non-union and resorption of the femoral neck. For information on apple core resorption of juvenile femoral neck fractures refer to Chapter 5.

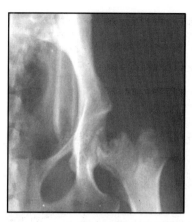

**9.16**

Old compression fracture of the left acetabulum and comminuted fracture of the femoral head.

### Coxofemoral luxation and subluxation

Luxation of the femoral head due to blunt trauma is common and can be diagnosed on VD and lateral views (Figure 9.17). In addition to trauma, animals with hip dysplasia are also predisposed to luxation. Small avulsion fragments of the head attached to the round ligament may be seen within the acetabulum. The femoral head is most commonly displaced craniodorsally, but can also be luxated dorsally, caudoventrally or medially when there is a central acetabular fracture. In chronic luxations, a pseudoarthrosis or periosteal reaction may develop on the adjacent shaft of the ilium.

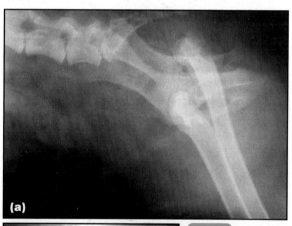

(a)

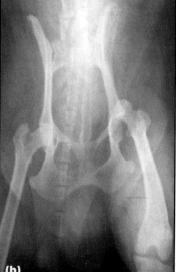

(b)

**9.17**

Dorsocranial luxation of the left femoral head. **(a)** Lateral oblique view. **(b)** VD extended view.

### Sacroiliac luxation and subluxation

Sacroiliac luxation or subluxation is a common injury, secondary to trauma in dogs and cats, and is often associated with pelvic fractures. If there are bilateral or ipsilateral pelvic fractures, cranial displacement of the pelvis is seen on lateral and VD views. The normal sacroiliac joint is radiolucent, especially when seen in profile on a slightly oblique VD view (see Figure 9.14). When abnormal, there is a step between the medial rim of the ilium and the sacral margin on the VD view.

## Congenital and developmental conditions

### Transitional vertebra

Transitional vertebrae are congenital and inherited anomalies that may occur anywhere in the spine, but are common at the lumbosacral region. The two most common forms are referred to as lumbarization of the first sacral segment and sacralization of the last lumbar vertebra. Transitional vertebrae can be bilaterally symmetrical or unilateral with pelvic asymmetry, and cause errors in interpretation of hip congruity due to pelvic tilting. In lumbarization the first sacral vertebra is separated and on the VD view there is an isolated spinous process of the anomalous vertebra with either a unilateral or bilateral wing-like transverse process. On the lateral view, there is a radiolucent disc space between S1 and S2. In lumbar sacralization, the transverse process of the last lumbar vertebra either fuses with the sacrum or articulates with the ilium on one or both sides (Figure 9.18).

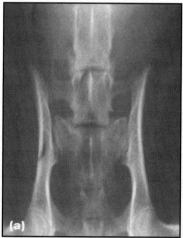

(a)

**9.18**

Transitional vertebra. **(a)** Cat with sacralization of L7. The right transverse process of L7 articulates with right ilium. **(b)** Dog with lumbarization of S1. The asymmetrical sacrum has a transverse process on the right that articulates with the ilium.

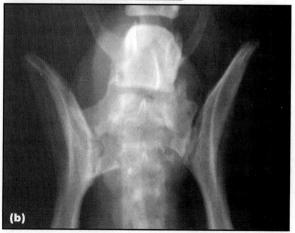

(b)

## Calcifying tendinopathy

A calcifying tendinopathy, such as bursitis calcarea, is a benign mineralization of a tendon(s) that is characterized by one or more smooth rounded mineralized bodies of varying size. They may be unilateral or bilateral and rarely cause any associated clinical signs. Common sites include:

- Tendon of the iliopsoas muscle (Figure 9.19)
- Tendon of the psoas minor adjacent to the iliopectineal eminence (Figure 9.19)
- Tendon of the gluteal muscle, usually the middle gluteal, near the major trochanter of the femur (Figure 9.20).

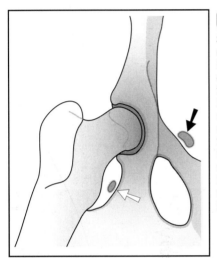

**9.19** Sketch of mineralized bodies (bursitis calcarea) in the tendon of the iliopsoas muscle (black arrow) and in the tendon of the psoas minor adjacent to the iliopectineal eminence (white arrow).

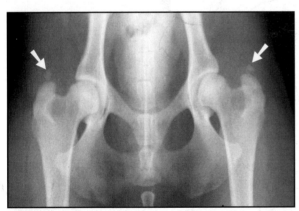

**9.20** Bilateral mineralization of the gluteal tendons (bursitis calcarea).

## Avascular femoral head necrosis

Spontaneous necrosis of the femoral head (Legg–Calvé–Perthes disease) is an inherited autosomal recessive trait that is most often seen in immature toy and small-breed dogs. Affected dogs are usually aged between 4 and 10 months and are often lame. Disuse muscle atrophy is present when chronic. The lesion is self-limiting and in cases when surgical resection of the femoral head and neck is not done, the osteonecrosis resolves with remodelling of the femoral head with secondary osteoarthrosis of the hip.

The earliest radiological findings may be subtle, with a slight radiolucency of the femoral head and a widened joint space. VD views, including a VD frog-leg view, are most helpful in identifying the earliest changes. As the necrosis progresses there is lysis and collapse of the femoral head. Later, there is osteoarthrosis with remodelling of the femoral head, resulting in coxa vara. These later changes can mimic hip dysplasia, especially if bilateral (Figure 9.21).

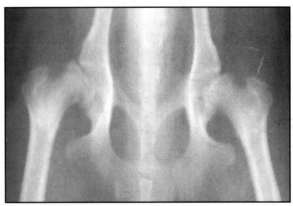

**9.21** Bilateral avascular femoral head necrosis with lysis and collapse of the heads and remodelling of the acetabula.

## Feline capital physeal dysplasia

Feline capital physeal dysplasia (metaphyseal osteopathy) is a cartilage disorder (dyschondroplasia) of the femoral capital physis with subsequent separation of the femoral head and neck, which mimics a traumatic capital physis fracture. Affected cats are usually less than two years of age, male, commonly obese and have a history of minimal or no trauma. The lesion in most cats is initially unilateral, but may occur later in the other hip. Radiologically, most are diagnosed on a VD hip view.

The lesion is characterized by separation of the femoral head and neck that otherwise appears normal (Figure 9.22). Later, there is osteolysis of the femoral neck and head, and a non-union develops with osteosclerosis and remodelling of the femoral neck and acetabulum. A similar lesion has recently been reported in dogs as 'slipped capital femoral epiphysis' (Moores *et al.*, 2004).

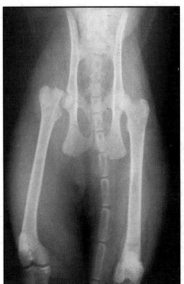

**9.22** VD view of a cat with capital physeal dysplasia with separation of the right femoral capital physis.

## Canine hip dysplasia

Hip dysplasia, an abnormal development of the hip, is reported to be the most common orthopaedic disease in the dog. It is a complex inherited disease with a polygenic and multifactorial aetiology. Estimates of heritability range from 0.2 to 0.6. Although, the true breed incidence is not known, all breeds of dogs are affected. It is well documented as being most common in the large and giant breeds with prevalence estimates ranging from 10% to 85% in many breeds. Increased bodyweight and rapid growth appear related to the development of hip dysplasia in dogs that are genetically predisposed. Although the hip is normal at birth, increased hip laxity is generally considered to be the cause of the subsequent radiological findings of femoral head subluxation/luxation or osteoarthrosis. As the osteoarthrosis advances the acetabulum may become shallow, the femoral head may change in shape, and the femoral neck may become irregular and thick due to osteophyte formation. Radiological changes commonly, but not always, progress with age. Hip dysplasia is usually bilateral, but it is not uncommon to have only unilateral disease.

The VD extended hip view is the standard view used in most countries for hip phenotype screening and for the diagnosis of hip dysplasia. Proper positioning and image quality are essential, and if not done correctly can lead to errors in radiological interpretation of normal *versus* abnormal hips (see Figure 9.9).

Asymmetry of the pelvis and hips is usually related to not keeping the head and body in a straight line. Radiographically pelvic symmetry is present when:

- The oburator foraminae are equal in size
- The ilial wings have the same diameter
- A line drawn through the caudal lumbar spinous processes continues through the pelvic symphysis.

The VD view is well documented as an insensitive method for detection of hip laxity (coxofemoral subluxation), a common radiological finding of hip dysplasia, and is age-dependent. In one study, only 16% of German Shepherd Dogs with confirmed hip dysplasia at 3.5 years of age had radiological changes visible when 6 months of age, and only 69% when 1 year of age (Jessen and Spurrell, 1972). The radiological findings of hip dysplasia (Figure 9.23) include:

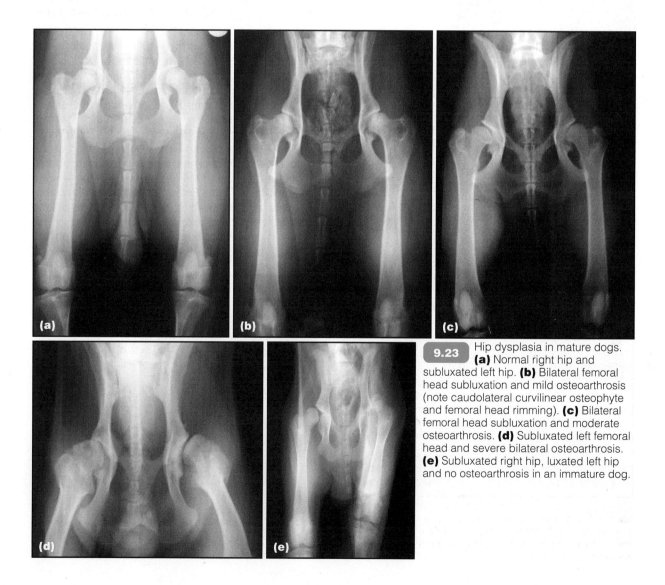

**9.23** Hip dysplasia in mature dogs. **(a)** Normal right hip and subluxated left hip. **(b)** Bilateral femoral head subluxation and mild osteoarthrosis (note caudolateral curvilinear osteophyte and femoral head rimming). **(c)** Bilateral femoral head subluxation and moderate osteoarthrosis. **(d)** Subluxated left femoral head and severe bilateral osteoarthrosis. **(e)** Subluxated right hip, luxated left hip and no osteoarthrosis in an immature dog.

**Chapter 9** The hip joint and pelvis

- Femoral head subluxation or luxation
  - Present when approximately 50% or more of the femoral head is not within the acetabulum or if the Norberg angle measurement is abnormal
- Osteoarthrosis
  - Remodelling of the femoral head and neck
  - Remodelling of the acetabulum
  - Periarticular osteophyte(s) on the margins of the femoral head and acetabulum
  - Osteophyte formation on the caudal aspect of the femoral neck, known as a caudolateral curvilinear osteophyte (CCO) or Morgan's line (Figure 9.24)
  - Osteophyte formation on the margin of the femoral head parallel to the physeal scar, which is known as femoral head rimming
  - Subchondral sclerosis of the acetabular margin.

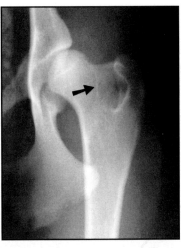

**9.24** VD view of the CCO (also referred to as Morgan's line) that is a finding of early osteoarthrosis (arrowed).

Measurement of the Norberg angle (Figure 9.25), a criterion for femoral head subluxation that is used by some evaluators, is determined by the intersection of a line extending between the centres of the femoral heads and a line extending cranially from the centre of the femoral head through the craniolateral acetabular margin. Most, but not all, normal hips in the dog have an angle of 105 degrees or more on a VD extended hip view

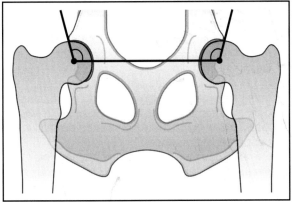

**9.25** Norberg angle measurement. On the VD extended hip view, it is the angle between a line connecting the femoral head centres and a line from the centre of the femoral head to the craniodorsal acetabular rim.

and 95 degrees or more in the cat. Values less than these indicate subluxation, with lower values indicative of the hip being more severely subluxated. The angle can be highly influenced by the position of the pelvic limbs, pelvic positioning and the amount of acetabular margin ossification which is age-dependent. The Norberg angle in dogs and cats has been shown not to correlate as well as the distraction index (DI) with regard to the subsequent development of osteoarthrosis.

***Hip control programmes:*** Independent systems for assessment of normal hips *versus* hip dysplasia have been developed in numerous countries throughout the world. Although, most use the VD extended hip view for the subjective evaluation of the hips, there are numerous differences in the scoring systems (Figure 9.26) and recommendations for breeding.

In Europe and many other countries of the world, there are various systems (e.g. British Veterinary Association (BVA)/Kennel Club (KC), Finland Kennel Club (SF), Fédération Cynologique Internationale (FCI), Swedish Kennel Club (SKK)), as well as different numbers and qualifications of the interpreters. In some countries that use the same system, there are also reported differences in the strictness of the same criteria that are used. In North America there are at least three control programmes (Ontario Veterinary College (OVC), Orthopedic Foundation for Animals (OFA) and University of Pennsylvania Hip Improvement Program (PennHIP®), in addition to the numerous veterinary radiologists and veterinary colleges that provide hip evaluations.

To illustrate some of the differences, details of the following hip control programmes can be compared:

- British Veterinary Association/Kennel Club Hip Dysplasia Programme
- Orthopedic Foundation for Animals
- PennHIP® (University of Pennsylvania Hip Improvement Program).

*British Veterinary Association/Kennel Club Hip Dysplasia Programme:*

- VD extended hip radiographs of dogs are voluntarily submitted by a veterinary surgeon for interpretation by two scrutineers who are appointed by the BVA. Each animal and radiograph must be properly identified and the radiograph must be of acceptable diagnostic quality.
- The minimum age for evaluation is 1 year with no upper age limit.
- A score for each hip, as agreed by the two scrutineers, is assigned based on a point system using nine radiological criteria. These include the Norberg angle, femoral head subluxation, shape of the acetabulum and osteoarthrosis changes. The greater the abnormality, the higher the score for each criterion.
- The minimum (best) score for each hip is 0 and the maximum (worst) is 53. The lower the score, the less the degree of evident hip dysplasia.

**127**

| FCI classification | Description | Country | | | | | | | | |
|---|---|---|---|---|---|---|---|---|---|---|
| | | **SF** Finland | **NL** The Netherlands | **D** Germany | **S** Sweden | **CH** Switzerland | **ZA** South Africa | **USA** OFA | **UK** * BVA (0–106) | |
| A1 | No signs of hip dysplasia (HD) | Ei-dysplasiaa 'hyvät' | Negatief geheel gaaf (1) | Kein Hinweis für HD | Utmärkt | Frei | 0 | Excellent (normal) | 0 | |
| A2 | No signs of HD | Ei-dysplasiaa | Negatief geheel gaaf (2) | Kein Hinweis für HD | U.A. | Frei | 0 | Good (normal) | 0–6 | |
| B1 | Transitional case | Rajatapaus | Transitional case | Übergangs-form (verdächtig für HD) | U.A. | Frei | 0 | Fair (transitional) | 6–12 | |
| B2 | Transitional case | Rajatapaus | Transitional case | Übergangs-form (verdächtig für HD) | I | I | I | Borderline (transitional) | 12–18 | |
| C1 | Mild HD | I | Licht positief (3) | Leichte HD | I | I | I | Mild | 18–24 | |
| C2 | Mild HD | I | Licht positief (3) | Leichte HD | I | I | I | Mild | 24–30 | |
| D1 | Moderate HD | II | Positief (3.5) | Mittlere HD | II | II | II | Moderate | 30–42 | |
| D2 | Moderate HD | II | Positief (4) | Mittlere HD | II | II | II | Moderate | 42–54 | |
| E1 | Severe HD | III | Positief (4) | Schwere HD | III | III | III | Severe | 54–66 | |
| E2 | Severe HD | IV | Positief optima forma (5) | Schwere HD | IV | IV | IV | Severe | >66 | |

**9.26**  Comparative international hip dysplasia grading schemes. Adapted from FCI, BVA and OFA data (the author does not accept responsibility for any inconsistencies that may be present in this figure). * = Author's placement of scores in FCI classification – guideline only. (Reproduced from Kirberger (1999) with permission from the publisher.)

- The numerical score for both hips (0–106) is then calculated and recorded for each animal. This score is then compared with others of the same breed (breed mean score) for a representation of the dog's hip status. Although not required, it is very important and highly recommended that all hip radiographs taken be submitted for scoring for a more accurate database of each breed.
- Using the individual dog's hip score and its breed mean score, veterinary surgeons can use this information to advise their clients on the dog's suitability for breeding. It is recommended that all breeders wishing to control hip dysplasia should breed only those animals with hip scores well below the breed mean score.

For further information contact the BVA at 7 Mansfield Street, London W1F 9NQ, England or www.bva.co.uk/public/chs/.

*Orthopedic Foundation for Animals:*

- VD extended hip radiographs are voluntarily submitted by the dog's owner for interpretation by three veterinary radiologists selected by the OFA who are diplomates of the American College of Veterinary Radiology. Each animal and radiograph must be properly identified and the radiograph must be of acceptable diagnostic quality.
- The minimum age for an official evaluation is two years. There is no upper age limit. Preliminary evaluations can be requested for dogs between four months and two years of age.
- Each dog's hips are scored subjectively into seven phenotypes: excellent normal; good normal; fair normal; borderline; mild dysplasia; moderate dysplasia; and severe dysplasia. The categories of mild, moderate and severe dysplasia are based on the subjective assessment of the degree of subluxation and osteoarthrosis present. The borderline category is those dogs where there is no clear consensus between normal or dysplastic features by the three radiologists. In follow-up radiographs of these cases more than six months later, about 50% of the dogs will be considered normal (usually fair normal) and 50% dysplastic.
- Dogs having a hip phenotype of excellent, good or fair are considered normal, but the dog's family phenotype is also important. For example, a dog with an excellent hip score, but with less than 75% of its brothers and sisters normal, is a poor breeding prospect.
- Owners may elect to have their animal's hip phenotype listed in an open registry in order for conscientious breeders to make educated decisions for the selection of breeding animals.

For further information contact the OFA at 2300 East Nifong Boulevard, Columbia, MO, 65201, USA or www.offa.org.

*PennHIP®:*

- PennHIP® requires three radiographic views (VD extended hip, distraction and compression views). Only certified PennHIP® veterinary surgeons and technicians may take the radiographs and must submit (not voluntary) the radiographs of all dogs examined.
- Each animal and radiograph must be properly identified and all radiographs must be of acceptable diagnostic positioning and quality.
- Hip dysplasia is diagnosed when there is osteoarthrosis present on the VD extended hip view.
- Joint laxity (passive) is determined quantitatively by comparing the compression and distraction views. For the compression view, the coxofemoral joints are compressed manually so that the femoral heads are fully seated in the acetabulum for maximum congruity. For the distraction view, a specially designed distraction device is placed between the femurs and the femurs are manually compressed against the device, creating a fulcrum to force the femoral heads laterally, in order to visualize the maximum amount of hip joint laxity. When the compression and distraction views are compared, any hip laxity is quantified by a quantitative unitless measure called the distraction index (DI) (Figure 9.27). The minimum amount of laxity is 0.0 DI (tightest hip) and a DI of 1.0 is the loosest hip.
- PennHIP® has identified DI thresholds for specific breeds, below which dogs are not at risk of developing osteoarthrosis. If laxity is present (greater than 0.3 DI), there is a direct relationship between the amount of laxity and the development of osteoarthrosis. Dogs with a DI of less than 0.3 are not at risk of developing osteoarthrosis.
- The DI has been shown to be the most heritable phenotypic trait for selecting dogs with the best hips compared to subjective phenotypic systems and the Norberg angle measurement (Figure 9.28).

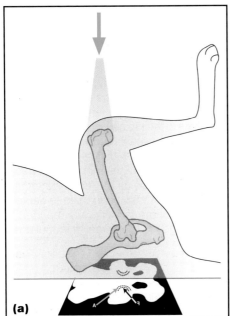

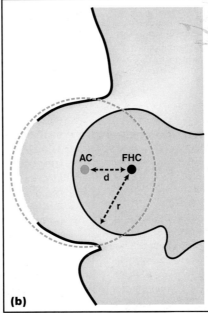

**9.27** PennHIP® scheme. **(a)** Schematic diagram of positioning for distraction and compression views. **(b)** The DI is determined by measuring the separation distance (d) of the femoral head centre (FHC) from the acetabular centre (AC) and dividing by the radius (r) of the femoral head.

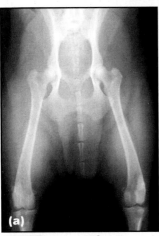

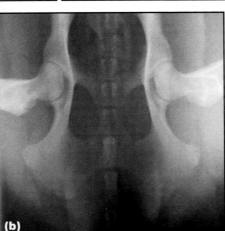

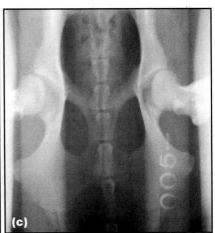

**9.28** PennHIP® radiographs. **(a)** Standard VD extended hip view of a 2-year-old dog's hips that had subjective diagnosis of excellent hips. **(b)** Compression view of hips of same dog. **(c)** Distraction view of hips of same dog. Both hips have increased laxity (looseness), more so in the right hip. Breeding from this dog was not recommended since the DI of the right hip had greater laxity than the mean for the breed.

Dogs with no osteoarthrosis and a DI that is less than the mean (tighter) for their breed should be considered for breeding, which will result in more rapid genetic change towards better hip phenotypes. If the hips appear normal subjectively, but the DI is more than the mean (looser hip), the offspring could have worse hip phenotypes.

• The minimum age for determining the DI is 16 weeks and it is accurate for predicting the dog's DI when older, and the animal's probability for developing osteoarthrosis (Figure 9.29).

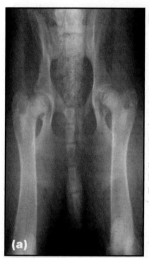

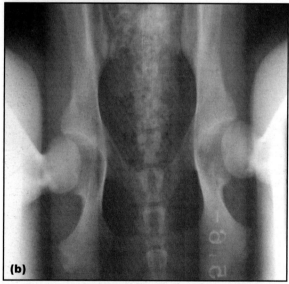

**9.29** Hip assessment in a 20-week-old dog. **(a)** The hips were considered normal for the dog's age on a standard VD extended hip view. **(b)** Distraction view of hips of same dog. The DI of both hips had much greater laxity than the mean for the breed (80% of the dogs in this breed have less laxity) and selection of this dog for breeding was not recommended.

• The DI has been shown not to be affected by hormone status (oestrus), physical activity or bodyweight.
• An individual dog's DI can be used as a breeding prospect criterion and the hip phenotype of its family is not as important as when using the subjective phenotype as a criterion.
• Owners may elect to have their animal's hip phenotype and DI listed in the PennHIP® open registry in order to assist breeders in making educated decisions for the selection of breeding animals.

For further information contact the University of Pennsylvania Hip Improvement Program at 20 Valley Stream Road, Suite 267, Malvern, PA 19355, USA or www.pennhip.org.

***Other hip dysplasia views:*** Several other radiographic techniques have been described that can demonstrate passive hip laxity, but they are not quantitative nor do they have a database sufficient to be of much value to breeders at this time for selecting breeding stock. One view described by Fluckiger (1999) is a stress radiographic technique, using a position similar to the clinical assessment of hip laxity (Ortolani manoeuvre). The dog is placed in dorsal recumbency with the femurs positioned at 60 degrees to the table top. The stifles are adducted and manually pushed craniodorsally during the exposure. This manual distraction is subjective with the measurement termed the subluxation index (SI). The SI then may be used for breeding recommendations.

Another view, called the dorsal acetabular rim (DAR) view, may aid in visualizing the dorsal acetabular rim, the weight bearing portion of the acetabulum and the caudal acetabular rim. In sternal recumbency the pelvic limbs are positioned cranially so that the femurs are parallel with the long axis of the body. The dog's thighs are pulled close to the torso and the stifles are flexed with the tibias at 90 degrees to the femur and the tarsi elevated. This results in the hip being rotated internally so that the X-ray beam passes through the iliac shafts. The DAR view, although reportedly helpful for visualizing osteophytes on the dorsocranial rim of the acetabulum, is not considered helpful by many veterinary radiologists. This view has also been used to demonstrate passive laxity, but the technique is reported to under represent changes to the dorsal acetabular rim and hip laxity in dogs.

#### Feline hip dysplasia

In cats the reported incidence of hip dysplasia amongst breeds ranges from about 6% to 32%, although lameness is less commonly seen than in the dog. The diagnosis is usually made on a VD extended hip view identical to the positioning used in dogs. The radiographic diagnosis is based on the presence of femoral head subluxation or luxation, remodelling of the femoral head and neck or presence of osteoarthrosis. Some clinicians may also use the Norberg angle measurement of approximately 95 degrees or higher as a criterion for normal. Most of the osteoarthrosis changes occur on the craniodorsal margin of the acetabulum (Figure 9.30).

Most feline hip control programmes use the subjective VD extended hip radiographic view. The procedures, radiographic techniques and reporting systems are the same as those used for the dog. The PennHIP® technique is identical to that performed in dogs but uses a specially designed distractor for cats. Similar to dogs, cats with the least amount of laxity (tight hips) are at less risk for developing osteoarthrosis.

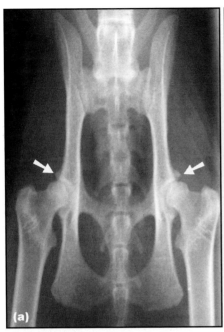
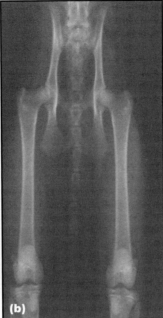
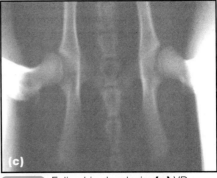

9.30 Feline hip dysplasia. **(a)** VD extended hip view showing bilateral hip dysplasia and osteoarthrosis (arrowed). **(b)** VD extended hip view of an apparently normal hip. **(c)** PennHIP® distraction view of the same cat as in (b) showing marked bilateral hip laxity.

### Osteochondrosis of the hip joint

Osteochrondrosis, as seen radiographically in the shoulder, elbow and other joints, is not recognized in the hip. Osteochondrosis has been shown in pathological studies to be present on the dorsolateral acetabular rim in dogs in association with hip dysplasia. However, there is no scientific evidence that hip dysplasia is caused by osteochondrosis.

### Radiological evaluation of surgical procedures and their complications

Radiological findings related to surgical procedures are highly variable and dependent on what procedure was undertaken. It is most helpful to take immediate postoperative radiographs for an instant assessment and as a baseline for subsequent follow-up films, especially when taken to monitor healing and complications. For comparison of radiographs taken at different dates, it is important that orthogonal views and equivalent technique be used. The exposure factors must be adjusted to accommodate changes in soft tissues, such as swelling or atrophy. Radiographs are necessary to evaluate fracture alignment, position and integrity of internal fixation devices, stability of the fracture site and the stage of healing.

The most common surgical procedures performed for disorders of the hip are:

- Triple pelvic osteotomy (TPO)
- Total hip replacement
- Femoral head resection.

Although most osteotomies heal rapidly, there are a significant number of reported postoperative complications. These include migration of screws, broken or non-supporting hemicerclage wire, pelvic narrowing, infection, decreased hip joint range of motion, progressive osteoarthrosis, plus nerve and soft tissue injury with constipation, stranguria or urethral obstruction.

With total hip replacement there are some additional complications besides implant failure and infection. These include femoral head luxation, aseptic loosening of implants, acetabular cup displacement, femoral fracture, extraosseous cement granuloma and an increased incidence of neoplasia in the hip later in life. Femoral head resection results in a pseudoarthrosis and has few complications, but infection, resorption of the femoral neck or a residual femoral neck bony spike causing pain, can occur (Figure 9.31).

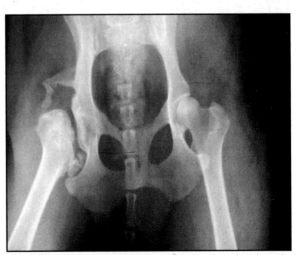

9.31 VD extended hip view of a dog that developed lameness several weeks after a right femoral head and neck resection. There was a low grade inflammatory process characterized by osteosclerosis, a periosteal reaction and several bone fragments.

### Infection

Osteomyelitis of the pelvis and hip is most common following a penetrating wound or as a postoperative complication. The radiological findings are usually a mixture of osteoblastic, osteolytic and osteosclerotic changes with adjacent soft tissue swelling. In the hip of an immature animal (open physes) there may be delayed development or rapid destruction of the femoral head and subsequent deformity of the hip (Figure 9.32). (For further information on osteomyelitis see Chapter 4.)

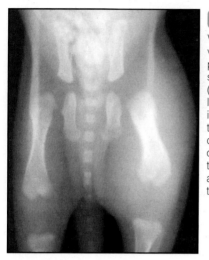

**9.32** VD extended hip view of a young puppy with septic arthritis (bacterial) of the left hip, resulting in destruction of the femoral capital epiphysis, osteomyelitis of the left femur and associated soft tissue swelling.

## Neoplasia

Although primary malignant neoplasms in the flat bones of the pelvis and hip are uncommon, they do occur. Radiologically they usually appear as aggressive lesions with poorly marginated osteolytic or osteoblastic changes, and an aggressive periosteal reaction (Figures 9.33 and 9.34). Most of the primary bone neoplasms are osteosarcomas, but less aggressive neoplasms (such as chondrosarcoma) do occur. Most other tumours involving the pelvis are from adjacent infiltrating soft tissue neoplasms (e.g. prostatic or urethral carcinoma) or multicentric neoplasms, such as lymphosarcoma, malignant histiocytoma and multiple myeloma. (For further information on neoplasia see Chapter 6.)

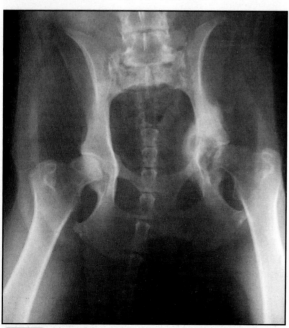

**9.33** Malignant neoplasm of the pelvis. Osteosarcoma arising from left acetabulum.

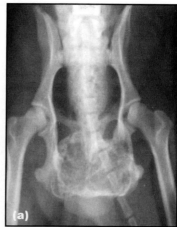
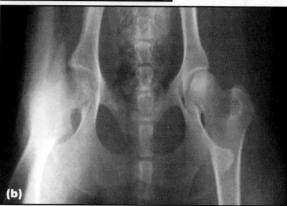

**9.34** Malignant neoplasms of the pelvis. **(a)** Chondrosarcoma of the ischia and pubic bones. **(b)** Synovial sarcoma of the right hip.

## Metabolic conditions

### Mucopolysaccharidosis

Mucopolysaccharidoses are a group of recessively inherited lysomal storage disorders in dogs and cats that result from metabolic deficits of different glycosaminoglycans. These different enzyme deficiencies cause a variety of abnormalities, many of which are visible radiologically. The abnormalities are bilateral and in the hip mimic those of canine and feline hip dysplasia. The abnormal radiological findings in the hip include coxofemoral luxation, deformity to the femoral head and acetabulum and osteoarthrosis (Figure 9.35) (see also Chapters 6, 12 and 16).

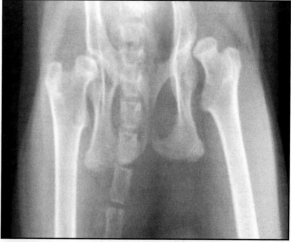

**9.35** VD extended hip view of a cat with mucopolysaccharidosis, which mimics hip dysplasia.

## Miscellaneous

### Anal gland gas or mineralization

Gas in the anal glands, resulting from abscessation, or mineralization due to chronic inflammation, may be seen summated upon the pubic or ischial bones of the pelvis on VD views and should not be misinterpreted as an osteolytic or osteoblastic lesion of the pelvis. Normal gas or bony foreign material in the descending colon and rectum can also be misinterpreted as a lesion.

### Osteoarthrosis

Besides the diseases discussed above, there are other conditions that can affect the hip joint. As with other synovial joints, there could be a joint effusion, loss of cartilage with remodelling of the subchondral bone, osteophyte formation and osteosclerosis. Additional conditions that can cause arthrosis include valgus or varus conformation defects of the pelvic limbs, immune-mediated arthropathies, infectious diseases (such as Lyme disease) and constitutional disorders (such as multiple epiphyseal dysplasia), congenital hypothyroidism (Figure 9.36) and other abnormalities of cartilage and bone development known as osteo-chondrodysplasias (Figure 9.37) (see also Chapters 3 and 6).

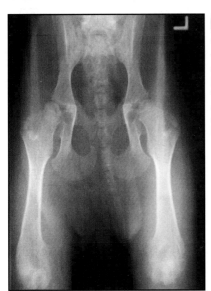

**9.36**
VD extended hip view of a young dog with hypoplastic femoral heads due to congenital hypothyroidism.

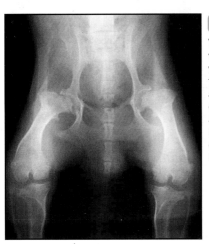

**9.37**
VD extended hip view of a dog with abnormal femoral heads and hips due to pseudo-achondroplasia, previously called epiphyseal dysplasia.

## References and further readings

Allan G (2002) Radiographic signs of joint disease. In: *Textbook of Veterinary Radiology, 4th edn*, ed. DE Thrall, pp 187–198. WB Saunders, Philadelphia

Craig LE (2001) Physeal dysplasia with slipped capital femoral epiphysis in 13 cats. *Veterinary Pathology* **38**, 92–97

Crawford JT, Manley PA and Adams WM (2003) Comparison of computed tomography, tangential view radiography and conventional radiography in evaluation of canine pelvis trauma. *Veterinary Radiology and Ultrasound* **44**, 619–628

Dennis R, Kirberger RM, Wrigley RH and Barr FJ (2001) Appendicular skeleton. In: *Handbook of Small Animal Radiological Differential Diagnosis*. pp. 50–52. WB Saunders, London

Fluckiger MA (1999) A radiographic stress technique for evaluation of coxofemoral joint laxity in dogs. *Veterinary Surgery* **28**, 1–9

Fordyce HH, Smith GK, Gregor TP and Biery DN (2001) Comparison of three methods to measure passive hip laxity in the dog. 12th International Radiology Association Meeting. *Veterinary Radiology and Ultrasound* **42**, 169 [Abstract]

Gibbs C (1997) The BVA/KC scoring scheme for control of hip dysplasia: interpretation of criteria. *Veterinary Record* **141**, 275–284

Hardie EM, Roe SC and Martin FR (2002) Radiographic evidence of degenerative joint disease in geriatric cats. *Journal of the American Veterinary Medical Association* **220**, 628–632

Jessen CR and Spurrell FA (1972) Radiographic detection of canine hip dysplasia in known age groups. In: *Proceedings of the American Veterinary Medical Association Symposium Hip Dysplasia*. pp. 93–98

Keller G (2003) The use of health databases and selective breeding – a guide for dog and cat breeders and owners. In: *Orthopedic Foundation for Animals Booklet. 4th edn*. Columbia, MO

Kirberger (1999) Hip dysplasia. In: *Proceedings of Hereditary Conditions in Dogs – a Dog Breeders Symposium*, pp. 9–25. Faculty of Veterinary Science, University of Pretoria, South Africa

Jezyk P (1985) Constitutional disorders of the skeleton in dogs and cats. In: *Textbook of Small Animal Orthopedics*, ed. CD Newton and DM Nunamaker, pp. 637–654. JB Lippincott, Philadelphia

Langenbach A, Giger U, Green P, Rhodes WH, Gregor TP, LaFond E and Smith GK (1998) Relationship between degenerative joint disease and hip joint laxity by use of distraction index and Norberg angle measurement in a group of cats. *Journal of the American Veterinary Medical Association* **213**, 1439–1443

Lanting FL (2005) *Canine Hip Dyplasia and Other Orthopedic Problems*. Los Perros Publishing Co., Miami

Mayhew PD, McKelvie PJ, Biery DN, Shofer FS and Smith GK (2002) Evaluation of a radiographic caudolateral curvilinear osteophyte on the femoral neck and its relationship to degenerative joint disease and distraction index in dogs. *Journal of the American Veterinary Medical Association* **220,** 472–476

Mayrhofer VE and Olensky G (1978) Bursitis calcarea im Hüftgelenksbereich beim Hunde. *Wiener Tierärztliche Monatsschrift* **65**, 193–199

Moores AP, Owen MR, Fewst D, Coe RJ, Brown PJ and Butterworth SJ (2004) Slipped capital epiphysis in dogs. *Journal of Small Animal Practice* **45**, 602–608

Morgan JP (2000) Hip dysplasia. In: *Hereditary Bone and Joint Diseases in the Dog*. pp. 109–208. Schlütersche, Hanover

Owens JM and Biery DB (1999) The coxofemoral joints and pelvis. In: *Radiographic Interpretation for the Small Animal Clinician*. pp. 85–91. Williams and Wilkins, Baltimore

Paster E, LaFond, E, Biery DN, Iriye A, Gregor TP, Shofer FS and Smith GK (2005) Estimates of prevalence of hip dysplasia in golden retrievers and rottweilers and the influence of bias on published prevalence figures. *Journal of the American Veterinary Medical Association* **226**, 387–392

Powers MY, Biery DN, Lawler DF, Evans RH, Shofer, FRS, Mayhew PD, Gregor TP, Kealy RD and Smith GK (2004) Use of the caudolateral curvilinear osteophyte as an early marker for further development of osteoarthritis associated with hip dysplasia in dogs. *Journal of the American Veterinary Medical Association* **225**, 233–237

Queen J (1998) Femoral neck metaphyseal osteopathy in the cat. *Veterinary Record* **142**, 152–162

Riser WH (1975) The dog as a model for the study of hip dysplasia. *Veterinary Pathology* **12**, 229–334

Riser WH (1985) Hip dyplasia. In: *Textbook of Small Animal Orthopedics*, ed. CD Newton and DM Nunamaker, pp. 953–980. JP Lippincott, Philadelphia

Schulz KS and Dejardin LM (2002) Surgical treatment of canine hip dysplasia. In: *Textbook of Small Animal Surgery, 3rd edn*. Ed. D Slatter, pp. 2029–2059. WB Saunders, Philadelphia

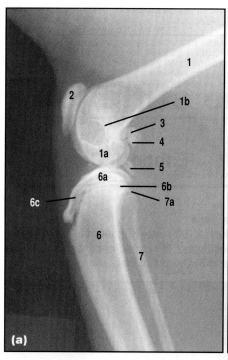

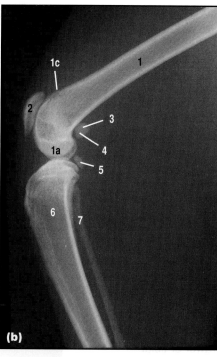

**10.3** ML views detailing the normal radiological anatomy of the stifle joint. **(a)** Skeletally immature cat. **(b)** Skeletally mature cat. 1 = Femur; 1a = Distal femoral epiphysis/femoral condyles; 1b = Distal femoral physis; 1c = Trochlear ridges; 2 = Patella; 3 = Lateral fabella (gastrocnemius); 4 = Medial fabella (gastrocnemius); 5 = Popliteal sesamoid; 6 = Tibia; 6a = Proximal tibial epiphysis; 6b = Proximal tibial physis; 6c = Tibial tuberosity; 7 = Fibula; 7a = Proximal fibular epiphysis. (Courtesy of C Gibbs.)

with a small foam wedge. A weighted radiographic aid, such as a sandbag, can be placed in the inguinal area of the opposite hindlimb, in order to keep it out of the area of interest. The cassette is placed under the stifle joint on the lateral aspect. The joint is palpated for normal landmarks, such as the apex of the patella, the tibial tuberosity and the medial and lateral femoral condyles. The primary beam is centred just cranial and distal to the medial condyle of the femur. The joint is usually kept in a semi-flexed position. The beam is collimated to include the distal femur, proximal tibia, patella, patellar ligament and caudal fascial planes.

### Caudocranial view

For a caudocranial (CdCr) view (Figure 10.4) the patient is placed in sternal recumbency; it may be useful to put the thorax in a cradle or place weighted

radiographic aids on either side of the thorax to support this area. The pelvic limbs are pulled caudally, the stifle joint to be radiographed is placed on the cassette and the body tilted very slightly to the same side as being radiographed. A wedge-shaped foam positioning aid may be used to support the distal limb. The primary beam is centred halfway between the femoral condyles and the caudal tibial plateau, using the landmarks described above.

### Horizontal beam caudocranial view

One advantage of taking a CdCr view in the horizontal plane (Figure 10.5) is that it is usually easier to obtain straight positioning of the joint. However, rotation of the X-ray tube is required and due regard must be paid to radiation safety. The patient is placed in lateral recumbency on the side opposite to the limb to be radiographed. The stifle joint under investigation will therefore be the uppermost limb and is placed on a

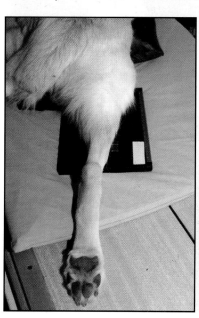

**10.4** Positioning for a CdCr view of the right stifle joint. The dog is placed in sternal recumbency and the thorax is supported with sandbags.

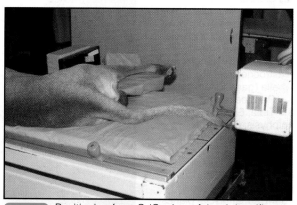

**10.5** Positioning for a CdCr view of the right stifle joint using a horizontal beam. The cassette is placed cranial to the affected stifle joint, which is elevated with a foam wedge. The X-ray tube is lowered to the level of the stifle joint and centred using the light beam diaphragm.

foam positioning aid. The cassette is placed cranial to the stifle joint and the primary beam is centred on the joint, as described previously for the CdCr view. It is important to move the X-ray tube to the correct film focal distance (approximately 100 cm) by measuring this distance from the stifle joint in the horizontal plane.

## Craniocaudal view

For a craniocaudal (CrCd) view (Figures 10.6 to 10.8) the patient is positioned in dorsal recumbency and both pelvic limbs are pulled caudally. It may be useful to put the thorax in a cradle or place weighted radiographic aids in both axillae to support this area. The patient can be tilted slightly to the opposite side of the stifle to be radiographed, which is placed on a square foam positioning aid for support, and the cassette is placed under the joint. The landmarks (described previously) are

palpated and the primary beam is centred halfway between the patella apex and the tibial tuberosity.

## Special views

### Craniodistal-cranioproximal oblique view

A craniodistal-cranioproximal oblique (CrDi-CrPrO) view (also known as a skyline view) of the patella (Figure 10.9) is useful for the general and surgical assessment of undisplaced and comminuted patellar fractures and patellar luxation. This view is usually obtained with a horizontal beam, with the patient in dorsal recumbency, the affected limb maintained in a flexed position and the radiographic cassette positioned proximal to the flexed joint. The primary beam is centred on the patella. (It is also possible is take a cranioproximal-craniodistal oblique (CrPr-CrDiO) view of the patella.)

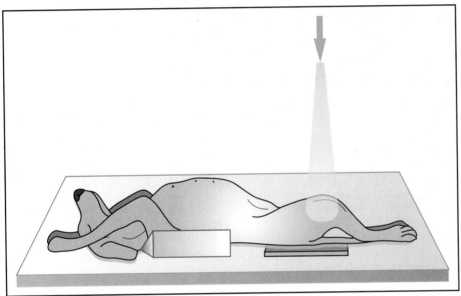

**10.6** Positioning for a CrCd view of the stifle joint. The dog is placed in dorsal recumbency, the cassette is placed under the stifle joint and the primary beam centred distal to the femoral condyles. It may be necessary to place a foam pad under the distal limb.

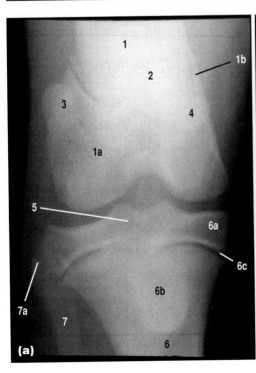
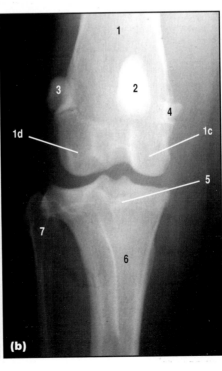

**10.7** CrCd views detailing the normal radiological anatomy of the stifle joint. **(a)** Skeletally immature dog (5 months old). **(b)** Skeletally mature dog. 1 = Femur; 1a = Distal femoral epiphysis; 1b = Distal femoral physis; 1c = Medial femoral condyle; 1d = Lateral femoral condyle; 2 = Patella; 3 = Lateral fabella (gastrocnemius); 4 = Medial fabella (gastrocnemius); 5 = Popliteal sesamoid; 6 = Tibia; 6a = Proximal tibial epiphysis; 6b = Tibial tuberosity; 6c = Proximal tibial physis; 7 = Fibula; 7a = Proximal fibular epiphysis.

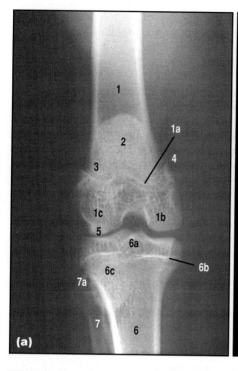
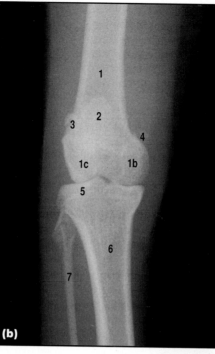

**10.8** CrCd views detailing the normal radiological anatomy of the stifle joint. **(a)** Skeletally immature cat (10 months old). **(b)** Skeletally mature cat. 1 = Femur; 1a = Distal femoral physis; 1b = Medial femoral condyle; 1c = Lateral femoral condyle; 2 = Patella; 3 = Lateral fabella (gastrocnemius); 4 = Medial fabella (gastrocnemius); 5 = Popliteal sesamoid; 6 =Tibia; 6a = Proximal tibial epiphysis; 6b = Proximal tibial physis; 6c = Tibial tuberosity; 7 = Fibula; 7a = Proximal fibular epiphysis. (Courtesy of C Gibbs.)

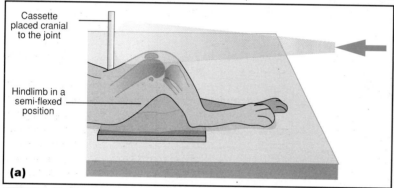
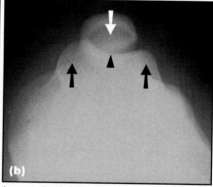

**10.9** Positioning and radiography of the stifle joint for a CrDi-CrPrO view of the patella. **(a)** The patient is placed in dorsal recumbency with the stifle joint flexed, the cassette is placed proximal to the joint and the X-ray beam is centred on the patella. **(b)** Radiograph of a normal stifle joint, showing the patella (white arrow), the medial and lateral trochlear ridges (black arrows) and the trochlear groove (arrowhead).

## Stress views

Stress radiography is most useful for establishing spatial derangements of the stifle, particularly secondary to collateral ligament injuries, and has wide applications in small animal radiography (Farrow, 1982). The most useful stress manoeuvres in the stifle joint are shear and wedge stress forces. It is important to achieve three-point bending with stress radiographs (Figure 10.10), and the limb proximal and distal to the stifle joint needs to be stabilized with radiolucent ties or tapes. It is important to compare both stifle joints when evaluating stress views.

## Closing wedge or tibial plateau levelling osteotomy procedure view

These surgical procedures require accurate measurement of the slope of the tibial plateau. It is therefore essential that the stifle and hock joints are parallel to the cassette. This is achieved by placing thin positioning aids under the ipsilateral coxofemoral joint and, where appropriate, under the stifle and hock joints. The X-ray

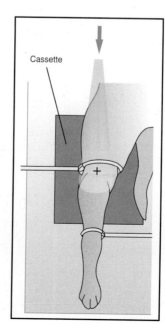

**10.10** Positioning for a stressed CrCd view of the right stifle joint to demonstrate a tear of the lateral collateral ligament. The patient is placed in dorsal recumbency, the cassette is placed under the stifle joint and the joint is subjected to a three-point stress by means of straps. The primary beam is centred (+) using the landmarks described in the text.

beam is centred over the stifle joint space at the level of the tibial intercondylar tubercles and is collimated to include the hock joint. The cranial and caudal limits of the medial tibial plateau, the tibial intercondylar tubercles and the centre of the talus are noted and the tibial plateau angle measured as detailed in Figure 10.11.

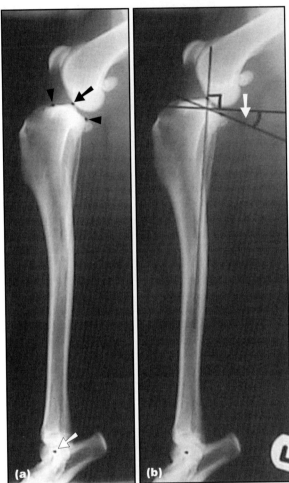

**10.11** ML views of a stifle and hock joint used for the measurement of the tibial plateau angle. Positioning for these radiographs must ensure that the medial and lateral femoral condyles are superimposed. **(a)** The cranial and caudal aspects of the tibial plateau (arrowheads), the tibial intercondylar tubercles (black arrow) and the centre of the talus (white arrow) are marked. **(b)** A line is drawn between the cranial and caudal aspects of the tibial plateau and another line drawn between the tibial intercondylar tubercles and the centre of the talus. At the point of intersection of both lines, a perpendicular line is drawn to the line connecting the talus. The resultant angle (arrowed) is the tibial plateau angle. (Courtesy of S Butterworth.)

## Physeal closure times

For information on physeal closure times see Chapter 3.

## Incidental findings

### Incomplete ossifications

Non-ossification of the medial fabella can be an occasional finding in the cat.

### Extensor fossa

The extensor fossa is a radiolucent defect on the lateral femoral condyle (see Figure 10.1), which corresponds with the origin of the long digital extensor tendon. It should not be confused with osteochondrosis, osteochondritis dissecans (OCD) or be associated with a ligament avulsion. It is a useful landmark to distinguish the medial and lateral condyles on ML views.

### Mineralized bodies of the stifle joint

There are four sesamoid bones (see Figures 10.1 and 10.3) associated with the stifle joints of dogs and cats (Mahoney and Lamb, 1996):

- The patella (within the insertion of the quadriceps femoris muscle located in the trochlear groove of the femur)
- Paired sesamoids (the fabellae) within the tendons of origin of the gastrocnemius muscle, located proximal to the caudal aspects of the medial and lateral femoral condyles
- The sesamoid within the popliteal muscle caudodistal to the lateral femoral condyle.

The patella and the fabellae (Figure 10.12) can be bipartite or multipartite occasionally, as the manifestation of a congenital abnormality. Bipartite and multipartite sesamoids are not associated with clinical signs and can be uni- or bilateral (Denny and Butterworth, 2000).

Pathological mineralized or calcified bodies found in or around the stifle joint can include avulsion fragments of the cruciate ligaments, the long digital extensor tendon, the gastrocnemius or popliteus muscles, fragmented sesamoids, joint mice associated with osteochondritis dissecans or osteoarthrosis, meniscal mineralization or synovial osteochondromatosis (see also Chapter 6 and under Abnormal radiological findings).

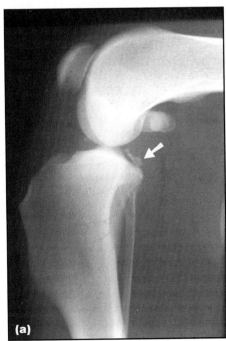

**10.12** ML views of canine stifle joints. **(a)** A multipartite popliteal sesamoid (arrowed). (continued) ▶

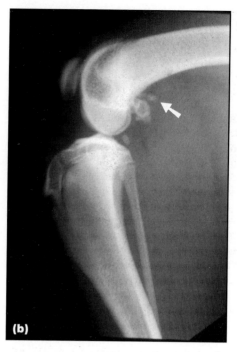

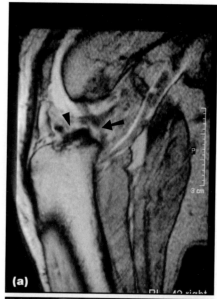

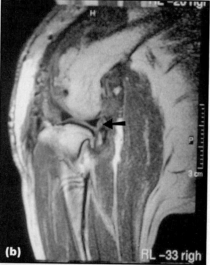

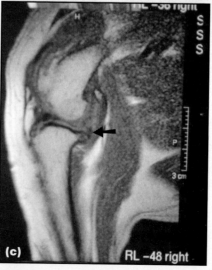

**10.12** (continued) ML views of canine stifle joints. **(b)** A multipartite fabella (arrowed).

## Contrast studies

Use of positive contrast arthrography has been reported in the diagnosis of canine cranial cruciate disease (Hay *et al.*, 1996); however, it is not used routinely.

## Alternative imaging techniques

### Magnetic resonance imaging

Low-field magnetic resonance imaging (MRI), including paramagnetic contrast arthrography studies, has been used to identify normal anatomical structures in the canine stifle joint (Baird *et al.*, 1998). To date it has mainly been used in military working dogs and experimentally (Widmer *et al.*, 1991; Banfield and Morrison, 2000). Its main application in practice is to identify medial meniscal and cranial cruciate ligament (CCL) tears. On T1-weighted images (Figure 10.13) synovial fluid has low signal intensity (dark) compared with the infrapatellar fat pad, which has a high signal intensity (bright). Articular cartilage has an intermediate signal intensity and is separated from trabecular bone by a dark line, representing subchondral bone. Menisci, fibrous joint capsules and ligamentous structures appear dark. In the true sagittal plane, the entire cranial and caudal cruciate ligaments can be seen within one image slice. The patella is visualized as an intermediate bright signal (trabecular bone) surrounded by a low intensity signal (cortical bone).

### Computed tomography

Computed tomography (CT) is not commonly used in veterinary practice for the diagnosis of stifle joint pathology. Its use has been reported in the diagnosis of a chronic long digital extensor tendon avulsion (Fitch *et al.*, 1997) and has been used for pre-surgical planning in the management of patellar luxation.

**10.13** T1-weighted MRI scans of a canine stifle joint. **(a)** Sagittal image showing a disrupted CCL (arrowhead) and a normal caudal cruciate ligament (arrowed). **(b)** Image lateral to the sagittal plane showing a normal lateral meniscus (arrowed). **(c)** Image medial to the sagittal plane showing an abnormal medial meniscus with the caudal part absent (arrowed).

## Ultrasonography

Ultrasonography is useful for assessing joint disease. Joint effusion, thickening of the joint capsule and cartilage defects can be identified by ultrasound examination (Kramer *et al.*, 1997). In one study (Gnudi and Bertoni, 2001) ultrasonography of the canine stifle was found to be useful in evaluating the presence of fibrous tissue within the joint due to repair processes, and for demonstrating the soft tissue pathological changes that were observed consequent to joint instability. Ultrasonography was not found to be an accurate test for cruciate rupture evaluation (Engelke *et al.*, 1997), identifying 20% of CCL ruptures when compared with cadaver findings (Gnudi and Bertoni, 2001). High frequency transducers (7.5–15 MHz) are recommended. Some experienced operators have a high success rate of identifying medial meniscal tears using a 15 MHz linear transducer (Cook, unpublished observations). The stifle should be positioned in maximum flexion during ultrasonography (Kramer *et al.*, 1999). The joint can be divided into different regions (suprapatellar, caudal, infrapatellar, medial and lateral) for examination.

## Scintigraphy

Scintigraphy has been used in assessing dogs with stifle osteoarthrosis (Innes *et al.*, 1996) but its main application is in lameness investigation, if there is suspicion of the stifle joint being involved but pain is not easily localizable to this joint (Schwarz *et al.*, 2004). Dogs are injected intravenously with technetium 99M methylene diphosphonate and then scanned immediately to obtain soft tissue phase images. Bone phase images are obtained 2.5–3.5 hours later. Both stifle joints are imaged for comparison (Figure 10.14).

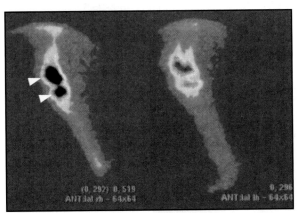

**10.14** Scintigraphic lateral left and right stifle bone phase scans. Note the increased uptake of isotope in the distal femur and proximal tibia (arrowheads) of the right stifle joint compared to the left stifle joint.

## Abnormal radiological findings

### Trauma

#### Fractures

*Patella:* Fractures of the patella are rare and may be transverse, longitudinal, apical or comminuted (Figure 10.15). An inability to extend the stifle may be seen in a patient with fracture of the patella or rupture

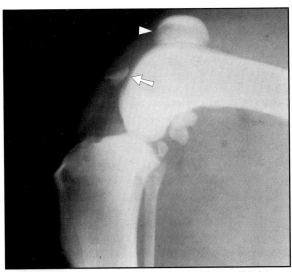

**10.15** ML view of a canine stifle showing a distal apical patellar fracture (arrowhead) with associated mineralized fragment (open arrow). Note the proximal displacement of the patella.

of the straight patellar ligament (Denny, 1985). ML and CdCr views are the most useful for confirming the diagnosis. A skyline view of the femoral trochlea and patella may be useful for surgical assessment and determining the extent of comminution. Old patellar fractures can be seen on standard stifle joint radiographs as an incidental finding in cats (Arnbjerg and Heje, 1993).

*Fabella:* Fractures of the fabellae are very uncommon and should be differentiated from the congenital bipartite or multipartite fabellae (see Figure 10.12). Multipartite or fragmented sesamoids are most commonly seen affecting the medial fabella, with Poodles and Fox Terriers appearing to be predisposed. Fractures of the lateral fabella have been reported in the dog (Houlton and Ness, 1993) and may be associated with avulsion of the lateral head of the gastrocnemius muscle (Muir and Dueland, 1994). The medial fabella is usually smaller than the lateral fabella in the cat. Two standard orthogonal views of the stifle will confirm the diagnosis, with a distinct radiolucent line likely to be evident in a fractured fabella compared with a roughened radiopaque outline of bipartite sesamoids.

*Tibial tuberosity avulsion:* Tibial tuberosity avulsion is usually seen in young dogs less than 8–10 months of age. Greyhounds and terriers appear to be predisposed. Another presentation of this injury is a Salter–Harris type II fracture of the proximal tibial physis (Figure 10.16). ML and CdCr views of both stifle joints will confirm this diagnosis. The radiological findings include displacement of the tibial tuberosity, approximately 1 cm proximal to the tibial plateau. There may be some speckled radiopaque mineralized particles at the distal aspect of the displaced fragment. This injury can be misdiagnosed in immature dogs due to the normal delayed ossification of the distal aspect of the tibial crest.

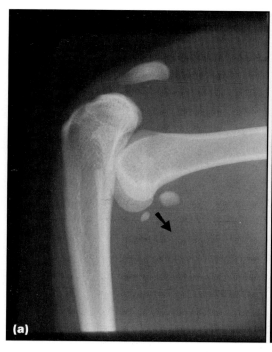
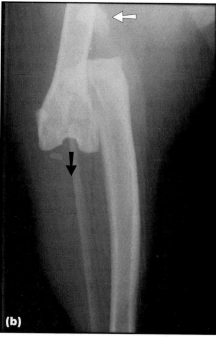

**10.20**
Stifle radiographs of a cat with severe ligamentous disruption.
**(a)** ML view.
**(b)** CrCd view. The femur is displaced caudodistally (black arrows) and laterally (open arrow), suggestive of collateral and cruciate injuries.

## Ligament injuries

***Cranial cruciate ligament:*** Rupture of the CCL is a very common injury in dogs, resulting in hindlimb lameness. Rupture of the CCL is a relatively uncommon condition in cats, but can occur in conjunction with damage to the collateral ligaments in cases of severe stifle disruption. Physical examination is essential in diagnosing CCL rupture but radiographic examination is useful in the diagnostic investigation of this condition. Standard orthogonal views are sufficient and help to exclude additional pathology. Certain surgical procedures (e.g. closing wedge osteotomy or tibial plateau levelling osteotomy) may require special views for planning the surgery.

The aetiopathogenesis of this condition is not known fully but most patients present acutely, following minor trauma. The presentation is associated with CCL rupture, secondary to chronic degeneration, known as 'cruciate disease'. Radiological findings with complete and partial ligament ruptures may range in severity from joint effusion, resulting in displacement of the infrapatellar fat pad and caudal fascial planes in the acute stage (Figure 10.21a), to severe osteophyte and enthesophyte formation on the trochlear ridges, proximal and distal patella, the fabellae and the tibial plateau (Figure 10.21b). The tibial eminence usually bisects the femoral condyles and can be cranially displaced in dogs with CCL rupture.

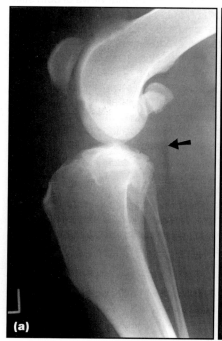
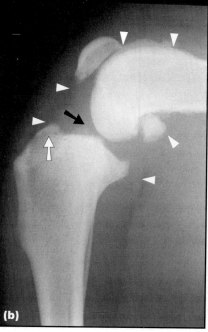

**10.21**
ML view of canine stifles with rupture of the CCL.
**(a)** Acute case. A marked joint effusion is present, obscuring the margin of the infrapatellar fad pad and displacing the fascial planes caudally (arrowed). **(b)** Chronic case. This radiograph is suggestive of rupture of the CCL due to the enthesophytes at the insertion point (open arrow) and associated osteoarthrosis, showing marked joint effusion (black arrow) and osteophytes (arrowheads) on the trochlear ridges, proximal and distal patella, tibial plateau and fabellae.

Certain young large-breed dogs can present with a purely traumatic rupture (Bennett *et al.*, 1988) and they can also avulse the bony insertion (most common) or origin of the ligament (Figure 10.22). Rupture of the CCL can result in medial meniscal tears in approximately 50% of cases at the time of injury. However, 'late meniscal tears' may occur in approximately 15% of cases and increased joint effusion may then be seen. It is important to perform other diagnostic tests, such as stifle arthrocenthesis and synovial fluid analysis, to differentiate this condition from joint sepsis.

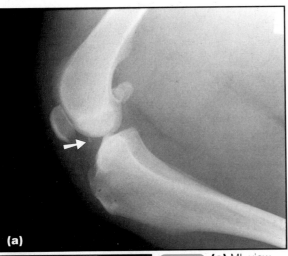

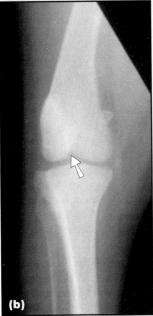

10.22 **(a)** ML view and **(b)** CrCd view of a canine stifle with an avulsion of the CCL showing a mild joint effusion and a mineralized intra-articular fragment (open arrow).

*Caudal cruciate ligament:* Rupture of the caudal cruciate ligament is an uncommon isolated injury in dogs and has been found in conjunction with medial collateral ligament tears. Standard orthogonal views of the stifle joint may reveal joint effusion, especially obliterating the caudal fascial planes, and avulsion fractures of the ligament at its femoral attachment site.

*Medial and lateral collateral ligaments:* Isolated rupture of a collateral ligament is rare but may occur in conjunction with a cruciate ligament rupture or stifle

disruption. Physical examination may reveal increased joint movement on the affected side. Standard orthogonal views and stressed CrCd or CdCr views are necessary to confirm these tears. Abnormal radiological findings include increased joint space width at the affected side and there may be avulsion fractures evident at the origin or insertion sites of the ligaments (Figure 10.23).

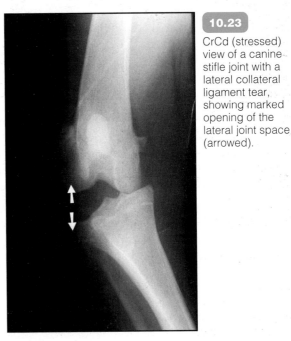

10.23 CrCd (stressed) view of a canine stifle joint with a lateral collateral ligament tear, showing marked opening of the lateral joint space (arrowed).

*Gastrocnemius and popliteus muscles:* Radiological findings associated with these injuries have been detailed in the previous section on traumatic avulsions.

*Patellar ligament rupture:* Rupture of the patellar ligament is an uncommon injury in dogs. Disruption of the extensor mechanism of the stifle will result in a severe mechanical lameness. The patellar ligament most commonly ruptures near its attachment on the apex of the patella or near its tibial attachment. A flexed ML view is the most useful in confirming this condition, revealing the patella to be proximally displaced in the femoral trochlea compared to the contralateral side (Figure 10.24).

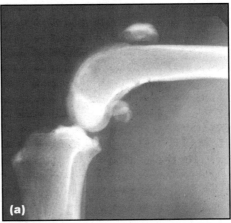

10.24 ML views of a stifle joint from a dog with a patellar ligament rupture. **(a)** Preoperative view showing marked proximal displacement of the patella. (continues) ▶

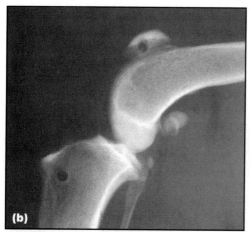

**10.24** (continued) ML views of a stifle joint from a dog with a patellar ligament rupture. **(b)** Postoperative view showing normal position of the patella. The circular radiolucent areas in the patella and tibial crest are where surgical implants have been passed.

### Quadriceps contracture

Quadriceps contracture occurs typically in juvenile dogs secondary to a distal femoral fracture, which has been managed with external coaptation. Contracture can occur over a number of weeks and will result in the stifle and hock being permanently locked in extension. Abnormal radiological findings will be related to severe disuse atrophy, with reduction of soft tissue mass around the stifle joint, proximal displacement of the patella and osteopenia of the femur and tibia compared with the contralateral side.

## Congenital and developmental conditions

### Congenital patellar luxation

The congenital form of patellar luxation is likely to be related to developmental abnormalities of the pelvic limb, resulting in malalignment of the quadriceps complex. The quadriceps complex consists of the quadriceps tendon, patella and patellar ligament. Malalignment of the quadriceps complex can result in medial or lateral patellar luxation; the degree of deformity associated with luxation can be graded in severity from Grades I–IV (Singleton, 1969). Congenital patellar luxation can be seen in small or toy-breed dogs (usually medial luxation) and in medium to large-breed dogs, e.g. Labrador Retrievers (medial or lateral luxation). A ventrodorsal (VD) view of the coxofemoral joints and femurs, as well as standard orthogonal and skyline views of the stifle, are necessary to assess and confirm the severity of this condition.

Abnormal radiological findings can include:

- A luxated patella on either side of the trochlear ridge (Figure 10.25)
- A shallow trochlear groove as well as bony abnormalities of the coxofemoral joints and femur (coxa vara, lateral bowing of the distal femur, retroversion of the femoral head and neck)
- A medial deviation of the tibia (Figure 10.25b).

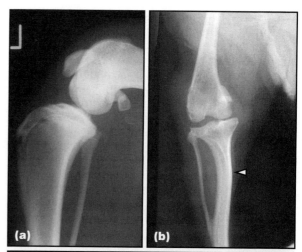

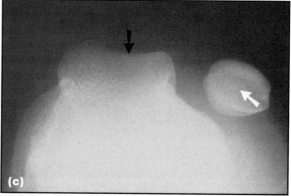

**10.25** Canine stifle, demonstrating the abnormal radiological findings associated with congenital medial patellar luxation. **(a)** ML view. Note the partial superimposition on the distal femur. **(b)** CrCd view. There is medial deviation of the proximal tibia (open arrowhead) and medial luxation of the patella. **(c)** Skyline view. The patella is displaced to the medial side of the trochlear groove (white arrow); the trochlear groove is shallow (black arrow).

Radiography may be helpful in ruling out other causes of stifle disease. In some long-standing cases of patellar luxation osteoarthrosis may be evident. Patellar subluxation can be found in medium to small-breed dogs, particularly the Bull Terrier breeds but radiography may not be rewarding in these cases.

### Idiopathic effusion

Idiopathic effusion (juvenile gonitis) has been historically reported in medium to large-breed dogs, such as the Boxer and Rottweiler, and commonly presents at 1–3 years of age. It may be bilateral and could be associated with rupture of the CCL. ML views may show increased intra-articular soft tissue opacity and displacement of the infrapatellar fat pad.

### Meniscal calcification and ossification

Meniscal calcification and ossification is rarely seen in dogs and is more common in cats, rodents and rabbits. It can be idiopathic but may also be secondary to trauma (ruptured CCL) or is found in osteoarthritic joints. Radiological findings may indicate the presence of an intra-articular mineralized radiopacity (Figure 10.26).

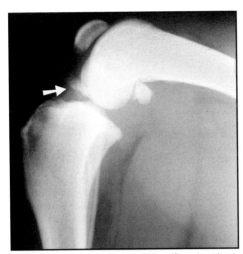

10.26  ML view of a canine stifle, showing mineralization and cranial luxation of a meniscus (arrowed).

## Genu valgum

Genu valgum occurs secondary to disturbance of a distal femoral or a proximal tibial physis. This disturbance allows the medial side of the physis to grow more rapidly than the lateral side, resulting in medial bowing of the distal femur and lateral deviation of the distal limb. The condition occurs in giant breeds (such as the Irish Wolfhound) at 4–5 months of age and tends to be bilateral. CdCr or CrCd views of the stifle will reveal medial bowing of the distal stifle and there may be lateral luxation of the patella (Figure 10.27) (see also Chapter 3).

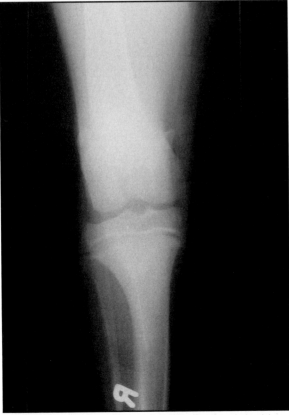

10.27  CrCd view of the right stifle of a 4-month-old Great Dane with a mild genu valgum. Note the mild lateral deviation of the distal limb.

## Osteochondrosis and osteochondritis dissecans

OCD is an uncommon cause of stifle lameness in the dog and has been reported in the cat (Ralphs, 2005). It can affect both medial and lateral femoral condyles. Radiological findings include flattening of the articular surface of one femoral condyle (usually the medial aspect of the lateral femoral condyle), a subchondral bone defect, possibly with adjacent sclerosis, and free mineralized fragments (joint mice) (Figure 10.28). ML views will demonstrate the condylar flattening; however, it is necessary to obtain a CdCr or CrCd view to determine which condyle is affected. It is necessary to adjust the exposure so that good trabecular detail of the femoral condyles is obtained.

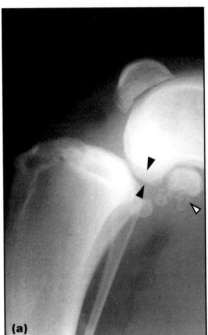

10.28

(a) ML view and (b) CrCd view of a canine stifle with OCD, showing evidence of flattened femoral condyles (arrowheads), intra-articular joint mice (open arrowhead), subchondral deficit of the articular surface of the lateral condyle (arrowed) and a joint effusion.

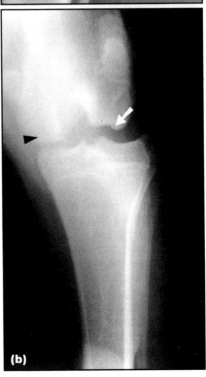

## Osteoarthrosis

Stifle osteoarthrosis is a very common condition in dogs, occurring less frequently in cats. It occurs most commonly secondary to partial and complete CCL rupture, with patellar luxation, and with trauma resulting in collateral ligament ruptures or articular fractures. Abnormal radiological findings (Figure 10.29) are predominantly enthesophyte formation of the joint capsule attachment on the proximal trochlear ridges, both femoral epicondyles, proximal and distal patella, fabellae, and popliteal sesamoid and osteophytes on the proximal tibia. Subchondral bone cysts can be seen in advanced osteoarthrosis of the stifle joint. The changes can vary in severity and do not correlate to the animal's clinical status. There may be radiological evidence of a joint effusion, which will obscure the infrapatellar fat pad and displace the caudal fascial planes (see also Chapter 6).

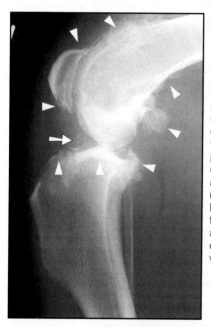

**10.29** ML view of a canine stifle with severe osteoarthrosis, showing osteophytes and enthesophytes on the tibia, the trochlear ridges, proximal and distal patella, and fabellae (arrowheads). Mineralized fragments (open arrow) and joint effusion are also visible.

## Infection

Septic arthritis of the stifle joint can occur:

- Secondary to joint arthrotomy
- Secondary to osteoarthrosis
- Following surgical repair of articular fractures
- Secondary to implant complications
- In association with acute haematogenous osteomyelitis.

The radiological changes associated with acute septic arthritis of the stifle include joint effusion, progressing to multiple subchondral lytic areas (Figure 10.30). Subchondral sclerosis and bony ankylosis may be seen in chronic cases. Fungal osteomyelitis (the most common causative agent in Europe is *Aspergillus*) can occasionally localize to the stifle joint. The most important differential diagnosis of septic arthritis is neoplasia, although immune-mediated polyarthropathies should also be considered. Synovial fluid analysis, in conjunction with synovial and bone biopsies of the affected area, is advised if the diagnosis is uncertain.

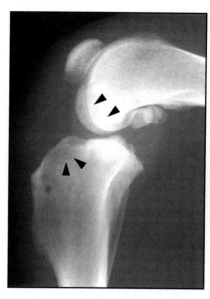

**10.30** ML view of a canine stifle with septic arthritis, secondary to surgery for a CCL rupture. Note the marked soft tissue swelling around the joint, a marked joint effusion and pinpoint radiolucencies in the femoral condyles and proximal tibia (arrowheads).

## Neoplasia

The stifle is a predilection site for synovial sarcoma. Abnormal radiological findings with this neoplasm can include marked soft tissue swelling, punctate areas of lysis in the distal femur and proximal tibia, and displacement of the patella by a soft tissue mass (Figure 10.31). Osteosarcoma can occur in the patella, distal femur or the proximal tibia (Figure 10.32). The main differential diagnoses with osteosarcoma are subchondral cysts, which may be seen in advanced osteoarthrosis and septic arthritis (See also Chapter 6).

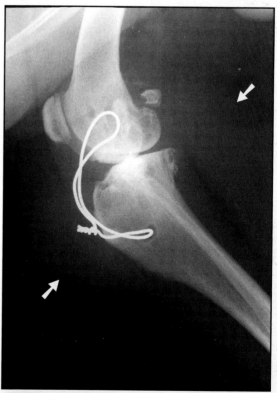

**10.31** ML view of a canine stifle with synovial sarcoma. Several 5 mm radiolucencies in the distal femur and proximal tibia are visible. Note also the marked soft tissue swelling around the joint (arrowed). The wire is from previous CCL surgery.

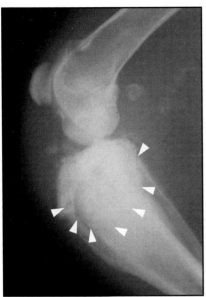

**10.32** ML view of a canine stifle with osteosarcoma of the proximal tibia, showing marked soft tissue swelling around the joint, mineralization of the soft tissues, increased radiopacity and irregularity of the proximal tibia (arrowheads). This is an unusual case as the patient is still skeletally immature and the neoplasm appears to enter the joint, which is rarely seen with osteosarcoma.

## Nutritional conditions

### Hypervitaminosis A

Hypervitaminosis A in adult cats develops in association with a diet based exclusively on raw liver. The stifle can be a predilection site for disease (after the elbow and spine) and is characterized radiologically by marked periarticular new bone formation at tendinous insertion points (see also Chapter 6).

## Miscellaneous conditions

### Synovial osteochondromatosis

Synovial osteochondromatosis is a condition seen occasionally in cats and, rarely, in dogs. Standard orthogonal radiographs reveal smooth intra- and periarticular mineralized bodies (Figure 10.33).

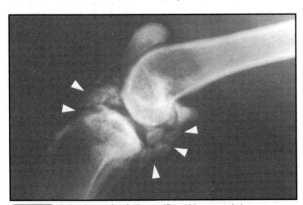

**10.33** ML view of a feline stifle with synovial osteochondromatosis, showing multiple smooth mineralized opacities located intra-articularly and periarticularly (arrowheads) in the synovium.

**Acknowledgements:** I would like to thank Mr John Conibear, Ms Tracy Dewey and Ms Fiona Skiera MRCVS for their assistance with the photographic and anatomical illustrations.

## References and further reading

Arnbjerg J and Heje NI (1993) Fabellae and popliteal sesamoid bones in cats. *Journal of Small Animal Practice* **34**, 95–98

Aron DN (1988) Traumatic dislocation of the stifle joint: treatment of 12 dogs and one cat. *Journal of the American Animal Hospital Association* **24**, 333–340

Baird DK, Hathcock JT, Rumph PF, Kincaid SA and Visco DM (1998) Low-field magnetic resonance imaging of the canine stifle joint: normal anatomy. *Veterinary Radiology and Ultrasound* **39**, 87–97

Banfield CM and Morrison WB (2000) Magnetic resonance arthrography of the canine stifle joint: technique and applications in eleven military dogs. *Veterinary Radiology and Ultrasound* **41**, 200–213

Bennett DT, Tennant B, Lewis DG, Baughan J, May C and Carter S (1988) A reappraisal of anterior cruciate ligament disease in the dog. *Journal of Small Animal Practice* **29**, 275–297

Denny H (1985) The canine stifle. II. Traumatic conditions. *British Veterinary Journal* **141**, 114–123

Denny HR and Butterworth SJ (2000) The stifle. In: *A Guide to Canine and Feline Orthopaedic Surgery, 4th edn*, pp. 512–553. Blackwell Science, Oxford

Engelke A, Meyer-Lindenberg A and Nolte I (1997) Ultrasonography of the stifle joint in dogs with rupture of the cruciate ligaments. *Deutsche Tierarztliche Wochenschrift* **104**, 114–117

Farrow CS (1982) Stress radiography: applications in small animal practice. *Journal of the American Veterinary Medical Association* **181**, 777–784

Fitch RB, Wilson ER, Hathcock JT and Montgomery RD (1997) Radiographic, computed tomographic and magnetic resonance imaging evaluation of a chronic long digital extensor tendon avulsion in a dog. *Veterinary Radiology and Ultrasound* **38**, 177–181

Gnudi G and Bertoni G (2001) Echographic examination of the stifle joint affected by cranial cruciate ligament rupture in the dog. *Veterinary Radiology and Ultrasound* **42**, 266–270

Hay CW, Aron DN, Roberts R, Stallings J and Brown J (1996) Evaluation of positive contrast arthrography in canine cranial cruciate ligament disease. *Veterinary and Comparative Orthopaedics and Traumatology* **9**, 10–13

Houlton JE and Ness MG (1993) Lateral fabellar fractures: a review of 8 cases. *Journal of Small Animal Practice* **34**, 349–352

Innes JF, Barr ARS, Patteson MW and Dieppe PA (1996) Scintigraphy in the evaluation of osteoarthritis of the canine stifle joint – relationship with clinical, radiographic and surgical observations. *Veterinary and Comparative Orthopaedics and Traumatology* **9**, 53–59

Kramer M, Gerwing M, Hach V and Schmike E (1997) Sonography of the musculoskeletal system in dogs and cats. *Veterinary Radiology and Ultrasound* **38**, 139–149

Kramer M, Stengel H, Gerwing M, Schmike E and Sheppard C (1999) Sonography of the canine stifle. *Veterinary Radiology and Ultrasound* **40**, 282–293

Mahoney PN and Lamb CR (1996) Articular, periarticular and juxta-articular calcified bodies in the dog and cat: A radiologic review. *Veterinary Radiology and Ultrasound* **37**, 3–19

Muir P and Dueland RT (1994) Avulsion of the origin of the medial head of the gastrocnemius muscle in a dog. *Veterinary Record* **135**, 359–360

Ralphs S (2005) Bilateral stifle osteochondritis dissecans in a cat. *Journal of the American Animal Hospital Association* **41**, 78–80

Schwarz T, Johnson VS, Voute L and Sullivan M (2004) Bone scintigraphy in the investigation of occult lameness in the dog. *Journal of Small Animal Practice* **45**, 232–237

Singleton WB (1969) The surgical correction of stifle deformities in the dog. *Journal of Small Animal Practice* **10**, 59–69

Vaughan LC (1979) Muscle and tendon injuries in dogs. *Journal of Small Animal Practice* **20**, 711–736

Widmer WR, Buckwalter KA, Braunstein EM, Visco DM and O'Connor BL (1991) Principles of magnetic resonance imaging and application to the stifle joint in dogs. *Journal of the American Veterinary Medical Association* **198**, 1914–1922

# 11

# Distal limbs – carpus and tarsus

## Graeme Allan and Robert Nicoll

## Indications

The following are some of the indications for radiography of the distal extremities:

- Lameness that can be related to a distal extremity
- Pain on manipulation or palpation of a joint or region
- Unexplained or unresolved swelling
- Signs of joint laxity
- Postural abnormalities, such as hyperextension of a joint or angular limb deformity (valgus or varus malformation)
- Suspected immune-mediated joint disease.

## Radiography and normal anatomy

### Radiography

#### Technique

Bones and joints of the distal extremities are radiographed using fine detail receptors and a low kVp technique. Ideally a kVp range between 45 and 60 should be selected. Fine detail screens and double emulsion film will usually provide adequate detail of small osseous structures but for added detail a single emulsion detail film and a cassette loaded with a single detail intensifying screen can be used. With this system the emulsion side of the film is placed against the single intensifying screen when the film is loaded into the cassette. A notch in the edge of the film facilitates identification of the emulsion side of the film in the darkroom.

#### Standardized terminology

The antebrachiocarpal and tarsocrural joints define a nomenclature barrier, with craniocaudal describing a caudally directed beam direction proximal to these joints and dorsopalmar and dorsoplantar describing the beam direction distally. The forepaw is the *manus* and the hindpaw the *pes*. Lateral and medial are used to describe the outer and inner sides of an extremity.

#### Positioning and labelling

Standard views are used when the joints are being radiographed. These, along with additional and special radiographic views, are summarized in Figure 11.1.

Care must be taken to identify medial and lateral aspects of the manus or pes if the region of interest within the radiograph does not include the carpus or tarsus, as differentiation of medial and lateral digits can be difficult

|  | Standard views | Special views |
|---|---|---|
| *Carpus and manus* | | |
| Antebrachiocarpal joint | DPa ML | DLPaMO DMPaLO ML flexed ML extended DPa medially stressed DPa laterally stressed |
| Carpus, carpometacarpus | DPa ML | DLPaMO DMPaLO ML flexed DPa medially stressed DPa laterally stressed ML extended |
| Manus | DPa ML | ML splayed toe |
| *Tarsus and pes* | | |
| Tarsocrural joint | PID ML | PILDMO PIMDLO ML flexed ML extended PID medially stressed PID laterally stressed DPI flexed skyline |
| Tarsus, tarsometatarsus | PID ML | PILDMO PIMDLO ML flexed ML extended PID medially stressed PID laterally stressed |
| Pes | PID ML | ML splayed toe |

**Note:** Dorsopalmar and plantarodorsal have been used to describe beam orientation for radiography of the distal extremities. Depending on user preference, palmarodorsal and dorsoplantar may be used interchangeably for these radiographic views.

**11.1** Radiographic views of the distal joints of the appendicular skeleton.

without the presence of differentiating anatomical structures in the field of view. Sedation or general anaesthesia may be required to position the patient optimally, particularly as affected regions may be painful due to underlying pathology. This is especially so with stress radiographs and lateral splayed toe radiographs.

## Standard views

***Dorsopalmar:*** A dorsopalmar (DPa) radiograph is taken with the patient in sternal recumbency and the forelimb extended with the palmar surface placed on the cassette. The primary beam is centred on the area of interest. A shallow foam padded trough placed beneath the elbow will assist in stabilizing and aligning the limb (Figure 11.2).

***Plantarodorsal:*** A plantarodorsal (PID) radiograph is taken with the patient in sternal recumbency and the hindlimb extended caudally with the dorsum placed on the cassette. The primary beam is centred on the region of interest. A shallow foam padded trough placed beneath the stifle will assist in stabilizing and aligning the limb (Figures 11.3 and 11.4). There will be occasions where the dorsoplantar (DPI) view is easier to acquire than the PID view.

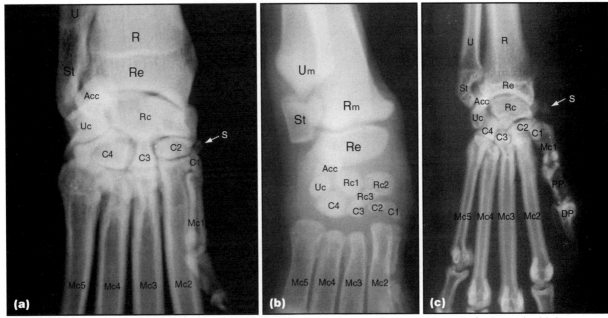

**11.2** **(a)** DPa view of a normal carpus in a mature dog. **(b)** DPa view of a normal carpus of a 2-month-old dog. **(c)** DPa view of a normal carpus of a mature cat. Acc = Accessory carpal bone; C1 = First carpal bone; C2 = Second carpal bone; C3 = Third carpal bone; C4 = Fourth carpal bone; DP = Distal phalanx of first digit; Mc (1–5) = Individual metacarpal bones; PP = Proximal phalanx of first digit; R = Radius; Rc = Radial carpal bone; Rc (1–3) = Three separate ossification centres that fuse to form the radial carpal bone; Re = Radial epiphysis; Rm = Radial metaphysis; S = Sesamoid bone in the abductor pollicis longus muscle; St = Styloid process of the ulna; U = Ulna; Uc = Ulnar carpal bone; Um = Ulnar metaphysis.

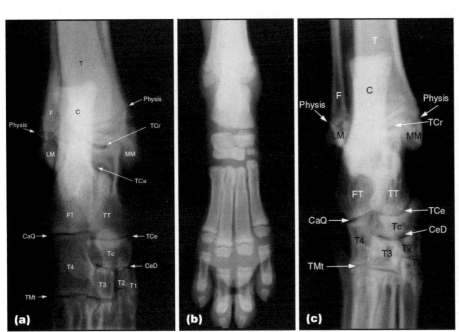

**11.3** **(a)** PID view of a normal tarsus of an immature dog. **(b)** PID view of a normal tarsus of a 2-month-old dog. **(c)** PID view of a normal tarsus of an immature cat. C = Calcaneus; CaQ = Calcaneoquartile joint; CeD = Centrodistal joint; F = Fibula; FT = Fibular tarsal bone; LM = Lateral malleolus; MM = Medial malleolus; T = Tibia; T1 = First tarsal bone; T2 = Second tarsal bone; T3 = Third tarsal bone; T4 = Fourth tarsal bone; Tc = Central tarsal bone; TCa = Talocalcaneal joint; TCe = Talocentral joint; TCr = Tarsocrural joint; TMt = Tarsometatarsal joint; TT = Tibial tarsal bone.

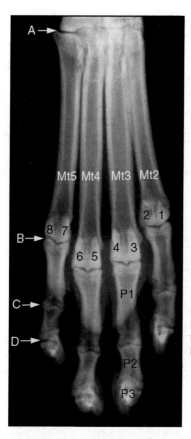

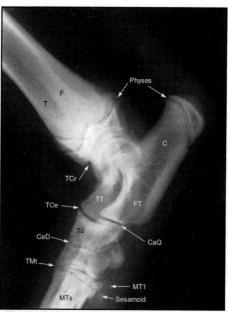

**11.4** PID view of a normal pes of a mature cat. 1–8 = Individual plantar metatarsophalangeal sesamoid bones; A = Tarsometatarsal joint; B = Metatarsophalangeal joint; C = Proximal interphalangeal joint; D = Distal interphalangeal joint; Mt2 = Second metatarsal bone; Mt3 = Third metatarsal bone; Mt4 = Fourth metatarsal bone; Mt5 = Fifth metatarsal bone; P1 = First phalanx; P2 = Second phalanx; P3 = Third phalanx.

**11.6** ML view of a normal tarsus of an immature dog. C = Calcaneus; CaQ = Calcaneoquartile joint; CeD = Centrodistal joint; F = Fibula; FT = Fibular tarsal bone; MT1 = First metatarsal bone; MTs = Metatarsal bones; T = Tibia; Tc = Central tarsal bone; TCe = Talocentral joint; TCr = Tarsocrural joint; TMt = Tarsometatarsal joint; TT = Tibial tarsal bone.

**Mediolateral:** A mediolateral (ML) radiograph is taken with the patient in lateral recumbency with the non-recumbent limb displaced so that it does not intercept the primary beam. The area of interest should be on and parallel to the cassette. The beam is centred on the area of interest (Figures 11.5 to 11.7).

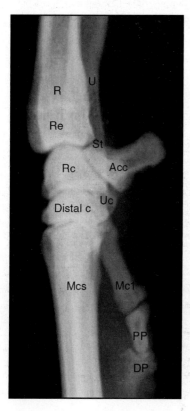

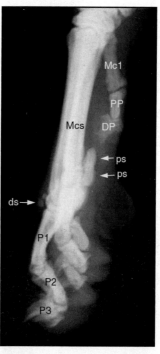

**11.5** ML view of a normal carpus of a mature cat. Acc = Accessory carpal bone; Distal c = Distal row of carpal bones; DP = Distal phalanx of first digit; Mc1 = First metacarpal bone; Mcs = Metacarpal bones; PP = Proximal phalanx of first digit; R = Radius; Rc = Radial carpal bone; Re = Radial epiphysis; St = Styloid process of the ulna; U = Ulna; Uc = Ulnar carpal bone.

**11.7** ML view of a normal manus of a mature cat. DP = Distal phalanx; ds = Dorsal metacarpophalangeal sesamoids; Mc1 = First metacarpal bone; Mcs = Metacarpal bones; P1 = First phalanx; P2 = Second phalanx; P3 = Third phalanx; PP = Proximal phalanx; ps = Palmar metacarpophalangeal sesamoids.

## Special views

**Lateral oblique:** Lateral oblique (PILDMO, DLPaMO) images may be taken with the limb positioned as for DPa or PID views. The area of interest is then obliqued so that the limb is aligned at approximately 45 degrees to the primary beam, which enters DL or PIL, and exits PaM (PIM) or DM, depending on whether it is a fore or hindlimb. Different users may prefer different angles of obliquity, but 45 degrees is the common angle used (Figures 11.8 and 11.9).

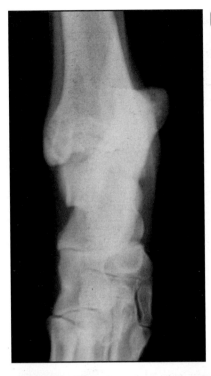

**11.8** PILDMO view of a canine tarsus. In this image the plantaromedial and dorsolateral aspects of the hock joint are visualized.

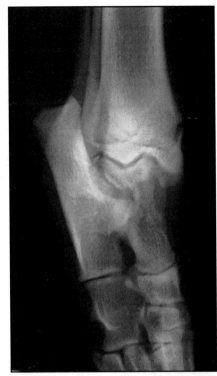

**11.10** PIMDLO view of a canine tarsus. In this image the plantarolateral and dorsomedial aspects of the hock joint are visualized.

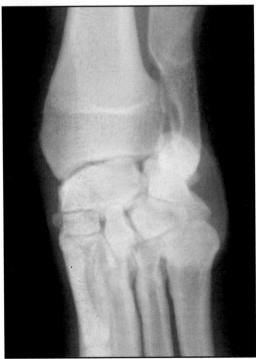

**11.9** DLPaMO view of a normal carpus of a mature dog. In this image the dorsomedial and palmarolateral aspects of the carpus are visualized.

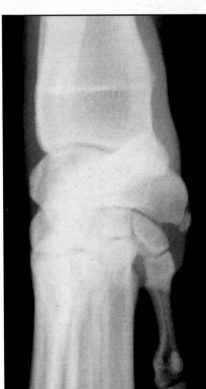

**11.11** DMPaLO view of a normal carpus of a mature dog. In this image the dorsolateral and palmaromedial aspects of the carpus are visualized.

*Medial oblique:* Medial oblique (PIMDLO, DMPaLO) images may be taken with the limb positioned as for DPa or PID views. The area of interest is then obliqued so that the limb is aligned at approximately 45 degrees to the primary beam, which enters DM (PIM) and exits DL (PaL or PIL), depending on whether it is a fore or hindlimb. Different users may prefer different angles of obliquity, but 45 degrees is the common angle used (Figures 11.10 and 11.11).

*Mediolateral maximally flexed:* Mediolateral maximally flexed (ML flexed) images are taken with the animal in lateral recumbency with the non-recumbent limb displaced so that it does not intercept the primary beam. The area of interest should be on and parallel to the cassette. The beam is centred on the joint of interest, which is maximally flexed. Flexion requires the use of tape and sandbags to maintain the joint in the desired position (Figure 11.12).

153

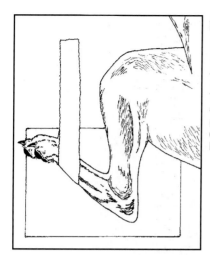

**11.12**
ML flexed view of a canine hock. Adhesive tape is used to hold the tarsocrural joint in a fully flexed position. (Courtesy of B Benshoof.)

*Mediolateral maximally extended:* Mediolateral maximally extended (ML extended) images are taken with the animal in lateral recumbency with the non-recumbent limb displaced so that it does not intercept the primary beam. The area of interest should be on and parallel to the cassette. The beam is centred on the joint of interest, which is maximally extended. Extension requires the use of tape and sandbags to maintain the joint in the desired position (Figure 11.13).

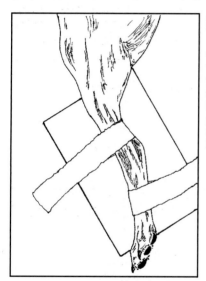

**11.13**
ML extended view of a canine tarsus. Adhesive tape is used to stabilize the hock in the extended position. (Courtesy of B Benshoof.)

*Stress views:* Stress radiographic views of the carpi and tarsi are used to illustrate joint instabilities or to disclose fractures, although care should be taken when fractures are suspected to minimize further displacement of fragments.

*Medially and laterally stressed dorsopalmar or plantarodorsal:* For DPa or PID medially and laterally stressed views the patient is positioned as for the DPa or PID view. The limb will need to be stabilized (tape, sandbags) to permit stress to be applied to the medial or lateral surface of the joint in question and to move the manus or pes laterally and medially. This will disclose any collateral joint laxity (Figure 11.14).

The application of stress requires the use of tape and sandbags to maintain the joint in the desired position (Figure 11.15).

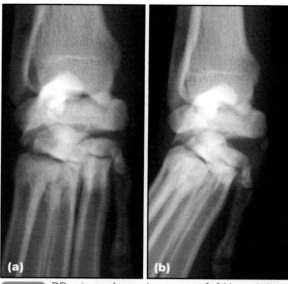

**(a)**   **(b)**

**11.14**   DPa views of a canine carpus. **(a)** Neutral view. There appears to be rotation of the distal row of carpal bones and opening of the medial aspect of the intercarpal articulation. **(b)** Stress applied to the medial aspect of the joint depicting intercarpal rotation and laxity.

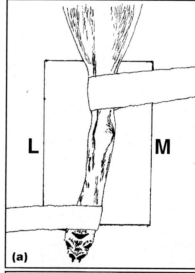

**(a)**

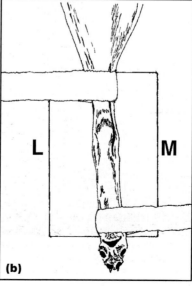

**(b)**

**11.15**
Set-up for the application of stress tarsal views. The tarsus is stabilized by adhesive tape. **(a)** Maximum stress is applied to the medial aspect of the tarsus. **(b)** Maximum stress is applied to the lateral aspect of the tarsus. (Courtesy of B Benshoof.)

*Other applications of stress during radiography:* Traction and rotation views are described in Chapter 6.

***Splayed toe mediolateral:*** ML splayed toe images are taken with the patient positioned in lateral recumbency, as for ML radiography. Tape is applied to the medial and lateral toes, which are pulled in a dorsal and palmar (plantar) direction, respectively. The use of adhesive tape simplifies the process, as the adhesive can be used to fix the toes to the cassette in the splayed position. This view enables each toe to be seen in isolation in the ML view (Figure 11.16). This view can also be used to disclose fractures that are difficult to see on routine DPa views (Figure 11.17).

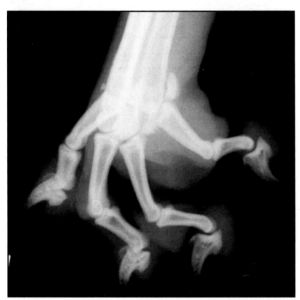

**11.16**   ML radiograph of the digits. The second and fifth digit have been taped in the splayed position to enable all phalanges to be seen individually.

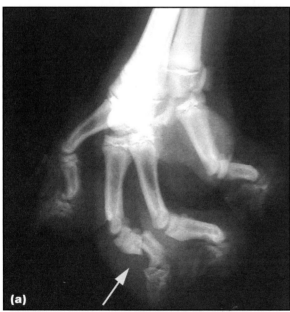

**11.17**   A juvenile dog with a transverse mid-diaphyseal fracture of P2. **(a)** ML view of a splayed toe radiograph. Arrow denotes the fracture. (Courtesy of Mountains Animal Hospital.) (continues) ▶

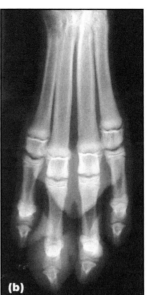

**11.17**
(continued) A juvenile dog with a transverse mid-diaphyseal fracture of P2. **(b)** PID view. Note that the phalangeal fracture is not visible in this view. (Courtesy of Mountains Animal Hospital.)

***Flexed dorsoplantar:*** Flexed dorsoplantar (DPI flexed) images are taken with the patient in dorsal recumbency. A foam pad 10–15 cm thick is placed beneath the tarsus and the tarsocrural joint is flexed so that the pes points towards the collimator of the X-ray machine, 15 degrees off the perpendicular. This flexed view permits a skyline view of the curved tarsocrural joint surfaces, avoiding superimposition of the calcaneus (Figure 11.18).

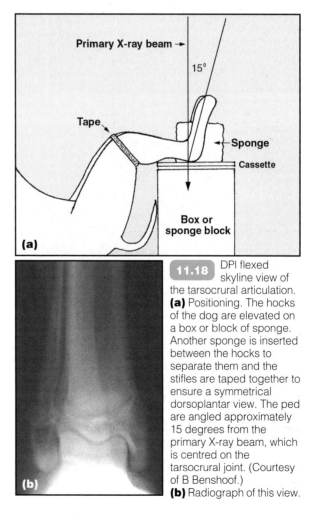

**11.18**   DPI flexed skyline view of the tarsocrural articulation. **(a)** Positioning. The hocks of the dog are elevated on a box or block of sponge. Another sponge is inserted between the hocks to separate them and the stifles are taped together to ensure a symmetrical dorsoplantar view. The ped are angled approximately 15 degrees from the primary X-ray beam, which is centred on the tarsocrural joint. (Courtesy of B Benshoof.) **(b)** Radiograph of this view.

## Normal anatomy

The joints of the carpi, tarsi and feet are diarthrodial joints. Opposing bones are lined with joint cartilage and in other places the joints are lined with synovium, which provides synovial fluid that lubricates each joint. The carpus, tarsus and the individual joints of the feet have a joint capsule and are supported by medial and lateral collateral ligaments. Intra-articular ligaments provide further support to the carpus and tarsus. Extra-articular tendons of various flexor and extensor muscles are located around the carpus and tarsus and on the dorsal and palmar/plantar surfaces of the joints of the feet. On the medial side of the carpus one of these tendons, that of the abductor pollicis longus muscle, contains a sesamoid bone that is usually clearly visible in most dogs and cats (Figure 11.19). On the plantar margins of the tarsometatarsal articulation there may be two sesamoids in dogs, one being the lateral plantar tarso-metatarsal bone and the other the intra-articular tarsometatarsal bone (Figure 11.20). Three sesamoid bones are seen adjacent to each metacarpo/metatarso-phalangeal joint (Figure 11.21).

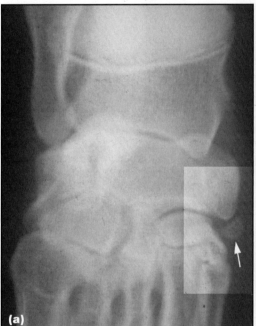
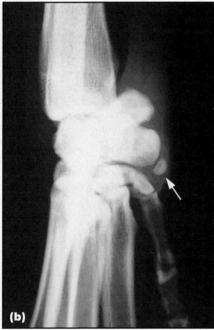

**11.19**
Carpal radiographs of a dog. The arrow points to the sesamoid bone in the tendon of the abductor pollicis longus muscle. **(a)** DPa view. **(b)** DMPaLO view.

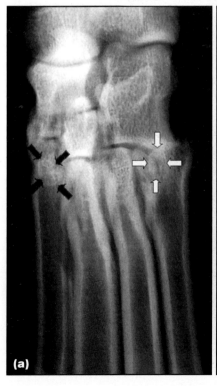
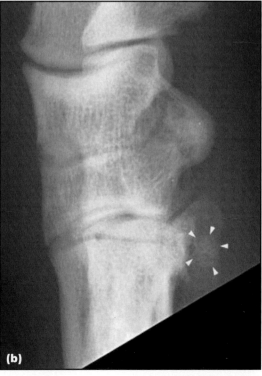

**11.20**
Tarsal radiographs in a dog depicting the two sesamoid bones on the plantar surface of the tarsometatarsal articulation. **(a)** PID view. The black arrows point to the intra-articular tarsometatarsal bone, which is medially located. The white arrows point to the lateral plantar tarsometatarsal bone. **(b)** ML view. One of the plantar tarsometatarsal sesamoids is defined by the white arrows.

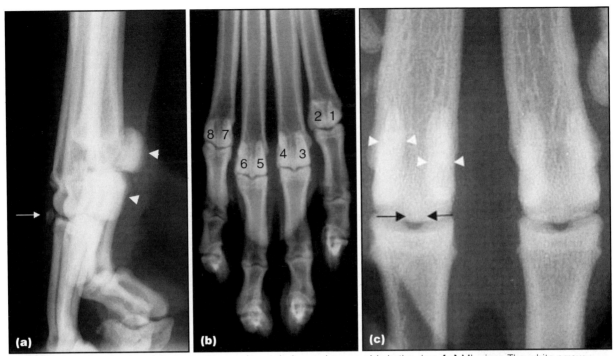

**11.21** Dorsal and palmar/plantar metacarpo/tarsophalangeal sesamoids in the dog. **(a)** ML view. The white arrow points to the single dorsal sesamoid bone located in the extensor tendons. The white arrowheads point to the palmar (plantar) sesamoids. **(b)** DPa/PID view. The palmar/plantar sesamoid bones are numbered from medial to lateral. **(c)** Close-up image of (b) demonstrating the margins of the paired palmar (plantar) sesamoid bones (white arrowheads) and the single dorsally located sesamoid (black arrows).

## Ossification centres and physeal closure
In most dogs and cats ossification centres appear and physes close at predictable times (see Chapter 3).

*Delayed appearance of ossification centres:* The common causes for delayed appearance of ossification centres are congenital disorders of enchondral ossification (as in Alaskan Malamute chondrodystrophy) or congenital disorders that affect the hormonal pathways that control bone growth (e.g. hypothyroidism and hypopituitarism) (see Chapter 3).

*Early closure of physes:* Normal physes are believed to close earlier in miniature dogs and later in giant breeds. The most common cause of early or premature closure of physes is trauma.

*Delayed closure of physes:* In cats, physeal closure may be delayed in gonadectomized animals when compared with intact animals. Consequently, the length of long bones (e.g. radius) is greater in gonadectomized cats, which demonstrate delayed physeal closure, than in gonadally intact animals. Age of gonadectomy is more critical in female cats (those that are gonadectomized prepubertally) than in male cats.

### Incidental findings

*Variation in number of bones:* Supernumerary digits (polydactyly; Figure 11.22) and aplasia of bones (Figure 11.23) are seen in the pes and manus of dogs and cats. In the pes, the dewclaw may be duplicated and in its most rudimentary form may be attached to the pes

by skin, without any other articular or osseous attachment. In some animals duplication of the entire first phalanx is encountered (see Figure 11.24).

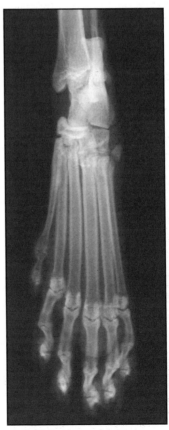

**11.22** PID view of the pes of a cat with supernumerary digits. There were six digits on each foot. (Courtesy of Forest Animal Hospital).

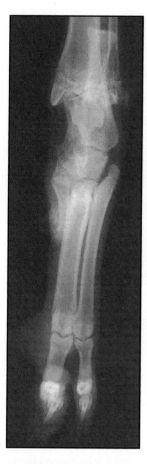

**11.23** PID view of a kitten with congenital absence of the medial pair of digits and their adjacent tarsal bones. (Courtesy of the Enfield Veterinary Hospital.)

*Variation in size and shape of bones:* Variation in the number of bones in the distal row of tarsal bones, and variation in the shape of the central tarsal bone are common in some breeds of dog (Rottweiler, Pyrenean Mountain Dog, Newfoundland, St. Bernard). The first tarsal and metatarsal bones may be fused, or the first metatarsal may be present as a separate, normally formed bone. Hypoplasia of individual bones or groups of bones also occurs sporadically (Figures 11.24 and 11.25).

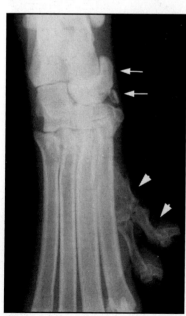

**11.24** PID view of the tarsus of a Bernese Mountain Dog. The arrows show the additional bones that are fused to the central tarsal bones. The arrowheads point to a paired dewclaw and a fused pair of first metatarsal bones. (Courtesy of C Bailey.)

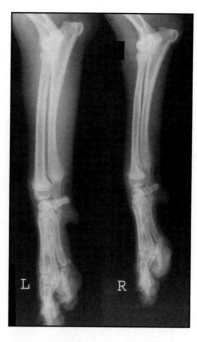

**11.25** ML view of the forelimbs of a dog with brachycarpo-metacarpalia. Note that the bones of the right forelimb (R) are smaller and shorter than those of the left forelimb (L).

*Mach bands:* The term Mach band originally described an optical illusion where a line or region of changed opacity was 'seen' at the junction of two different opacities. In radiology the term has been applied to the dark line that runs along the edge of a curved osseous surface, which is superimposed on another curved osseous surface. These are commonly seen in the feet, when the cortices of the metacarpal or metatarsal bones are seen superimposed on a radiograph (Figure 11.26).

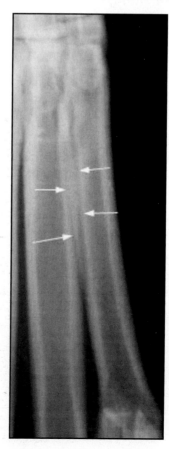

**11.26** DPa view. Mach bands seen where two metacarpal bones are superimposed (arrowed).

## Contrast studies

Positive contrast fistulography has been described for use in the distal limb as a means of detecting foreign bodies associated with draining sinuses, but has limited practical use. A negative result does not rule out the presence of foreign body (see Chapter 1).

## Alternative imaging techniques

The complexity of the cuboidal joints (carpus and tarsus) combined with their inherent dependence upon structural support of ligaments, tendons and joint capsules can make radiological detection of subtle bony and fibrous tissue injuries difficult. In situations where routine and stress radiographic examinations fail to define the cause of lameness adequately, alternative imaging modalities can be used.

### Computed tomography

While rarely indicated for use in the manus or pes, computed tomography (CT) does provide advantages over radiography in evaluation of the carpus and tarsus. Subtle fractures and osteochondral defects not evident in radiographs may be diagnosed with CT examinations (Figure 11.27). In addition, software manipulation of the data acquired during CT examination allows three dimensional reconstructions of complex fractures and virtual disarticulation to evaluate individual bones.

### Magnetic resonance imaging

Although use is currently limited in clinical practice due to cost and accessibility, magnetic resonance imaging (MRI) provides exquisite detail of the soft tissues

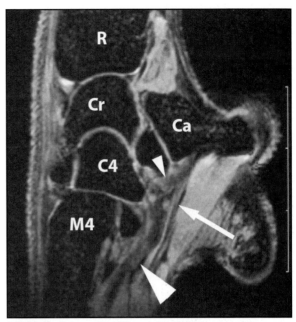

**11.28** Parasagittal T2-weighted MR image of the normal carpus of a Coon Hound. The accessorioquartile ligament (small arrowhead) is evident, extending from the accessory carpal bone (Ca) dorsodistally to the palmar margin of the fourth carpal bone (C4). The accessoriometacarpal (arrowed) and palmar carpometacarpal (large arrowhead) ligaments are also evident, extending distally to the palmar metacarpal bones (M4). (Courtesy of KA Johnson.)

supporting the distal limbs (Figure 11.28). The identification and characterization of tendon and ligament injuries is possible using this modality. Similarly, early detection of chondral lesions and non-deforming bone injuries (bone bruises and non-displaced fractures) is possible with MRI.

**11.27** A retired racing Greyhound with a slab fracture of the third tarsal bone. **(a)** Flexed ML view showing osteophyte formation on dorsal margin of the distal intertarsal joint. Additional views could not reveal the fracture.
**(b)** Parasagittal plane CT image of the tarsus. Contiguous 2 mm thick images were viewed with bone windows. The tibia (Ti), talus (Ta), central tarsal bone (Tc) and third tarsal bone (T3) were identified proximal to the metatarsus. On the dorsodistal margin of the central tarsal bone a periarticular osteophyte was evident (arrowhead). The dorsal slab fragment (arrowed) was separated from the third tarsal bone by a thin hypodense fracture line with minimal displacement. (Courtesy of KA Johnson.)

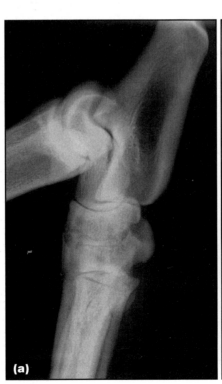

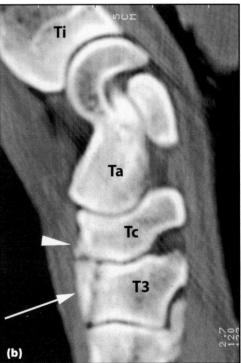

## Scintigraphy

In rare instances where localization of lameness cannot be made, scintigraphic examination may be utilized. Differentiation between serendipitous and significant radiological lesions may be possible using angiographic, soft tissue and bone phases of the study. Appendicular degloving, crushing or shearing injuries may result in complete or segmental loss of vascular supply (Figure 11.29), with the distal limb being more vulnerable. Scintigraphy may be used to determine the viability of bone and soft tissues in these injuries.

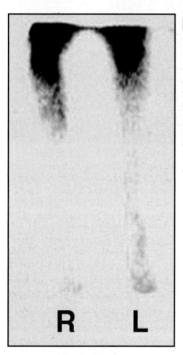

**11.29**

Soft tissue phase scintigram of the extremities of a dog using technetium-99M. Relative hypovascularity is present in the right extremity, which was involved in a degloving injury.

## Ultrasonography

Ultrasonographic examination may be used to evaluate tendon and ligament injuries as well as to detect foreign bodies within soft tissues. In practice, the small amount of soft tissue overlying the bones of the distal limbs limits the use of diagnostic ultrasonography to high resolution imaging. The irregular contours limit transducer contact unless a flexible standoff pad is used. Injuries involving the insertion of the Achilles apparatus upon the calcaneal tuberosity are most commonly evaluated.

## Abnormal radiological findings

### Trauma

#### Fractures and avulsions

Articular and periarticular fractures are common in the bones and joints of the feet. They may involve avulsion of a malleolus or tuberosity where a tendinous or capsular insertion is involved. Intra-articular fractures of individual carpal or tarsal bones may be induced by direct trauma or by stress during athletic activity. Because the extent of soft tissue injury is difficult to assess using standard views, stress views have been developed so that the extent of both bony and soft tissue injury can be fully assessed.

### Salter–Harris fractures that affect joints

Physeal fractures (classified as Salter–Harris type III or IV) are fractures that, when complete, enter the adjacent joint space (see Chapter 5). Physes are located at the ends of the long bones adjacent to the carpi and tarsi, the distal end of the metacarpal and metatarsal bones and the proximal end of P1 and P2. The proximal metacarpal and metatarsal physes are closed at birth, so rarely present a clinical problem, but their distal physis and the adjacent proximal physes of P1 and P1 are prone to injury as their closure is later.

Non-displaced physeal injuries (Salter–Harris type V) may require serial radiographic examination for identification. Additionally, injuries that result in angular limb deformities proximal to the carpus (see Chapter 3) and tarsus may lead to aberrant stress loads on developing bones or supporting ligaments, and subsequent osteoarthrosis.

### Sprains and loss of tendon support

Complete rupture of supportive ligaments results in loss of stability, which, if not entirely evident on physical examination (Figure 11.30), can usually be demonstrated in stress radiographs.

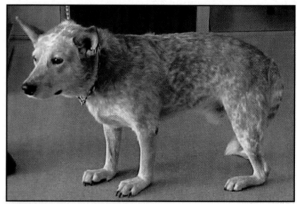

**11.30** A middle-aged Cattle Dog cross-breed with hyperextension of both carpi and tarsi.

Incomplete tear or sprain of ligaments can be more difficult to identify radiologically. In acute injuries, soft tissue swelling may be detected. Over time, fibrosis may persist and therefore remain evident as a soft tissue swelling. In many instances, enthesophytes may form at the site of origin or insertion of the damaged ligaments. Mineralization of scar tissue within torn fibrous tissues may also develop, and within ligaments will usually follow the course of the affected structure. Acute exacerbation of chronic desmopathies commonly occurs, resulting in a mixture of soft tissue swelling and mineralization at the site of injury. In the distal limbs such changes commonly affect collateral ligaments of the injured phalanges, the metacarpo(tarso)phalangeal joints, and the cuboidal joints.

The presence of mineralization and swelling alone is not sufficient to reach a diagnosis as these radiological changes can persist beyond the time of pain (Figures 11.31 to 11.33). For instance, Greyhounds with radiological evidence of mineralization of the shorter collateral ligament of the radio-carpal articulation may have no signs of lameness. Similarly, the presence of enthesophytes at the site of origin of the plantar ligaments and fibrocartilage of the tarsometatarsal joint (on the plantarodistal aspect of the calcaneus) or of the palmar ligaments (on the distal margin of the accessory carpal bone) must be correlated with evidence of significant pain on palpation and hyperextension of the adjacent joint. (For further information on sprains and loss of tendon support see Chapter 6.)

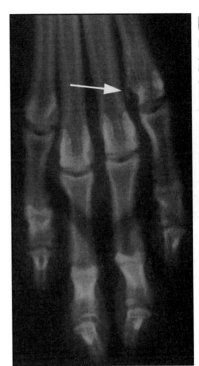

**11.33**
DPa view of digits. An enthesophyte on the axial surface of a metacarpal bone (arrowed) signifies a chronic injury to the medial metacarpophalangeal collateral ligament of the manus of a dog. (Courtesy of Coreen Avenue Veterinary Clinic).

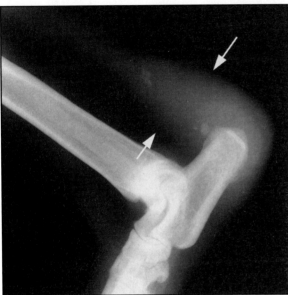

**11.31**   ML tarsal view of a dog. There is thickened soft tissue proximal to and around the calcaneus (arrowed). Within the thickened soft tissue foci of calcification are evident; these changes represent a chronic tendinopathy of the tendons of insertion of the Achilles tendon. (Courtesy of Petersham Veterinary Hospital.)

### Luxations and high-rise syndrome

Traumatic luxation of the joints of the distal extremities is commonly encountered. When destabilization of the radio-carpal joint or tarsocrural joint is the result of a fractured malleolus or styloid process, simple reduction and stabilization of the joint can usually be achieved by reducing and stabilizing the fractured osseous support. The aptly named 'high-rise' syndrome, seen more commonly in cats than in dogs and so-called as it describes the injuries sustained after an animal falls from a tall building, presents a variety of injuries that includes carpal hyperextension (Figure 11.34).

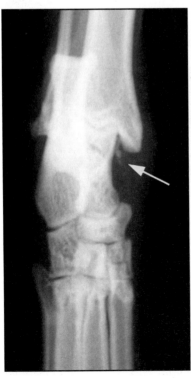

**11.32**   DPl view of cat tarsus. A fine line of soft tissue calcification (arrowed) is the result of avulsion of the origin of the medial collateral ligament from the medial malleolus. (Courtesy of Sylvania Veterinary Hospital.)

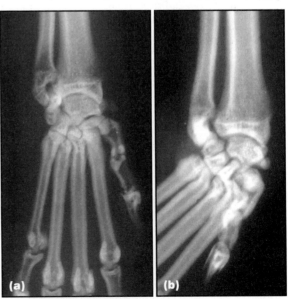

**11.34**   Feline carpus with ligamentous injuries. **(a)** DPa looks normal. **(b)** DPa view illustrating medial instability induced by stress radiography. (Courtesy of the Kippax Veterinary Hospital.) (continues) ▶

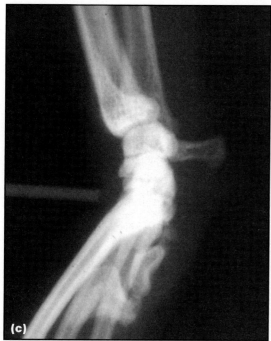

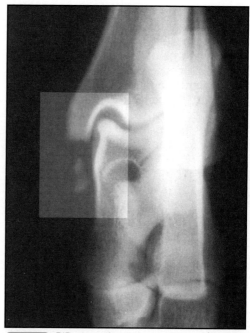

**11.34**   Feline carpus with ligamentous injuries. **(c)** ML view with palmar instability induced by stress radiography. (Courtesy of the Kippax Veterinary Hospital.)

**11.36**   PID view of the tarsus of a racing Greyhound. There is mineralization within soft tissues on the medial aspect of the joint, representing avulsion of the medial collateral ligament of the joint.

### Disorders of racing dogs

Racing dogs (e.g. Greyhounds) are subject to activity-specific injuries to the bones and joints of the extremities. Common foot injuries, such as cuts, penetrating wounds and foreign bodies, and bruises often require survey radiography to rule out more important problems. Nail bed infections (paronychia) may be superimposed on painful conditions, such as phalangeal fractures or luxations. Flexor tendon desmopathies and low grade hyperextension injuries represent a series of conditions that can be evaluated with sensitive imaging modalities, such as ultrasonography and MRI.

Radiography (Figures 11.35 and 11.36) is used to evaluate carpal and tarsal injuries, such as slab and compression fractures of the carpal bones, which are common track injuries. Another common injury is luxation of a digit (sprung toe). The more insidious metacarpal stress osteitis that is seen in racing Greyhounds can lead to comminuted fractures of the affected bone if not detected and treated. Stress osteitis is prevalent in the metacarpi, and is always more serious in the metacarpal bones of each manus nearest to the centre of the track (Figure 11.37); when dogs race in an anticlockwise direction, it is Mc5 of the left manus and Mc2 of the right manus that will be preferentially affected. If affected animals are not rested, osteitis will appear in other metacarpals with descending frequency in metacarpals that take less stress.

**11.35**

Comminuted fracture of the central and fourth tarsal bones of a racing Greyhound. **(a)** ML view. **(b)** PID view.

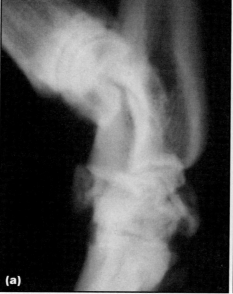

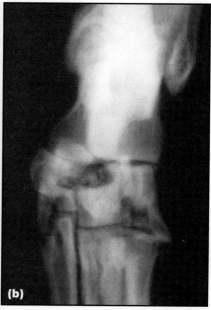

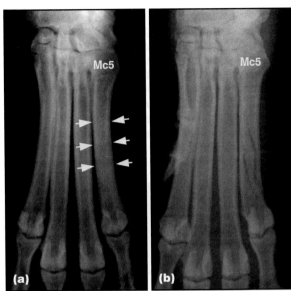

**11.37** DPa views of the left metacarpal region of a racing Greyhound, trained and raced running in an anticlockwise direction. **(a)** Note the increased osseous opacity in the diaphysis of the fifth metacarpal bone (Mc5; arrowed), which represents a region of stress osteitis in the left forelimb. **(b)** A comminuted fracture of Mc5. (Courtesy of Gladesville Veterinary Hospital.)

## Achilles apparatus

The most common injuries affecting the Achilles tendon of small animals are a consequence of direct trauma. Usually, the affected region is the distal tendon or the site of insertion on the calcaneal tuberosity. Tears may be partial or complete, and either acute or chronic, although the latter frequently present as acute exacerbation of a chronic problem. Diagnosis is usually made clinically, but radiographs may assist in defining the involvement of the calcaneus (avulsions or fractures) as well as provide evidence of chronicity, seen as dystrophic mineralization within the tendon (see Figure 11.31). Ultrasonographic examination of affected tendons may assist in differentiating tendon and peritendinous injuries, and assessing response to therapy (Figure 11.38).

## Congenital and developmental disorders

### Conformational anomalies

Congenital conformational anomalies, such as lateral rotation of the tarsus or metatarsus (prevalent in Great Danes, St. Bernards, Bernese Mountain Dogs, Italian Spinones and Rottweilers), is a recognized conformational disorder. There appears to be a high correlation between the presence of metatarsal rotation and variations in the anatomy of the first digit.

### Carpal flexural deformity

Attributed to asynchronous development of the feet and flexor tendons, carpal flexural deformity is recognized by the curled toes and flexed digits that are visible in affected individuals. The condition affects puppies in the first year of life (Figure 11.39). From a radiological perspective the feet appear normal.

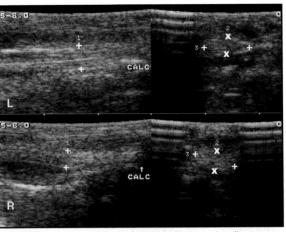

**11.38** Ultrasonogram of the Achilles tendon (between + and X) imaged in sagittal and transverse planes. The left tendon appears normal in both planes. Fibres within the tendon appear as hyperechoic linear echoes in the sagittal plane and stippled echogenic foci in the transverse plane. The right tendon is thickened and its margins are less well defined. There are less linear echoes in the sagittal plane and stippled foci are less echoic in the transverse plane, indicative of damaged (torn) fibres. CALC = Calcaneus.

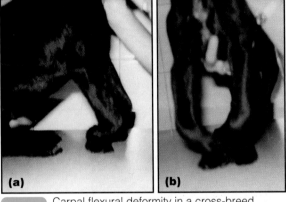

**11.39** Carpal flexural deformity in a cross-breed puppy. **(a)** Side view. **(b)** Front view.

### Supernumerary or missing bones

For information on supernumerary and missing bones, see Incidental findings above.

### Osteochondritis dissecans

Osteochondritis dissecans (OCD) occurs in the tarsocrural joint, being located on either the medial (most frequently) or lateral trochlear ridge of the talus. When located on the medial ridge it manifests radiologically as a crescent-shaped subchondral bone fragment adjacent to the medial ridge. An important accompanying sign is increased width of the medial tarsocrural joint space. OCD manifests a different appearance on the lateral side, where it develops as an oblique osteochondral fracture through the lateral condyle. This fragmentation of the lateral ridge produces a large osseous 'joint mouse' within the lateral side of the tarsocrural joint (Figures 11.40 and 11.41). If left untreated OCD will lead to severe osteoarthrosis.

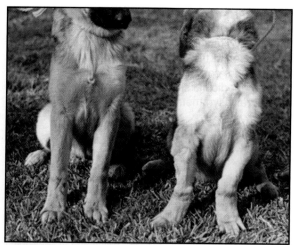

**11.45** German Shepherd Dog litter mates. The dog on the left has normally formed and straight legs. The dog on the right has chondrodystrophoid malformation of both forelimbs.

In the same way, physeal trauma involving the distal radius, ulna or tibia is capable of resulting in angular deformities of the carpi or tarsi (see also Chapters 3 and 8). When the ulna fails to grow in synchrony with the radius because of retained cartilage cores in the distal ulna, the consequences mirror those seen with retarded ulnar growth due the distal ulnar physeal trauma (Figure 11.46).

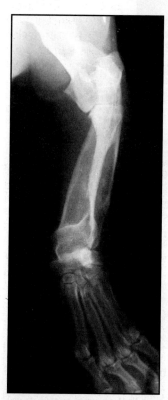

**11.46**

CrCd/DPa view of a forelimb of a chondrodystrophoid dog with short ulna syndrome. Valgus displacement of the carpus and manus is evident as a result of angulation of the distal radius and loss of lateral stability, which is usually provided by the styloid process of the ulna.

## Sesamoid disease

There are 12 sesamoid bones in each foot, located on the dorsal (single) and palmar/plantar (paired) surfaces of the metacarpo- and metatarsophalangeal joints. There are also a single carpal and two tarsal sesamoid bones (see Figures 6.2, 11.19 and 11.20).

Fragmented or multipartite metacarpophalangeal sesamoids may represent osteonecrosis of a sesamoid or congenital sesamoid fragmentation. Metacarpophalangeal sesamoid fragmentation (Figure 11.47a) is regarded as a potential cause of lameness in dogs, particularly in the Rottweiler (Read *et al.,* 1992), where it occurs predominantly in sesamoids 2 and 7 of the manus. However, clinical significance can be attributed to the presence of fragmentation only if pain is localized to the sesamoid or if some other imaging modality, such as scintigraphy (Figure 11.47b), indicates that the lesion is active. Clinically, quiescent multipartite sesamoids may be serendipitously present in a limb that has another cause of lameness. Sesamoid fractures are seen from time to time, the latter being described in racing Greyhounds and other large dogs (Davis *et al.,* 1969).

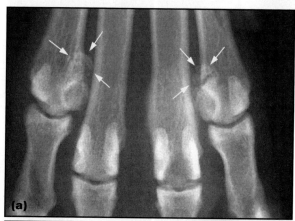

(a)

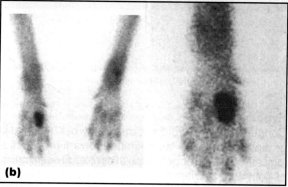

(b)

**11.47** **(a)** DPa view. Fragmentation of the palmar metacarpophalangeal sesamoids numbers 2 and 7 (arrowed) is evident on this radiograph of a manus. **(b)** A scintigraphic study of the same dog shows increased activity in the distal end of the third metacarpal bone, without demonstrable increase in isotope uptake in the fragmented sesamoid bones. Interpretation: healing callus or osteitis. (Courtesy of Gladesville Veterinary Hospital.)

## Arthrosis

### Osteoarthrosis

Osteoarthrosis is a degenerative arthropathy that may affect individual or multiple joints. In the feet osteoarthrosis is recognized in the interphalangeal, metacarpophalangeal, metatarsophalangeal, carpometacarpal, tarsometatarsal, intercarpal, intertarsal, antebrachiocarpal and tarsocrural articulations. Its aetiopathogenesis may be idiopathic or age-related, conformational, functional or the result of trauma. The radiological signs of osteoarthrosis are most commonly represented by periarticular osteophytes and enthesophytes (see Chapter 6), which sometimes produce an ankylosing arthropathy. Generally, the underlying cortical and articular surfaces appear normal. There may be a history of trauma (e.g. sprain injury) or, more commonly, signs of osteoarthrosis develop without any knowledge of a predisposing cause. Periarticular osteophyte formation is the predominant radiological change in these cases.

### Immune-mediated arthrosis

***Non-erosive polyarthropathies:*** Disorders, such as systemic lupus erythematosus, produce lameness characterized by an effusive polyarthropathy that is non-erosive. Their principal radiological abnormality is soft tissue swelling around multiple joints, due to synovial thickening and synovial effusion. It should be noted that in the early stages of the disease process, the erosive polyarthropathies develop similar changes prior to radiological evidence of subchondral bone erosion.

### Erosive polyarthropathies

*Canine rheumatoid arthritis:* Rheumatoid arthritis is an immune-mediated erosive polyarthropathy seen in dogs. Affected animals initially have signs of a non-erosive polyarthropathy, but gradually periarticular and subchondral erosive changes develop. Typically, the distal joints of the extremities are first affected, and the best examples of erosive polyarthropathy are generally seen in the carpi (Figure 11.48) and tarsi. The relentless progression of rheumatoid arthritis leads to ligamentous weakness so that in severely affected animals joint laxity may produce a plantigrade stance and lateral deviation of the feet (Figure 11.49).

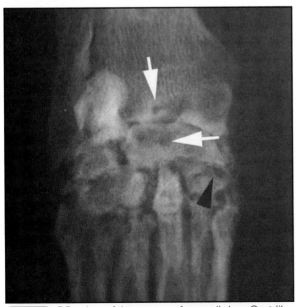

**11.48** DPa view of the carpus of a small dog. Cyst-like lucencies (white arrows) and subchondral erosion (black arrowhead) indicate an erosive arthropathy. (Courtesy of the Department of Veterinary Clinical Science, Bristol.)

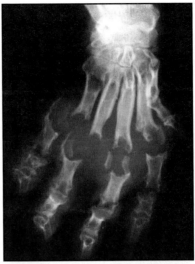

**11.49** DPa view of an erosive polyarthropathy due to rheumatoid arthritis in a dog showing advanced destruction of the metacarpophalangeal joints and, to a lesser extent, the interphalangeal joints. (Courtesy of Hornsby Veterinary Hospital.)

*Feline rheumatoid arthritis and feline chronic progressive polyarthropathy:* Rheumatoid arthritis and chronic progressive polyarthropathy are proliferative and erosive polyarthropathies seen in cats. Young male cats (generally younger than five years) are mainly affected by disorders that include fever, malaise, inappetence and lameness. Initially, painful joint swelling, muscle wasting and lymphadenopathy may be detected, with the joints most affected being those of the extremities of the appendicular skeleton, particularly the carpus and tarsus. Progressive changes include periosteal proliferation on bones around affected joints (Figures 11.50 and 11.51). Where erosive changes develop around and within joints, the condition may be referred to as the feline version of rheumatoid arthritis if a positive test for rheumatoid factor is returned.

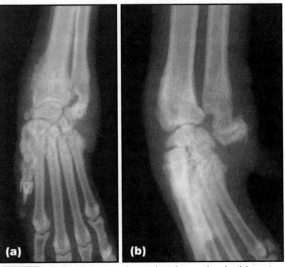

**11.50** Feline progressive polyarthropathy. In this cat soft tissue swelling surrounds the carpus. Periosteal proliferation is noted on the distal radius, the accessory carpal bone and the proximal ends of the metacarpal bones. **(a)** DPa view. **(b)** DLPaMO view. (Courtesy of The University Veterinary Centre, Sydney.)

167

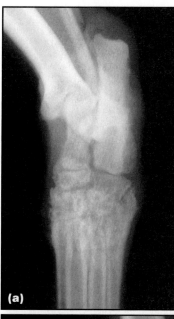

(a)

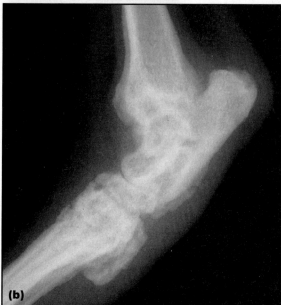

(b)

**11.51**

Chronic progressive polyarthropathy in the tarsus of a cat. Soft tissue swelling is present around the tarsus and periosteal new bone formation is noted on the distal tibia, calcaneus and distal rows of tarsal bones as well as the proximal ends of the metatarsal bones. **(a)** PID view. **(b)** ML view. (Courtesy of The University Veterinary Centre, Sydney.)

## Nutritional disorders

### Hypervitaminosis A

Excessive dietary intake of vitamin A (found in high levels in liver) leads to a clinical syndrome of hypervitaminosis A in cats within a few months. Affected animals are stiff and cannot ambulate or jump normally. Radiologically, an ankylosing spondylopathy and polyarthropathy are the predominant findings. These changes are most commonly seen in the cervical vertebral column and affecting the more proximal joints of the appendicular skeleton, but may be seen in the distal joints (see also Chapters 6, 7, 8 and 16). Because the joint changes mimic changes seen in osteoarthrosis, care should be taken to distinguish the two conditions.

### Hyperparathyroidism

Generalized skeletal under-mineralization is a feature of the various forms (primary, renal, nutritional) of hyperparathyroidism (see also Chapters 3, 6 and 16). In young actively growing animals, the paradox of

metaphyseal opacity due to normal enchondral ossification contrasts with the surrounding relative osteolucency, which is a result of active mineral resorption (Figure 11.52).

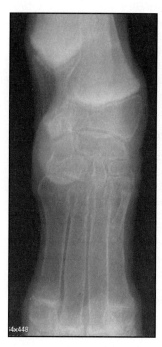

**11.52**

DPa view of osteopenia in a dog with nutritional secondary hyperparathyroidism. In the metaphyseal zones new bone formation continues, resulting in relative increased bone opacity, but elsewhere under-mineralization and reduction in cortical thickness is evident due to active bone resorption. (Courtesy of The University Veterinary Centre, Sydney.)

### Rickets

Rickets is due to a lack of vitamin D. There is normal production of the physeal cartilage but concurrent failure of metaphyseal ossification by the process of enchondral ossification. The result is that the physes grow wider than normal (Figure 11.53). The adjacent metaphyseal bone is present as an opaque margin of bone that is wider than normal, and may be saucer shaped. These changes may be seen at any physis but are always most dramatic in the distal radius and ulna (see also Chapter 3).

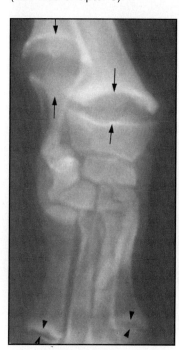

**11.53**

DPa view of the expansion of physeal cartilage (arrowed) and malformation of the zones of calcification. Provisional ossification of the metaphyses is evident in the distal radius and ulna and in the distal metacarpal physeal regions in this dog with rickets.

## Infection

### Osteomyelitis and septic arthritis/pododermatitis

Infection most commonly develops in the distal limb as a consequence of penetrating trauma or open fractures. However, infection from haematogenous spread of micro-organisms can also occur in the bones of the carpus, tarsus, manus and pes. Differentiation of direct inoculation from haematogenous infection is usually possible based on history and physical examination (Figures 11.54 to 11.57).

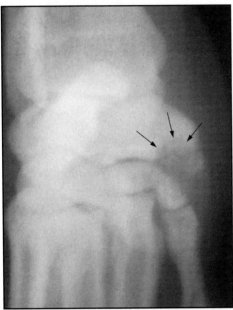

**11.54** D15°MPaLO view of a dog with bacterial septic arthritis, which has eroded the distal margin of the radial carpal bone (arrowed). (Courtesy of Vineyard Veterinary Hospital.)

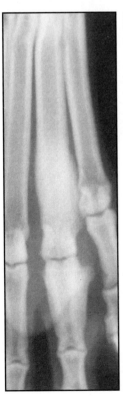

**11.55** DPa view of a focal region of increased bone opacity and expansion by periosteal proliferation in the distal metacarpus and in P1 of the digit of a dog. This was caused by bacterial osteomyelitis. (Courtesy of Vineyard Veterinary Hospital.)

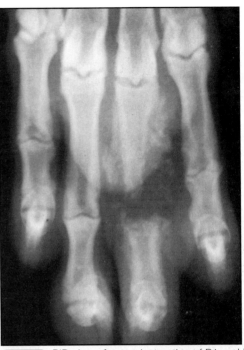

**11.56** PID view of osteodestruction of P1 and P2 of the digit of a dog. There is soft tissue mineralization around these bones caused by fungal osteomyelitis. (Courtesy of Baulkham Hills Veterinary Hospital.)

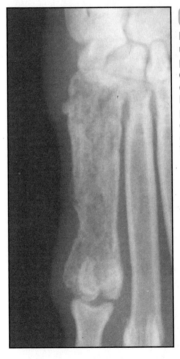

**11.57** DPa view of an unstructured mixed pattern of lucency and opacity in an expanded metacarpal bone caused by a pyogranulomatous osteomyelitis. (Courtesy of Sylvania Veterinary Hospital.)

Paronychia (inflammation of the nail bed) may result in extension of infection into the distal phalanx and distal interphalangeal joint. It might be a consequence of loss of the protection afforded by the nail, although, disease of the nail bed may result in loss of the nail and subsequent trauma to the distal phalanx. Differentiation of inflammatory disease from neoplasia based on the underlying aetiology of soft tissue swelling associated with a digit cannot be made on radiological changes alone; a definitive diagnosis requires a biopsy.

## Neoplasia

### Subungual squamous cell carcinoma or other neoplasms

Neoplasms of the nail bed and digit may be benign or malignant and cannot be adequately differentiated by radiological features alone (Voges *et al.,* 1996). Radio-logical distinction of neoplastic and inflammatory aetiologies of swollen digits, with or without extension of the disease process into the adjacent phalanx, is not possible, although lesions that demonstrate osteolysis of the distal phalanx are more likely to be associated with malignant neoplasms (Figures 11.58 and11.59).

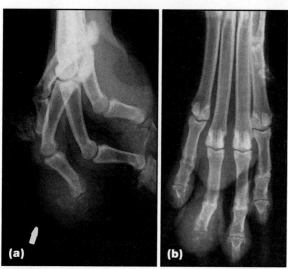

**11.58** Soft tissue swelling surrounding P2 and P3 of the fourth digit of a dog with subungual squamous cell carcinoma. P3 is osteolucent and malformed. **(a)** ML splayed toe view. **(b)** DPa view. (Courtesy of The University Veterinary Centre, Sydney.)

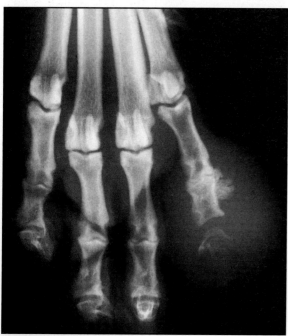

**11.59** DPa view of digital soft tissue swelling and destruction of P3 in a dog with subungual neoplasia. New bone proliferation is present on P2 of the second digit. (Courtesy of Bradbury Veterinary Clinic.)

### Lung–digit syndrome

Lung–digit syndrome is peculiar to the cat and can result in metastasis of primary pulmonary neoplasms to the digit. Many affected cats present with lameness and a lesion of one or occasionally more digits, and are subsequently found to have pulmonary carcinoma (Figure 11.60) (Gottfried *et al.*, 2000). Radiological features of the digital lesions include a mixed lytic or proliferative lesion of one or more phalanges.

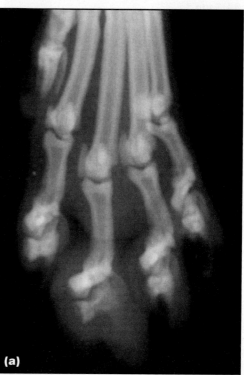

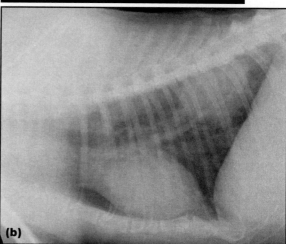

**11.60** Lung–digit syndrome in a cat. **(a)** D15°MPaLO view of a distal thoracic limb. Soft tissue swelling surrounds P2 and P3 of the third digit, representing a metastatic neoplasm. **(b)** Lateral thoracic radiograph. A well defined soft tissue mass is present in the left caudal lung of this cat. It was a primary bronchogenic carcinoma.

### Primary joint neoplasms

Primary joint neoplasms occur less commonly in the digits than in the larger joints of the appendicular skeleton (Figure 11.61; see also Chapter 6).

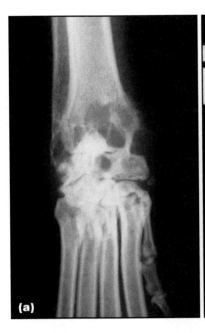
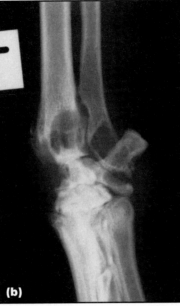

**11.61** Lucent foci of bone destruction present in the distal radius, ulna, and in the ulnar and radial carpal bones of a dog with synovial sarcoma. **(a)** DPa view. **(b)** Pa15°MDLO view. (Courtesy of Allpets Veterinary Hospital.)

## Miscellaneous

### Panosteitis

Panosteitis is a polyostotic disorder of long bones seen mostly in the young skeleton (< 24 months), but which occurs sporadically up to five years of age (see also Chapter 3). It is seen in dogs of large and giant breeds. Many bones may be affected at different stages of the condition but the distribution is random, with the exception that lesions are likely to be found near nutrient foramina. The lesions are always located in medullary or cancellous bone, and consist of variably defined opaque zones of bone within the medulla of long bones. Panosteitis may be seen in the metatarsal or metacarpal bones (Figure 11.62). Care must be taken to distinguish panosteitis from haematogenously disseminated osteomyelitis due to systemic bacterial or fungal infection.

### Hypertrophic osteopathy

This is a bony disease that affects dogs and cats. At various times called hypertrophic osteoarthropathy or hypertrophic pulmonary osteoarthropathy, this disorder produces symmetrical periosteal proliferation on long bones (see also Chapter 4). Typically it first manifests in the feet but progressively extends proximally to affect any or all long bones. Clinically, the feet are swollen and may feel oedematous. New bone, often in a palisade configuration, is a response to periosteal vascular connective tissue proliferation, mediated by humoral stimulation originating from a distant focus of disease. In the majority of cases the stimulation arises from intrathoracic mass lesions, but extrathoracic disorders such as prostatic masses, pregnancy and pyometra have also been implicated in the aetiology (Figure 11.63).

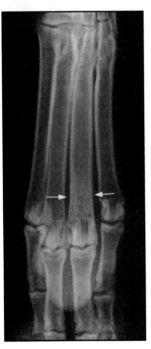

**11.62** PID view of a focal region of increased opacity of cancellous bone at the distal end of the metacarpal bone in a young dog (arrowed) with panosteitis. (Courtesy of The University Veterinary Centre, Sydney)

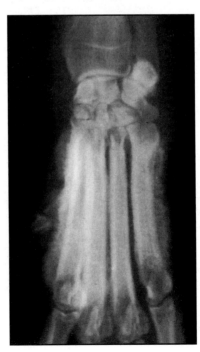

**11.63** DPa view of new bone in a palisade configuration seen on the metacarpal bones of a dog with hypertrophic osteopathy.

## Calcinosis circumscripta

Ectopic calcification of soft tissues, sometimes called tumoral calcinosis, has been identified in a variety of locations and may be seen around joints of the extremities. In these locations it is of doubtful clinical significance unless it is of sufficient size to inhibit function, or has inadequate soft tissue protection to protect the joints from trauma or pressure injuries (Figure 11.64; see also Chapter 1).

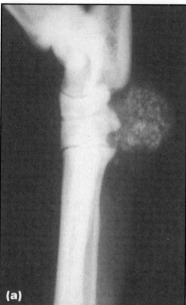

**11.64** Soft tissue mineralization on the plantar surface of the tarsus of a dog with calcinosis circumscripta. **(a)** ML view. **(b)** PID view. (Courtesy of The University Veterinary Centre, Sydney.)

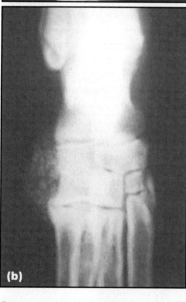

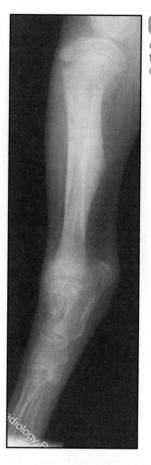

**11.65** ML view showing the presence of disuse osteopenia distal to the healing tibia fracture in a dog.

## Osteopenia

Osteopenia can develop rapidly in juvenile animals when a limb is immobilized. Relative bone opacity is reduced and cortical thinning is evident when affected limbs are compared with contralateral structures (see also Chapter 2). When immobilizing the distal limb of a juvenile the practitioner should be prepared for signs of disuse osteopenia after 10–14 days (Figure 11.65). Generalized osteopenia is also recognized, being mediated by disorders such as hyperparathyroidism (primary or secondary), mucopolysaccharidosis and hypervitaminosis A.

## References and further reading

Abeles V, Harrus S, Angles JM, Shalev G, Aizenburg I, Peres Y and Aroch I (1999) Hypertrophic osteodystrophy in six Weimaraner puppies associated with systemic signs. *Veterinary Record* **145**, 130–134

Allan G (2002) Radiographic signs of joint disease. In: *Textbook of Veterinary Diagnostic Radiology, 4th edn*, ed. DE Thrall, pp. 187–207. WB Saunders, Philadelphia

Crawley AC, Yogalingam G, Muller VJ and Hopwood JJ (1998) Two mutations within a feline mucopolysaccharidosis type VI colony cause three different clinical phenotypes. *Journal of Clinical Investigation* **101**, 109–119

Davis PE, Bellenger CR and Turner DM (1969) Fractures of the sesamoid bones in the Greyhound. *Australian Veterinary Journal* **45**, 15–19

Fitch RB and Beale BS (1998) Osteochondrosis of the canine tibiotarsal joint. *Veterinary Clinics of North America: Small Animal Practice* **28**, 95–113

Gottfried SD, Popovitch CA, Goldschmidt MH and Schelling C (2000) Metastatic digital carcinoma in the cat: a retrospective study of 36 cats (1992–1998). *Journal of the American Animal Hospital Association* **36**, 501–509

Malik R, Dowden M, Davis PE, Allan GS, Barrs VR, Canfield PJ and Love D (1995) Concurrent juvenile cellulitis and metaphyseal osteopathy: an atypical canine distemper syndrome? *Australian Veterinary Practitioner* **25**, 62–67

Newell SM, Mahaffey MB and Aron DN (1994) Fragmentation of the medial malleolus of dogs with and without tarsal osteochondrosis. *Veterinary Radiology and Ultrasound* **35**, 5–9

Read RA, Black AP, Armstrong SJ, MacPherson GC and Peek J (1992) Incidence and clinical significance of sesamoid disease in Rottweilers. *Veterinary Record* **130**, 533–535

Resnick D and Niwayama G (1983) Entheses and enthesopathy: anatomical, pathological and radiological correlation. *Radiology* **146**, 1–9

Sjöström L and Håkanson N (1994) Traumatic injuries associated with lateral collateral ligaments of the talocrural joint. *Journal of Small Animal Practice* **35**, 163–168

Voges AK, Neuworth L, Thompson JP and Ackerman NI (1996) Radiographic changes associated with digital, metacarpal and metatarsal tumours, and pododermatitis in the dog. *Veterinary Radiology and Ultrasound* **37**, 327–335

# 12

# Skull – general

## Ruth Dennis

## Indications

Indications for skull radiography are mainly for investigation of clinical signs relating to different parts of the head, but in some cases systemic metabolic disease affecting bone may be best seen in the skull. Typical clinical signs include:

- Deformity, swelling or discharging sinus
- Trauma to the head area
- Ear disease (including vestibular syndrome)
- Proptosis
- Pain in the head area
- Problems with jaw movement, including open-mouth jaw locking
- Suspected metabolic disease that may involve the skull
- Signs referable to nasal disease (see Chapter 13)
- Signs referable to dental disease (see Chapter 14).

Neurological signs suggesting brain or cranial nerve disease are less likely to produce radiographic changes and are usually better investigated using magnetic resonance imaging (MRI) (or computed tomography (CT) if MRI is not available), although radiography could be used as an initial screening tool.

## Radiography and normal anatomy

The skull is a complex structure, comprising about 50 bones, teeth, cartilage and soft tissues, and thus superimposition of other features over the area of interest is often hard to avoid. However, the skull is symmetrical and so comparison of the two sides is helpful. Many different radiographic views are described, demonstrating various parts of the skull, and most require heavy sedation or general anaesthesia of the patient. A high detail film/screen combination should be used and a grid is not necessary even in the largest dogs. Dental non-screen film is helpful for radiography of teeth and for the nasal cavity and mandibles in smaller patients. Accurate centring and collimation is important to minimize geometric distortion and optimize radiographic definition.

## Radiography

### Laterolateral view

For a laterolateral view the patient is positioned in lateral recumbency and the head is placed in a true lateral position with the mid-sagittal plane parallel to the table top, using radiolucent foam wedges placed under the nose and mandibles (Figure 12.1). Good positioning is best achieved if the neck and thorax are also padded into a lateral position and the head and neck reasonably extended. Centring and collimation depend on the area of interest, which may be the whole skull or a defined area such as the cranium. The laterolateral radiograph provides a useful overview of the skull and pharynx, although, there will be superimposition of bilateral structures, such as the nasal cavities, frontal sinuses, maxillae, mandibles and ear structures (Figure 12.2).

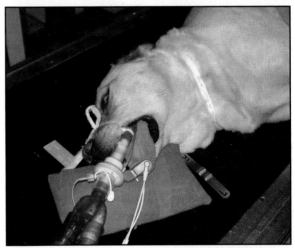

**12.1** Positioning for a lateral view of the skull in a dog. A radiolucent foam wedge has been placed under the nose and rostral mandible in order to achieve accurate skull positioning.

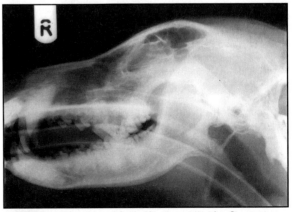

**12.2** Normal lateral skull radiograph of a German Shepherd Dog.

## Dorsoventral and ventrodorsal views

For the dorsoventral (DV) radiograph the patient is placed in symmetrical sternal recumbency with the head extended and the hard palate parallel to the cassette (Figure 12.3). It is usually necessary to raise the cassette from the table surface slightly on a rectangular pad or wooden block. Sticky tape may be a helpful way of restraining the head on the cassette, and a sandbag placed gently over the neck may be required in patients that are not fully anaesthetized.

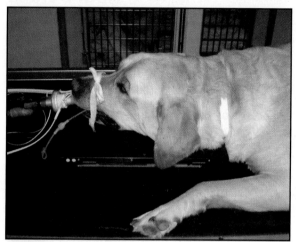

**12.3**  Positioning for a DV view of the skull in a dog. The cassette has been slightly raised from the table on a small rigid box.

For the ventrodorsal (VD) radiograph the patient is placed in dorsal recumbency, usually in a trough. The head is extended so the hard palate is parallel to the cassette, which is placed on the table top (Figure 12.4).

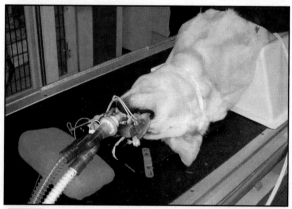

**12.4**  Positioning for a VD view of the skull in a dog. The dog is restrained in symmetrical dorsal recumbency using a rigid trough and sandbags.

The endotracheal tube should be removed before exposure if midline structures are of interest. Centring and collimation again depend on the area under investigation. It is important that positioning is symmetrical, which can be surprisingly difficult.

The DV/VD radiograph is particularly helpful for comparison of bilateral structures, such as the frontal sinuses, orbits, temporomandibular joints (TMJs) and ear structures (Figure 12.5). It is also useful for

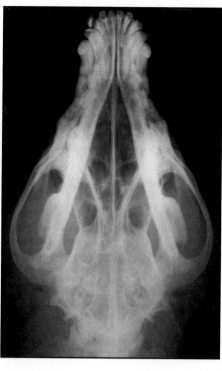

**12.5**  Normal DV skull radiograph of a Labrador Retriever.

examining the nasal septum and vomer bone and the cribriform plate. However, the lateral parts of the nasal cavities are obscured by the mandibles. The DV and VD radiographs are very similar, except that slightly more of the nasal cavity may be seen on the VD projection.

## Left or right 30 degree dorsal-right or left ventral oblique and left or right 30 degree ventral-right or left dorsal oblique views ('lateral oblique')

Oblique lateral views are used to skyline certain parts of the skull. The projection used depends on the area of interest, viz. left dorsal-right ventral oblique (LeD-RtVO), right dorsal-left ventral oblique (RtD-LeVO), left ventral-right dorsal oblique (LeV-RtDO) and right ventral-left dorsal oblique (RtV-LeDO). It is usually helpful to obtain right and left-sided views at similar degrees of obliquity for comparison. The degree of obliquity used depends on the area under investigation and the conformation of the patient's head, but a rotation of about 20–30 degrees is usually sufficient to separate superimposed structures adequately. The patient normally lies in lateral recumbency with the side of interest closest to the table and the head rotated towards the DV position for the dorsolateral cranium, frontal sinus, maxilla and upper dental arcade, and towards the VD position for the TMJs, tympanic bullae, mandibles and lower dental arcade (Figures 12.6 and 12.7). If the teeth are under investigation, it may be helpful to hold the mouth open with a gag to reduce superimposition.

The oblique lateral radiograph may often be obtained with the patient conscious or sedated, and this may be all that is required for an oblique 'lesion-orientated' view of a large swelling. In conscious patients only rotation of the head towards the DV position is possible.

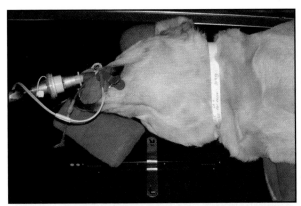

**12.6** Positioning for a lateral oblique (Le30°V-RtDO) radiograph of the skull in a dog. From the lateral position the head is rotated towards the VD position, in order to skyline the mandible and tympanic bulla closest to the cassette. Rotating the head towards the DV position is used to profile the dependent frontal sinuses.

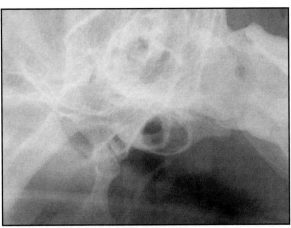

**12.7** Normal oblique lateral view of a tympanic bulla in a Springer Spaniel. Note that this view is generally unsatisfactory for the TMJ (see Figures 12.8 and 12.9) due to obliquity of the joint.

## Dorsoventral intra-oral view

A DV intra-oral view is used to demonstrate the nasal cavities without superimposition of the mandibles, and also gives a useful overview of the maxillary teeth ( see Chapter 13). As well as the nasal cavities, composite nasal septum and vomer shadow and teeth, this view may also demonstrate parts of the frontal sinuses, the medial walls of the orbits and the cribriform plate, depending on the animal's conformation.

## Ventral 20 degree rostral-dorsocaudal oblique view ('open-mouth VD')

A ventral 20 degree rostral-dorsocaudal ('open-mouth VD' V20°R-DCdO) view is an alternative to the DV intra-oral, and has the advantage of showing structures located more caudally and laterally, although it is technically more challenging to obtain (see Chapter 13).

## Ventrodorsal intra-oral view

The VD intra-oral view is used to demonstrate lesions affecting the ramus of the mandible and for an overview of the mandibular teeth. The patient is placed on their back and the film inserted, corner first, into the mouth, preferably between the tongue and the jaw.

## Left or right 20 degree rostral-right or left caudal oblique views ('tilted-up lateral or sagittal oblique')

A left or right 20 degree rostral-right or left caudal oblique ('tilted-up lateral or sagittal oblique' Le20°R-RtCdO or Rt20°R-LeCdO) view is used for the TMJs, which are seen more clearly than they are on a lateral oblique radiograph. The patient is placed in lateral recumbency with the side of interest facing down (although, normally both sides will be radiographed). From a true lateral position of the head, the nose is elevated by 10–30 degrees using a triangular foam wedge (Figure 12.8). A larger elevation is required in brachycephalic than in dolichocephalic animals. Elevating the nose brings the joint space of the dependent TMJ into a vertical position, parallel to the X-ray beam, and it is therefore seen much more clearly (Figure 12.9) than on an oblique lateral view. In animals with open-mouth jaw locking, radiographs should be obtained with the mouth both closed and open.

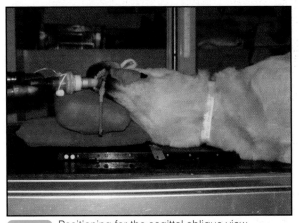

**12.8** Positioning for the sagittal oblique view (Le20°R-RtCdO) for the right TMJ. Elevation of the nose brings the TMJ that is closer to the table into a vertical position so that the joint space can be seen clearly.

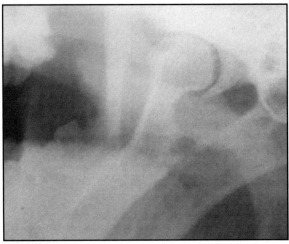

**12.9** Normal appearance of the TMJ on a sagittal oblique view.

## Rostrocaudal and caudorostral closed-mouth views (RCd and CdR closed mouth)

Rostrocaudal (RCd) radiographs are used to skyline the cranium and frontal sinuses (see Chapter 13) and also to evaluate the foramen magnum. With the animal in dorsal recumbency the occipitoatlantal joint is flexed so that the hard palate is roughly vertical to the cassette; a greater degree of flexion is required for the cranium than for the frontal sinuses. The exact angle of flexion depends on the animal's conformation, especially the size of the frontal sinuses, and is assessed by looking at the shadow cast on the cassette by the light beam diaphragm. The head may be restrained using tapes and sandbags, although a perspex frame (AG Donald Engineering Services, Scotland) will give much better stability (Figures 12.10 and 12.11). Care must be taken not to occlude the endotracheal tube during positioning.

An alternative view for the frontal sinuses is the horizontal beam caudorostral (CdR) view (see Chapter 13).

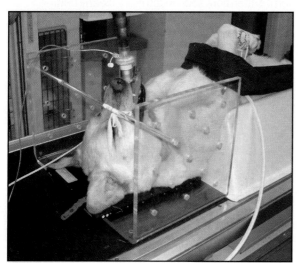

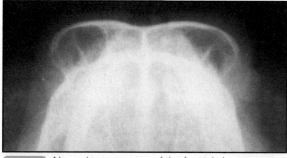

**12.10** Positioning for the RCd view of the frontal sinuses and cranium, using a perspex positioning frame. A greater degree of flexion is required to profile the cranium than the frontal sinuses.

**12.11** Normal appearance of the frontal sinuses on a RCd view.

### Rostrocaudal open-mouth view

A RCd open-mouth view is mainly used for examination of the tympanic bullae, which can both be seen and therefore compared with each other. Positioning is as for the closed-mouth view with flexion of the head, but the mouth is held open using a gag, tapes or a perspex frame (Figures 12.12 and 12.13). The tongue is placed against the lower jaw and it is wise, although not essential, to remove the endotracheal tube before exposure. Again, exact positioning varies with head conformation and several different techniques are described, but the hard palate and beam should form an angle of about 30

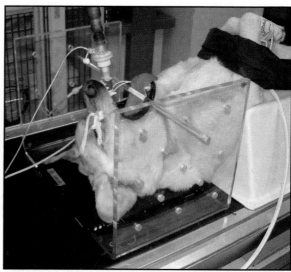

**12.12** Positioning of the head for the open-mouth RCd view of the tympanic bullae. For the purposes of photography the endotracheal tube remained in place, although, it is preferable to remove it before making the radiographic exposure in case of superimposition over the bullae.

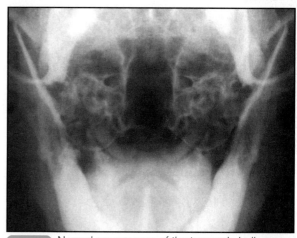

**12.13** Normal appearance of the tympanic bullae on an open-mouth RCd view.

degrees to each other (either with the perpendicular X-ray beam bisecting the open mouth or with the hard palate vertical and the beam slightly angled).

This view has also been advocated for demonstration of the dens in animals with possible atlantoaxial subluxation, but clearly where instability exists such severe flexion of the head is likely to be hazardous.

### Rostral 10 degrees ventral-caudodorsal oblique view for feline tympanic bullae

Since the open-mouth RCd view is rather hard to obtain in cats because of the small size of their mouths, an alternative (rostral 10 degree ventral-caudodorsal oblique (R10°V-CdDO) view) is described, which avoids the need to open the mouth. The cat is placed in dorsal recumbency with the occipitoatlantal joint gently flexed so that the mandible is about 10 degrees less than vertical (Figures 12.14 and 12.15). Centring the vertical beam just ventral to the nares will show the large feline bullae ventral to the skull base (Hofer *et al.*, 1995).

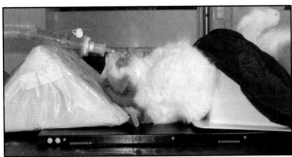

**12.14** Positioning of the head for the R10°V-CdDO view of the tympanic bullae in a cat.

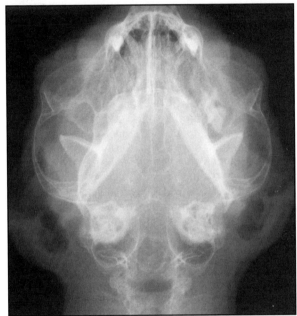

**12.15** Normal appearance of the feline tympanic bullae using the R10°V-CdDO view. The bullae are imaged caudal to the cranium and are, therefore, seen with less superimposition of other structures.

### Dental projections

A number of special projections exist for more precise evaluation of the teeth as required in dentistry and are described in Chapter 14 (see also *BSAVA Manual of Canine and Feline Dentistry*).

### Normal anatomy

#### General

***Dogs:*** The radiographic appearance of the skull varies greatly between breed types. The canine skull can be divided into three broad types with respect to conformation:

- Dolichocephalic (long-nosed)
- Mesaticephalic (cranium and nose of roughly equal length)
- Brachycephalic (short-nosed).

In dolichocephalic and mesaticephalic breeds the following main anatomical structures can easily be identified (see Figures 12.2 and 12.5):

- Cranium with sagittal crest and external occipital protuberance
- Cranial base and sphenoidal sinus
- Frontal sinuses
- Nasal cavities
- Composite nasal septum and vomer bone
- Nasal, maxillary and ethmoidal turbinates
- Cribriform plate
- Maxillae and maxillary recesses
- Zygomatic arches
- Teeth
- Hard and soft palates
- Mandibles (ramus and body)
- TMJs
- Tympanic bullae.

Pharyngeal and laryngeal structures can be seen clearly on a lateral radiograph. Several variations are present in brachycephalic dogs (and to a lesser extent in brachycephalic cats) (Figure 12.16) including:

- Domed and thin cranium, lacking an obvious sagittal crest
- Ventrally directed cribriform plate
- Reduced or absent frontal sinuses
- Shortened nasofacial area with crowded maxillary teeth
- Curved mandibles, which are relatively longer than the maxillae, resulting in an inferior prognathus
- Small and thick-walled tympanic bullae
- Increased soft palate and peripharyngeal soft tissue
- Excessive submandibular soft tissue (muscle mass)
- Caudally displaced hyoid apparatus.

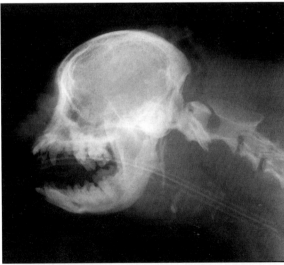

**12.16** Normal appearance of the skull and pharynx in a severely brachycephalic dog (Boston Terrier).

Many brachycephalic dogs have some degree of hydrocephalus, albeit subclinical. The cranium tends to be thin and rather featureless, and the fontanelles and cranial suture lines may remain open. In some other breeds (Pitbull Terrier, West Highland White Terrier and Bullmastiff) the cranium may appear very thick.

*Cats:* The feline skull varies much less in its appearance between breeds, and has several notable features compared with dogs (Figures 12.17 and 12.18). The tentorium ossium cerebelli (a shelf of bone between the cerebral hemispheres and the cerebellum) is prominent on lateral radiographs, as are the ethmoturbinates, although the nasal cavity itself is somewhat reduced. On the DV view the zygomatic arches curve markedly laterally and bear large post-orbital processes. The tympanic bullae are large and thin-walled, with a fine shelf of bone dividing them into dorsolateral and ventromedial compartments.

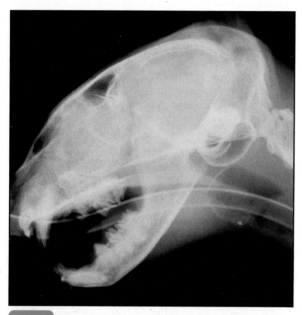

**12.17** Normal lateral skull radiograph of a cat.

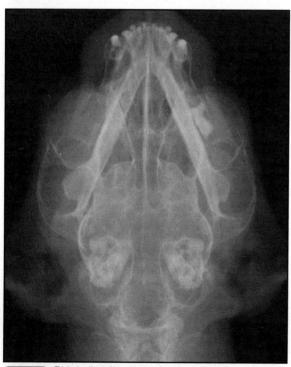

**12.18** DV skull radiograph of a cat, which is essentially normal except for the absence of numerous premolars and molars.

## Temporomandibular joints

The TMJs consist of a laterally elongated condyle, which is part of the mandible, and a concave fossa formed by the temporal bone. The joint is capable of considerable lateral sliding motion and a prominent retroarticular process on the caudal part of the fossa prevents caudal subluxation. A thin articular disc provides congruency between the bones and facilitates movement. On the DV radiograph the joint can be seen to lie in a slightly oblique transverse plane; the joint space is directed rostromedially to a degree which varies with skull conformation, being more oblique in brachycephalic dogs. Because of this slight obliquity the joint space is only clearly seen on the sagittal oblique view, in which the dependent TMJ is positioned vertically, parallel to the X-ray beam (see Figure 12.9).

## The ears

The temporal bone consists of petrosal, tympanic and squamous parts. The anatomy of the petrous temporal bones and tympanic bullae is complex but pathology is usually unilateral, and so comparison of the two sides (on symmetrical RCd and DV or comparable oblique lateral radiographs) is very helpful in recognizing deviations from normal. In the cat, the tympanic bulla is divided into two unequal parts by a fine bony shelf. On the DV/VD and RCd radiographs, air may be seen within the external ear canals and calcification of the aural cartilage is an occasional incidental finding in older dogs.

## Contrast radiography

### Sialography

Sialography is an infrequently performed technique that is used to outline the salivary glands and ducts. Its main indication is to confirm the side and gland of origin of a salivary mucocele where this is not apparent clinically. It can also be used to show gland morphology in the case of suspected salivary gland disease, or to show obstructions or ruptures of salivary ducts.

The opening of the salivary duct is cannulated with a very small catheter or blunted 25 gauge needle, and a small amount (0.5–1 ml) of an iodine-containing water-soluble contrast medium injected. Although ionic media have been recommended it is probably preferable to use a non-ionic contrast medium, as the lower osmolarity of this type of medium means that it is less irritant to the tissues and that radiographic contrast and definition persist for longer.

The parotid salivary duct opens on a small papilla on the buccal mucosa at the level of the fourth premolar tooth, and the zygomatic duct about 1 cm more caudally. The mandibular and sublingual ducts may have a common opening at a papilla lateral to the rostral end of the frenulum; when they open separately the sublingual duct's papilla is slightly caudal to that of the mandibular duct. The sublingual duct is most often implicated in disease. The ducts are small and difficult to cannulate; if cannulation proves impossible the contrast medium may be injected directly into the mucocele, which is then massaged to distribute the contrast medium within the saliva. Both lateral and DV radiographs should be obtained.

Normal salivary ducts are narrow and well defined tubular structures of fairly even diameter, branching within the gland. The mandibular and lingual glands show fairly uniform opacification whereas the parotid and zygomatic glands have a rather less well defined and lobulated appearance.

### Positive contrast ear canalography
Canalography can be used to assess the status of the tympanic membrane prior to topical medication if it cannot be inspected visually (Trower *et al.*, 1998). About 5 ml of non-ionic, iodine-containing positive contrast medium (around 150 mg/ml) is infused into the ear canal. Subsequent presence of contrast medium within the bulla, best seen on an open-mouth RCd radiograph, shows that the tympanic membrane is breached. However, false negatives may occur due to impedance of flow of contrast medium by the tissue and debris that obscured visual examination.

### Dacryorhinocystography
Dacryorhinocystography uses iodinated positive contrast medium to outline the nasolacrimal duct. It is technically rather difficult and results can be disappointing, but it may be used to demonstrate nasolacrimal duct occlusion, rupture and involvement or otherwise in maxillary lesions. The technique is described in Chapter 13.

### Sinography
Positive contrast medium is instilled via a catheter into a discharging sinus in order to attempt to show its direction and extent. In the head it is most often used to demonstrate communication between a sinus tract and a diseased tooth, and in the pharyngeal area for investigation of suspected foreign bodies, although these are more reliably imaged using MRI. Sinography is described more fully in Chapter 1.

## Alternative imaging techniques

### Ultrasonography

#### Ocular and orbital ultrasonography
Ultrasonography is well established as a most helpful tool for investigation of ocular and orbital disease, although its successful use in this area requires considerable expertise. Indications for ocular ultrasonography include cases where the eye cannot adequately be examined visually due to eyelid swelling, third eyelid protrusion or ocular media opacities such as corneal oedema, cataract or intra-ocular haemorrhage. Ultrasonography should be performed prior to cataract surgery to check that no detached retina is present to render the eye persistently blind. It is also used to assess the size of the globe, usually by comparison with the opposite eye. Ultrasonography can be used as part of the investigative process for suspected orbital disease, especially when radiographs are unremarkable.

The eye is best scanned in the conscious patient, as rotation of the eyeball may occur under anaesthesia. The direct corneal contact method provides the best images, and is surprisingly well tolerated by most patients after instillation of a topical anaesthetic into the eye. Ultrasonography may also be performed through the eyelids or the skin lateral to the eye. A high frequency transducer of at least 7.5 MHz is required, ideally with a built-in stand-off.

The normal globe is spherical and anechoic except for small curvilinear hyperechoic lines, representing the corneal surfaces, the iris, the front and back of the lens and the caudal wall of the globe. The ciliary bodies may also be identified, and the optic nerve head is sometimes seen as a small depression at the back of the eye. In the normal eye only structures that are perpendicular to the ultrasound beam (such as the centre of the cornea and lens) are visible whereas the curving lateral margins of the globe and lens are not visible since ultrasound waves from these areas are not reflected back to the transducer. Within the orbit extra-ocular muscles may be seen as spindle-shaped, hypoechoic bands interspersed with hyperechoic fat. The orbital soft tissues form a cone shape, bounded medially and dorsally by a shadowing, echogenic line created by the frontal bone. The optic nerve is infrequently seen.

### Other uses of cranial ultrasonography
If a persistent fontanelle is present, ventricular size can be seen rather crudely in animals with suspected congenital hydrocephalus. A high-frequency, sector-scanning transducer with a small contact area is required. The ventricles are seen as anechoic areas surrounded by echogenic brain parenchyma. However, unless the ventricles are grossly enlarged a diagnosis of hydrocephalus cannot be made with confidence due to the fact that large lateral ventricles are a common incidental finding in many dogs of small or dome-headed breeds. Ultrasonography can also be used to examine the brain during surgical procedures, but this is a rather specialized technique.

Swellings of the head in general may be examined and ultrasound-guided fine needle aspirates taken. The main value of ultrasonography here lies in its ability to differentiate solid soft tissue and fluid-filled areas. Although ultrasonography has not been traditionally used for imaging bony structures, it can be used to show the surface of bone in cases of traumatic or neoplastic disruption, and has been shown to be surprisingly accurate at detecting fluid and soft tissue within the bony tympanic bulla. Likewise, the fact that ultrasound waves do not pass readily through air is used to advantage in laryngeal ultrasonography in which masses, cysts and vocal fold paralysis can be detected.

### Computed tomography
CT produces cross-sectional 'slice' images of the area under investigation. The primary images are normally in the transverse plane and must be reformatted into other planes; in older scanners this causes some loss of resolution but this is much less of a problem with the newer spiral CT scanners. CT is based on conventional radiography in that images are produced by differential absorption of an X-ray beam by tissues of different composition and thickness, but unlike radiography, differentiation between fluid and soft tissue is possible and some information about internal soft tissue architecture

is also discernable. After image acquisition, which takes only a few seconds, post-processing of the digital information produces images that emphasize either bone or soft tissue. This is achieved by altering the window level and width of the many grey shades in the resulting image. Radiographic iodinated contrast media can be administered intravenously and vascular structures will opacify; this is helpful for the detection of areas of inflammation and damage to the blood–brain barrier.

Although the soft tissue resolution is greatly inferior to that produced by MRI, bone detail is excellent and CT is extremely sensitive for detecting subtle areas of osteolysis, new bone formation and soft tissue mineralization (Figure 12.19). Areas of haemorrhage will appear opaque or hyperdense. CT is thus an excellent tool for imaging many diseases affecting the skull, such as frontonasal, cranial and orbital neoplasms, nasal conditions and middle ear disease. Additional advantages include the rapid scanning time and the ability to use conventional anaesthetic and monitoring equipment, which make it a more suitable imaging tool for animals with head trauma.

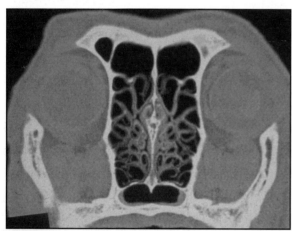

**12.19** Normal CT scan of the nasal cavity of a dog at the level of the orbits. The image is optimized for bone. (Courtesy of the Glasgow University Veterinary School.)

### Magnetic resonance imaging

MRI is currently more widely available than CT for veterinary patients in the UK, despite being a newer technology. Images are produced using a combination of magnetism and radio waves, creating cross-sectional images based on the distribution and molecular binding of the protons in hydrogen nuclei. The soft tissue contrast and resolution of the images is far greater than with CT, although it is less sensitive at detecting changes involving bone (Figure 12.20). Paramagnetic contrast media given intravenously will show areas of inflammation and blood–brain barrier breakdown as with CT, a change known as 'contrast enhancement'. The main advantages of MRI lie in its excellent soft tissue resolution and in the ability to acquire primary images in any plane. Disadvantages include the much longer scanning time required (usually at least 30–45 minutes for a thorough head study) and the need to keep conventional anaesthetic and monitoring equipment out of the stray magnetic field

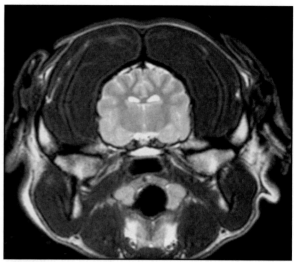

**12.20** Normal MRI scan of the brain of a dog at the level of the TMJs. This is a T2-weighted scan, i.e. fluid is bright.

created by the scanner. With the exception of brain disease, CT and MRI are probably equally helpful for imaging diseases of the skull; for brain disease MRI is vastly superior.

### Scintigraphy

Scintigraphy is of little relevance to imaging of the skull. Its main indication might be as part of a whole body bone scan using Technetium 99M to screen for skeletal metastases, although these would be unusual in the skull. The use of scintigraphy for detection of brain neoplasms has been described but has been superseded by CT and MRI. Single-photon emission CT (SPECT) and positron emission tomography (PET) are used in human medicine to combine metabolic and structural information, and are being used experimentally in dogs.

## Abnormal radiological findings

Radiography of the skull is usually performed in response to clinical signs, which can be attributed to a particular part of the head, for example nasal discharge, proptosis, an oral mass, craniofacial swelling or vestibular signs. For each area, a particular combination of radiographic views is helpful whilst others may be unnecessary. Radiography and radiology of diseases affecting the head can therefore logically be considered according to the clinical signs.

### Cranium and brain

The most useful radiographic views are lateral, RCd, DV/VD and lesion-orientated oblique to skyline areas of deformity.

#### Trauma

*Cranial fractures:* Fractures to the cranium are usually the result of a road accident, horse kick or significant fall. They are uncommonly seen as the temporal muscle provides a significant protection to the cranium in most breeds, and animals with severe injuries are unlikely to survive and be candidates for veterinary attention. Most cranial fractures are seen in cats and in toy breeds of dog as they have relatively thin cranial bone and overlying muscle.

Animals that survive the trauma often have non-displaced or minimally displaced fractures. These are usually seen as fine radiolucent lines, which must be differentiated from suture lines in young animals or in toy dogs (Figure 12.21); fracture lines will be asymmetrical whilst suture lines will be seen on both sides of the cranium. Oblique cranial radiographs may be needed to show areas of depression, and where bone fragments overlap sclerotic lines will be seen. In recent fractures there will be overlying soft tissue swelling, and subcutaneous emphysema in the absence of a skin wound indicates that the fracture also involves the frontal sinus or nasal cavity. A subperiosteal haematoma may occur following single or repeated episodes of lesser trauma to the calvarium, for example a dog that persistently crawls beneath a gate. Such lesions are seen as soft tissue swellings, which later form new periosteal bone, and are typically located in the sagittal or nuchal crest region.

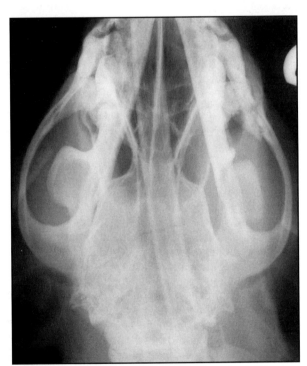

**12.21** DV radiograph of a non-displaced cranial fracture in a Hungarian Vizsla that had fallen into a quarry. A narrow, radiolucent line runs obliquely across the cranium and was not visible on other views. The dog was stuporous and blind, and MRI showed severe cranial contusion. However, the patient went on to make a full recovery.

CT and MRI are required to detect intracranial damage, such as brain contusion and haemorrhage between the brain and the cranium; the latter may require emergency surgery (Figure12.22).

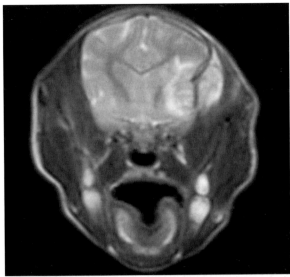

**12.22** Transverse T2-weighted MR image of the cranium of a 9-week-old Jack Russell Terrier puppy that had been bitten on the head by another dog and was showing neurological signs indicating left forebrain damage (falling to the right, right-sided menace deficit and right-sided conscious proprioceptive deficits). A depressed cranial fracture is visible with an abnormal hyperintense signal from the adjacent brain parenchyma and temporal muscle, indicating oedema and haemorrhage, but there is no subdural haemorrhage. The puppy recovered with conservative treatment.

### Congenital and developmental conditions

*Hydrocephalus:* Severe congenital hydrocephalus may produce radiographic changes, although the physical appearance of the animal is likely to be just as suggestive. The cranium is abnormally domed, with rostral and lateral bulging of the calvarium (Figure12.23). The fontanelle and suture lines remain open and the cranium has a homogenous opacity with a reduction in its normal 'copper-beaten' appearance. This is the result of flattening of the bony jugae (ridges) on the internal surface of the cranial bones, which normally accommodate the gyri and sulci of the brain.

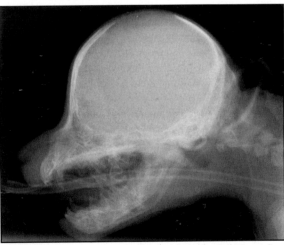

**12.23** Severe congenital hydrocephalus in a 7-week-old Staffordshire Bull Terrier X puppy. The cranial vault is grossly enlarged with large open fontanelles and absence of normal bony calvarial markings. (Courtesy of the Minster Veterinary Practice, York.)

Clinically significant hydrocephalus is likely to be gross, with massive dilatation of the ventricular system and thinning of the brain parenchyma. It is easily detected with MRI and CT, and the use of ultrasonography if the fontanelle remains open. However, many dogs of small and dome-headed breeds have quite large lateral ventricles without showing clinical signs. This is likely to be due to mild, subclinical hydrocephalus, which has been selected for in the breeding of dogs with a particular head conformation. Likewise, asymmetry of the lateral ventricles seen on MRI or CT is a common finding and in the absence of a midline shift does not indicate dilatation or compression of either ventricle.

Acquired hydrocephalus occurs secondary to obstruction of the caudal flow of cerebrospinal fluid (CSF), usually as a result of brain inflammation or neoplasia. No radiographic signs result and ultrasonography is not likely to be possible. MRI is the best modality for demonstrating both the hydrocephalus and the underlying lesion.

*Occipital dysplasia:* In recent years it has been recognized that a slight malformation of the occipital bone can lead to reduction in size of the caudal fossa and crowding of the foramen magnum by the cerebellum, preventing free flow of CSF from the ventricular system into the spinal subarachnoid space. This in turn may lead to syringohydromyelia (dilatation of the central canal of the spinal cord and dissection of fluid into the cord parenchyma) and occasionally mild obstructive hydrocephalus. MRI is required for diagnosis (Figure 12.24); although in severe cases enlargement of the cervical spinal cord may be evident on myelography (see Chapter 16). The condition is extremely common in the Cavalier King Charles Spaniel and is seen sporadically in other small dogs; it has some similarities with Chiari syndrome in humans. Clinical signs of neck pain and head and neck hyperaesthesia occasionally result but the severity of the clinical signs has no correlation with the degree of syringohydromyelia and the condition is often subclinical.

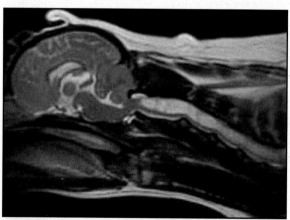

**12.24** Sagittal T2-weighted MR image of the skull and cervical spine of a 2-year-old Cavalier King Charles Spaniel with occipital dysplasia and severe syringohydromyelia ('Chiari' syndrome). The caudal fossa of the skull is small, resulting in crowding of the foramen magnum by the cerebellum and brainstem, which in this dog has also caused mild obstructive hydrocephalus. (CSF in the ventricles and spinal cord appears bright on T2-W images.)

Formerly, occipital dysplasia was diagnosed when an enlarged or 'keyhole'-shaped foramen magnum was identified on a RCd view of the skull. It is likely, however, that this was not due to a true skull defect but was due to thinning of the central bony sulcus of the caudal fossa, or to the replacement of bone by a fibrous band. The relationship of these radiographic bony changes to occipital dysplasia is unclear.

**Neoplasia**

*Brain neoplasia:* Brain neoplasms rarely produce radiographic changes or detectable metastases. However, many feline intracranial meningiomas provoke overlying hyperostosis (thickening and sclerosis of the calvarial bones) that can often be seen radiographically (Figure 12.25). The affected bones appear thicker and of increased radiopacity than normal, a change which is best seen on the RCd view. Such findings are pathognomonic for meningioma.

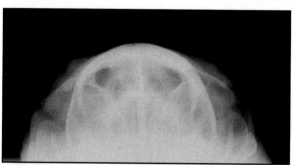

**12.25** RCd view of the cranium of a 12-year-old Domestic Short-haired cat with seizures. The left side of the calvarium (on the right of the image) is thickened and shows increased radiopacity compared with the left. MRI revealed a large meningioma with hyperostosis of the overlying bone.

*Cranial neoplasia:* Most cranial neoplasms are malignant, although, differentiation between benign and malignant bone disease cannot be made radiographically. Malignant neoplasms are most likely to be osteosarcomas, chondrosarcomas or multilobular osteochondrosarcomas (synonyms include chondroma rodens; multilobular chondroma, osteoma, osteosarcoma or tumour of bone; calcifying or juvenile aponeurotic fibroma; cartilage analogue of fibromatosis) for which the cranium is a predilection site. Benign osteomas and osteochondromas are rare in small animals. Cranial neoplasms usually show both unstructured new bone formation and underlying osteolysis, although new bone often predominates and may mask underlying bone loss (Figure 12.26). Lesion-orientated oblique projections to skyline the area of greatest external deformity are likely to be the most informative views. The appearance of multilobular osteochondrosarcoma is usually characteristic, showing a well defined mass with a dense pattern of coarse, granular ossification and little or no osteolysis. Bone neoplasms occasionally affect the sphenoid bones ventral to the brain but are hard to see radiographically. MRI or CT are required to show the

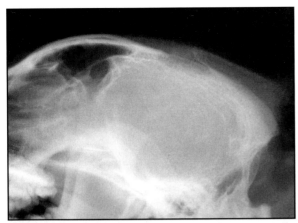

**12.26** Lateral radiograph of a cranial osteosarcoma in a 5-year-old cross-bred dog. A focal area of osteolysis with overlying shallow new bone production is visible in the dorsal midline but no information about possible inward extent is given.

internal extent of cranial neoplasms, which may be large (Figure 12.27). When neoplasia is suspected a search for metastases should be made, although cranial malignancies are less likely to spread than those in the appendicular skeleton.

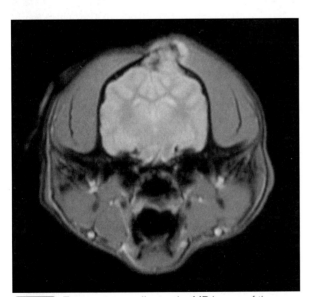

**12.27** Transverse gradient echo MR image of the same dog as in Figure 12.26. On this image, mineralized tissue is black. It can be seen that the osteosarcoma has completely breached the bone and is causing slight compression of the adjacent brain, although inward extent is much less than is often the case with such neoplasms. The lesion was surgically resected.

## Metabolic conditions

*Acromegaly in cats:* Acromegaly (hypersomatotrophism) occurs in cats secondary to a functional adenoma of the pars distalis of the pituitary gland, and may be associated with insulin-resistant diabetes. Affected cats are usually neutered males of middle to older age. Radiographic signs include thickening of the calvarium, mandibular prognathism, spondylosis and osteoarthrosis. Myocardial hypertrophy may lead to

left-sided heart failure and is best assessed using echocardiography. Pituitary enlargement is seen in 90% of cases using MRI.

*Mucopolysaccharidosis:* Mucopolysaccharidoses (MPSs) are rare lysosomal storage diseases that affect both cats and dogs. The most severe form is MPS VI, which is inherited as an autosomal recessive condition in Siamese cats. Affected cats have a characteristically short, broad face. A wide spectrum of bony radiographic changes occur, including an abnormal nasal turbinate pattern, severe spinal epiphyseal dysplasia, pectus excavatum, hip dysplasia and hyoid hypoplasia. The spinal changes are similar to those seen with hypervitaminosis A (see Chapter 16).

### Miscellaneous

*Idiopathic calvarial hyperostosis:* Young Bullmastiffs of either sex and between five and ten months of age occasionally develop idiopathic calvarial hyperostosis seen as marked thickening of the frontal and parietal bones. In severe cases obvious pain and swelling of the head is detected and systemic changes of fever, depression, nasal discharge and lameness are seen. Radiographs show marked thickening and increased radiopacity of the calvarium (Figure 12.28), and limb changes similar to metaphyseal osteopathy have also been reported. In addition, CT and MRI show dramatic bone thickening, which may be internal as well as external. The condition resembles craniomandibular osteopathy and human infantile cortical hyperostosis, and is self-limiting at skeletal maturity. Since the canine condition has been recognized only in the Bullmastiff, a genetic aetiology is likely.

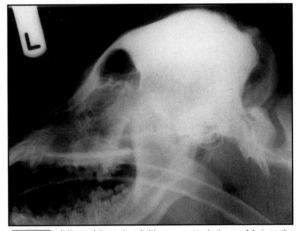

**12.28** Idiopathic calvarial hyperostosis in an 11-month-old Bullmastiff bitch. The frontal, parietal and occipital bones are massively thickened and radiopaque, and the volume of the cranial vault appears to be reduced.

### Orbit

The most useful radiographic view is the DV/VD, due to superimposition of the orbits over each other and over other structures on the lateral projection. Lateral oblique, RCd and DV intra-oral views are helpful to look for extension of orbital disease into the frontal sinuses or nasal cavity.

### Neoplasia

Orbital neoplasia usually results in a slow progressive proptosis without significant associated pain. Several scenarios are possible: neoplasms may arise within the orbit and remain confined to the orbital soft tissue; or they may erode beyond the orbit into the cranial cavity, frontal sinuses or nasal area; or they may erode from the cranial cavity, frontal sinuses or nasal area into the orbit. Neoplasms that are confined to the orbital soft tissues do not produce radiological changes in the skull, whereas those involving the normally aerated areas of the nose and sinuses show opacification of affected areas and varying degrees of osteolysis (Figure 12.29). Opacification of the frontal sinuses is often the result of trapped fluid rather than neoplastic extension and so radiography may overestimate the extent of the disease, although it does indicate that the neoplasm has spread beyond the orbit. Minor intracranial extension may be impossible to see radiologically. The presence of radiographic changes implies that the neoplasm is quite extensive and the prognosis is poor. In the absence of radiological changes (and if surgical treatment is planned) MRI or CT should be performed to check that the disease is indeed confined to the orbit (Figure 12.30).

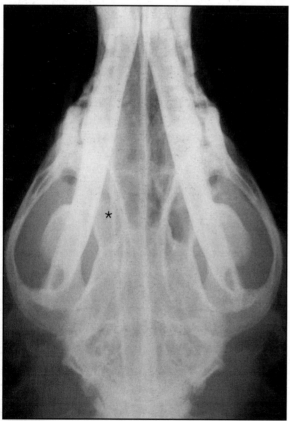

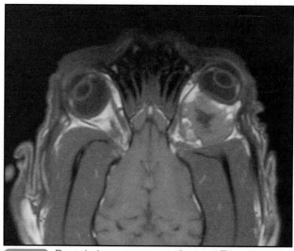

**12.30** Dorsal plane, contrast-enhanced T1-weighted MR image at the level of the orbits, in a 12-year-old Labrador X with proptosis. A discrete irregular mass is seen in one orbit, displacing the globe rostrally and compressing the normal orbital fat (bright areas) and muscle (dark bands). The opposite orbit is normal.

Orbital masses may be visible with ultrasonography, and usually appear hypoechoic relative to surrounding orbital fat (Figure 12.31). Frontal bone osteolysis may also be evident as an irregularity in the normally curved and smooth echogenic line that represents the frontal bone. If orbital neoplasia is suspected, thoracic and abdominal imaging should also be performed in a search for possible metastases.

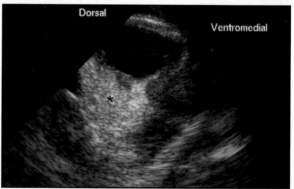

**12.31** Ultrasonogram of an orbital mass in a 10-year-old Domestic Short-haired cat with proptosis. A well defined, hypointense mass (*) is seen in the ventromedial part of the orbit, outlined dorsally by echogenic orbital fat.

### Infection

*Orbital inflammation and abscessation:* Radiographs are likely to be normal in cases of inflammatory orbital disease as the changes will probably be confined to the soft tissues. Ultrasonography is insensitive for diffuse cellulitis, but abscesses should be visible as discrete hypoechoic to anechoic areas surrounded by an echogenic 'capsule'. The orbit is likely to be very painful in such patients and in order to perform ultrasonography the animal may require sedation or even general anaesthesia. MRI is the ideal way of imaging an inflamed

**12.29** DV skull radiograph of a 13-year-old crossbred dog with neoplasia involving the right orbit and caudal nasal cavity (seen on the left of the image). The right frontal sinus is opacified (*), which suggests either fluid trapping or neoplastic extension. Identifying such changes radiographically shows that the lesion is already extensive and that further imaging techniques are not necessary.

orbit·as the soft tissue changes are easily seen and the opposite orbit can usually be used as a control. Cellulitis causes a diffuse increase in signal intensity on T2-weighted images in the normally hypointense extra-ocular muscles, and ill defined contrast enhancement will be apparent on post-contrast T1-weighted scans. Abscesses create discrete areas of hyperintense or hypointense signal on T2-weighted and T1-weighted images, respectively, and peripheral contrast enhancement will be evident. CT will produce less detailed images but soft tissue swelling, foci of fluid accumulation and diffuse opacification with intravenous contrast media may be seen. However, orbital abscesses may be hard to differentiate from zygomatic sialoceles with imaging. Zygomatic sialoceles are rare, but may occur secondary to trauma in the area.

*Orbital foreign bodies:* Orbital foreign bodies will only be visible radiologically if they are radiopaque, e.g. ballistics and certain types of glass (Figure 12.32). Production of two or more radiographs made from different angles will show that the material is in the region of the orbit, but it may be impossible to know whether the foreign body is within or outside the globe. Plant material, such as wood and grass awns, will produce no radiological changes.

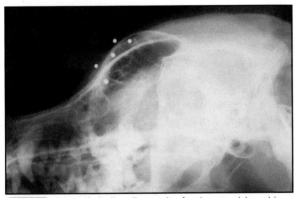

**12.32** Lateral skull radiograph of a 4-year-old working Labrador Retriever which presented with severe ocular haemorrhage. Several pieces of lead shot are seen in the frontal area, although even with multiple radiographic projections it is difficult to know whether any of them are within the eye. Ultrasonography would be required for this since metal objects produce artefacts with both CT and MRI.

Ultrasonography will usually allow visualization of the foreign body as an abnormal echogenic structure with distal acoustic shadowing or reverberations, depending on its physical nature, and is better than radiography for precise localization of the material. Associated abscessation may also be seen. However, MRI is the most accurate way of identifying foreign material within the orbit and any associated soft tissue inflammation.

## Maxillae and mandibles

The most useful radiographic views are DV or VD intra-oral as appropriate and oblique laterals (right dorsal-left ventral and left dorsal-right ventral).

## Trauma

*Fractures of the maxilla, mandible and zygoma:* Fractures of the maxilla, mandible and zygoma will usually displace these bones and thus they are readily recognizable radiographically, provided that appropriate radiographic views are obtained (Figure 12.33). The normal mandibular symphysis may be fibrous and therefore radiolucent, especially in cats, and should not be mistaken for a symphyseal separation. Likewise, the oblique suture line in the zygomatic arch should be recognized as a normal feature. Maxillary fractures extend into the nasal cavity and subcutaneous emphysema may result. Injuries to either the mandible or maxilla may involve teeth, resulting in secondary periodontal disease (see Chapter 14). Fracture of the premaxilla has been reported as causing caudal displacement of a canine tooth into the nasal cavity, resulting in upper respiratory signs. Multiple fractures of the zygoma with inward displacement and subsequent malunion can affect jaw movement by impinging on the ramus of the mandible; this is more likely in the dog than in the cat in which the zygoma curves more laterally. Severe periodontal disease, neoplasia and demineralization due to hyperparathyroidism may all lead to pathological fractures, especially of the mandible, and so radiographs of apparently spontaneous fractures should be examined carefully for signs of possible pre-existing bone rarefaction.

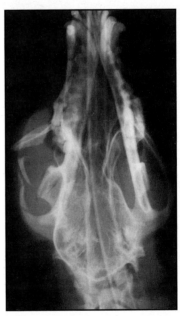

**12.33** Oblique DV view of the head of an English Pointer which had been kicked by a horse. Multiple fractures of the caudal maxilla and zygoma are seen, together with a fracture of the mandibular coronoid process and soft tissue emphysema.

## Neoplasia

Oral neoplasms are relatively common, comprising about 6% of all canine and 3% of feline cancers. The most common types in dogs are fibrosarcomas, squamous cell carcinomas and malignant melanomas; less commonly osteosarcomas and basal cell tumours (acanthomatous epuli) as well as benign fibromas, osteomas and epulides occur. Neoplasms arising from dental tissue are unusual and are described in Chapter 14. In the cat, squamous cell carcinomas are most common and are possibly associated with grooming carcinogens, such as tobacco smoke, from the coat.

Oral neoplasms have a range of radiographic appearances ranging from those which are almost entirely osteolytic to those which are productive; most will show a combination of features (Figure 12.34). However, no radiographic appearance is characteristic for any of the histological types, which means therefore that this cannot be differentiated on radiographs. Most, but not all, malignant oral neoplasms produce bony changes but these may also occur with some benign oral masses. The main value of radiography, therefore, lies in planning biopsy sites or margins for surgery or radiotherapy.

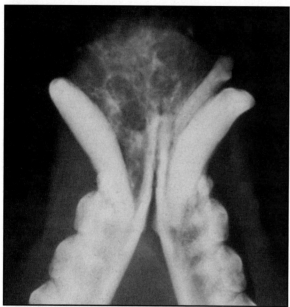

**12.34** Rostral mandibular neoplasm in an 11-year-old Labrador Retriever. There is extensive destruction of both rostral mandibles with loss of five incisors and displacement of the remaining incisor and one of the canine teeth. Chaotic, spicular new bone extends into an overlying area of soft tissue swelling. The histological diagnosis was acanthomatous epulis, although the radiographic changes are non-specific for tumour type.

Osteolysis is usually diffuse and poorly circumscribed but varies greatly in its extent and may even mimic focal periodontal disease. New bone production tends to be unstructured, although a Codman's triangle may be seen at the edge of the lesion due to periosteal elevation. Other radiographic signs of an oral neoplasm include:

- Soft tissue swelling
- Displacement or erosion of tooth roots
- Tooth loss (which may be iatrogenic as early neoplasms often mimic gingivitis).

The differential diagnosis for an oral neoplasm may be severe osteomyelitis of the jaw, but this is less common in small animals. Oral neoplasms uncommonly metastasize but nevertheless radiography of the thorax should be performed.

CT and MRI are excellent means of assessing the extent of an oral neoplasm if maxillectomy or mandibulectomy is proposed, as they are much more sensitive for bone infiltration than are radiographs. CT is very sensitive for osteolysis or new bone production, whilst MRI shows bone invasion as a reduction in the normally very bright signal of fat in the bone marrow.

## Metabolic conditions

*Hyperparathyroidism:* This is usually secondary to dietary calcium deficiency or to hypocalcaemia resulting from renal disease. Nutritional secondary hyperparathyroidism causes osteopenia, predominantly in the spine and appendicular skeleton and is described in Chapter 3. Bone changes due to renal secondary hyperparathyroidism, however, occur mainly in the skull, resulting in the clinical condition 'rubber jaw' in which the mandibles become soft and pliable. This condition is rather unusual and most often arises in young dogs with congenital renal dysplasia, although it occasionally occurs in older dogs and cats with acquired chronic renal disease. Radiographically, the lesions are most dramatic in the younger animal because of the rapid bone turnover that occurs at this age.

The appearance on skull radiographs is of osteopenia relative to the teeth and soft tissues, which appear unusually prominent (Figure 12.35). Demineralization of the mandibles and maxillae occurs, especially around the tooth roots, with loss of the lamina dura; there are also ill defined radiolucent haloes around the teeth giving the impression of teeth that are displaced or 'floating' in soft tissue. The osteopenia results in a coarse, lace-like trabecular bone pattern, which in advanced cases may affect the cranium as well as the jaw bones. Fibrous dysplasia of the nasal turbinates together with demineralization of the surrounding bones results in an abnormally prominent turbinate pattern, and in some cases respiratory signs may occur due to nasal obstruction.

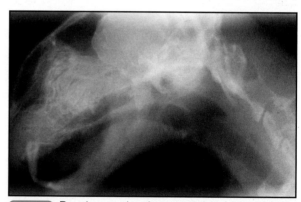

**12.35** Renal secondary hyperparathyroidism ('rubber jaw') in an aged Siamese cat with renal failure. There is reduced opacity and poor definition of the skull bones compared with the soft tissues, and the nasal turbinates are abnormally prominent. Dental loss may be related to age but could also be the result of alveolar bone resorption.

If renal secondary hyperparathyroidism is suspected, appropriate blood and imaging tests should be performed to investigate renal structure and function. Calcification of soft tissues, such as gastric rugae and some blood vessels, may be evident on radiography and ultrasonography in advanced cases.

## Miscellaneous

***Craniomandibular osteopathy:*** Craniomandibular osteopathy ('lion jaw') is a non-neoplastic, proliferative bone disease that affects the skull and occasionally long bones in adolescent dogs of about three to eight months. It is primarily seen in Highland Terriers, most notably the West Highland White Terrier. Scottish and Cairn Terriers are also predisposed to the condition, but other breeds of dog are sporadically affected. The aetiology is not known, except in the West Highland White Terrier, in which an autosomal recessive inheritance has been recognized.

The typical location and appearance of the rather florid new bone production, together with the age of the dog and the clinical signs, usually mean that diagnosis is straightforward. Periosteal new bone, often 'palisading' (at right angles to the underlying cortex), usually forms on the mandibles and tympanic bullae (Figure 12.36). The severity and extent of the changes vary greatly between dogs, and the new bone may be symmetrical or asymmetrical (even unilateral) in distribution. The cranium and frontal bone are occasionally affected, and craniomandibular osteopathy confined to the frontal bone and resulting in exophthalmos has been reported (Dennis *et al.*, 1993). Clinical signs of pain, pyrexia and jaw swelling may be seen, and mechanical interference with jaw movement occurs if new bone on the bullae impinges on the TMJs. These signs usually follow an undulant clinical course and become self-limiting at skeletal maturity, when the new bone remodels. Collars of paraperiosteal new bone may occasionally be seen adjacent to the distal radius and ulna in dogs affected with craniomandibular osteopathy. The limb lesions may resemble metaphyseal osteopathy (see Chapter 3) but without evidence of underlying metaphyseal radiolucency.

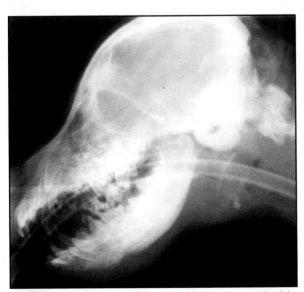

**12.36** Craniomandibular osteopathy in a 4-month-old West Highland White Terrier. Florid periosteal new bone production is visible in the mandibles and tympanic bullae. This new bone is already starting to remodel as it appears mainly solid, without the characteristic 'palisading' appearance.

***Cystic maxillary lesions:*** A number of different conditions may result in the formation of cystic or pseudocystic lesions in the maxilla (Featherstone and Llabres Diaz, 2003). Nasolacrimal duct cysts may be congenital or acquired, secondary to nasolacrimal duct obstruction. Epithelial cysts, cholesterol granulomas, maxillary giant cell granulomas and epidermoid cysts have also been reported in dogs. The radiographic appearance is similar for all, with a spherical radiolucent area in the maxilla surrounded by a fine radiopaque bony margin (Figure 12.37). Dacryorhinocystography can be employed to look for connection or otherwise with the nasolacrimal duct, and ultrasonography may be possible if there is a defect in the overlying bone.

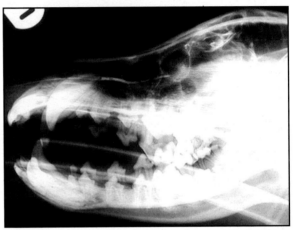

**12.37** Cystic maxillary lesion in a 1-year-old Labrador Retriever with a facial swelling near the medial canthus of the right eye. A 15 mm diameter radiolucent structure with a fine bony wall is seen rostral to the orbit. Dacryorhinocystography has been performed and shows that the structure does not communicate with the nasolacrimal duct. The histological diagnosis was of epithelial cyst formation. (Reproduced from Featherstone and Llabres Diaz (2003) with permission of the *Journal of Small Animal Practice*.)

## Temporomandibular joints

The most useful radiographic views are the sagittal oblique (Le20°R-RtCdO or Rt20°R-LeCdO) with the mouth closed, and open, the DV and the lateral oblique (Le30°D-RtVO or Rt30°D-LeVO).

### Trauma

The TMJs are rather susceptible to luxations and fractures secondary to impact to the mandibles, especially in cats. The clinical signs of drooling and malocclusion with lateral displacement of the mandible and inability to close the mouth are highly suggestive of TMJ trauma, which may be unilateral or bilateral. Unfortunately, the area is hard to radiograph in cats, although loss of symmetry of the TMJs is suggestive. A perfectly straight DV radiograph is the most helpful view for unilateral injury, as the relationship between the mandibular condyles and the fossae on the two sides can be compared. When a luxation is present the condyle is usually luxated rostrodorsally and the joint space widens. The mandible is displaced towards the opposite (unaffected) side. The sagittal oblique radiograph may be hard to obtain and to interpret, but should be examined for fractures of the condyle, fossa or retroarticular process (Figure 12.38).

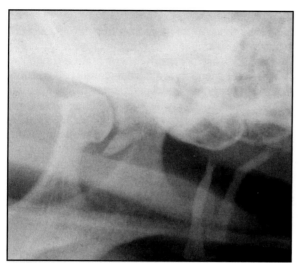

**12.38** Mildly displaced fracture of the retroarticular process of the TMJ in the same dog as shown in Figure 12.33, an English Pointer that had been kicked by a horse and sustained severe zygomatic arch fractures. The TMJ fracture did not seem to be associated with clinical signs, although may have predisposed the joint to degenerative change.

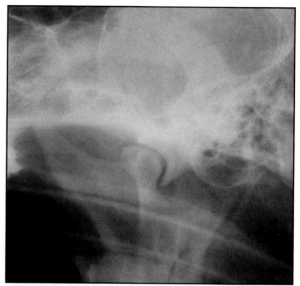

**12.39** TMJ dysplasia in a 1-year-old Irish Red Setter with open-mouth jaw locking. Although in this dog the retroarticular process appears of normal size, the rostral part of the mandibular fossa and condyle are slightly flattened (compared with the normal TMJ, see Figure 12.9).

In cats especially, uni- or bilateral TMJ ankylosis may occur following trauma, such as a road traffic accident or a fall when the cat lands on its chin. This may be either a bony articular ankylosis, resulting from callus formation, or a soft tissue ankylosis due to mineralization or fibrosis, secondary to haemarthrosis. The animal shows progressive difficulty in mouth-opening and eating, resulting in weight loss. Radiographs may show new bone crossing the joint or bridging the space between the mandibular coronoid process and the zygomatic arch.

### Congenital and developmental conditions

***Temporomandibular joint dysplasia:*** TMJ dysplasia is an uncommon condition seen in young Irish Red Setters and Basset Hounds in which laxity of one or both TMJs results in open-mouth jaw locking, usually when the animal yawns. When the mouth is opened widely, abnormal movement at the affected TMJ causes displacement of the mandible to the opposite side, allowing the coronoid process to become trapped lateral to the zygoma and preventing the mouth from closing.

Radiographs may show bony changes in the form of a flattened condyle, shallow fossa and hypoplasia of the normally prominent retroarticular process (Figure 12.39). On the DV view the joints may be angled more obliquely than normal in a rostromedial direction. Performing the sagittal oblique radiograph with the mouth both closed and open may show subluxation of the mandibular condyle, resulting in widening of the TMJ space. However, the bony changes may not be dramatic, as the primary cause is predominantly a laxity of the collateral ligaments of the joint exacerbated by increased mobility of the mandibular symphysis. CT is an excellent means of visualizing the bony conformation of the TMJs.

### Neoplasia

Neoplasms arising in the TMJ itself are rare, but the joint may be affected by neoplasia of other parts of the temporal bone or by extension of local soft tissue neoplasms, including those of the salivary glands. The radiographic appearance will usually be of an aggressive, mixed bone lesion, combining both osteolysis and unstructured new bone formation (Figure 12.40). Surrounding soft tissue swelling may occlude the external ear canal. Osteomyelitis should be considered as a possible differential diagnosis, although the radiographic appearance is not usually as severe as with neoplasia; extension from the adjacent tympanic bulla is the likely cause and so there will usually be concurrent signs of severe ear disease. A search for distant metastases

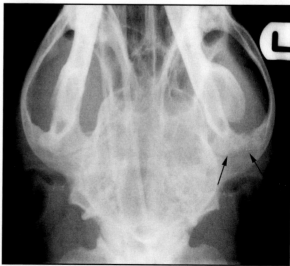

**12.40** Soft tissue neoplasia (myxosarcoma) involving the TMJ of an 11-year-old Labrador Retriever with ipsilateral proptosis. The radiograph demonstrates osteolysis of the TMJ (arrowed).

should be made using radiography and ultrasonography, and if negative a biopsy will be required for a definitive diagnosis.

CT and MRI can both be used to demonstrate the extent of pathology involving the TMJ, although in the case of malignant neoplasia this is of academic rather than practical interest.

### Arthrosis

Osteoarthrosis of the TMJ may occur idiopathically in older animals or be secondary to trauma or middle ear disease. New bone on the tympanic bulla in young dogs with craniomandibular osteopathy may also affect the TMJ. The radiographic signs of TMJ arthrosis are narrowing of the joint space, subchondral sclerosis and periarticular osteophyte formation.

### External, middle and inner ear

The most useful radiographic projections are RCd open-mouth (dog) and R10°V-CdDO (cats), DV/VD and lateral obliques (Le30°D-RVO or Rt30°D-LVO).

### Neoplasia

*Aural and nasopharyngeal polyps:* Benign inflammatory polyps may arise in the middle ear of young cats, and extend either into the external ear canal or through the Eustachian tube into the pharynx, where they form nasopharyngeal masses. Whilst the former are readily recognized on otoscopy, the clinical signs of nasopharyngeal polyps may be less clear and include stertor and nasal discharge. A straight lateral radiograph will show the polyp as a discrete soft tissue mass dorsal to the soft palate, which may be displaced ventrally (Figure 12.41). The cranial margin of the polyp is usually unclear but the caudal margin is outlined by air in the pharynx. Radiographic signs of middle ear disease (see below) are usually present and indicate the bulla of origin. Nasopharyngeal masses in both dogs and cats may rarely be caused by lymphoma, and in such cases bony bulla changes are less likely to be seen, although there may be an increased opacity within the bulla itself.

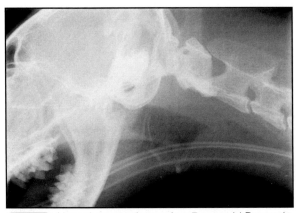

**12.41** Nasopharyngeal mass in a 7-year-old Domestic Short-haired cat with stertor and nasal discharge. A discrete soft tissue mass is visible in the nasopharynx, outlined caudally by air. Although more commonly benign lesions arise in the middle ear, this mass was found histologically to be a lymphoma.

*Other neoplastic lesions:* Neoplasms involving the ear usually arise in the soft tissues and involve, secondarily, the bony ear structures, especially the bullae. Squamous cell carcinoma and ceruminous gland carcinoma are the most common, and result in an aggressive, mixed osteolytic/proliferative bone lesion with surrounding soft tissue swelling (Figure 12.42). The adjacent TMJ or the cranium may also be involved in the lesion. Primary temporal bone neoplasms, such as osteosarcoma, occur less commonly. Severe osteomyelitis or previous bulla osteotomy may give rise to a similar appearance. CT and MRI are sensitive techniques for demonstrating such lesions, although cannot be relied upon to differentiate neoplasia from severe osteomyelitis.

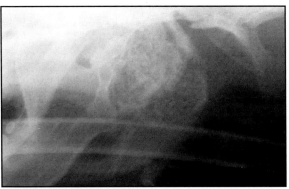

**12.42** Extensive, aggressive bone lesion affecting the tympanic bulla of an 8-year-old Golden Retriever, which was due to a ceruminous gland adenocarcinoma. The normal architecture of the bulla is completely lost and replaced by unstructured new bone over a wide area.

### Infection

*External, middle and inner ear disease:* Although radiography is not required to diagnose external ear disease, the signs of discharge and soft tissue swelling occluding the ear canal may be seen radiographically. Extensive, unilateral or asymmetrical calcification of ear cartilage may occur, although, moderate and symmetrical changes are quite common incidental findings in older dogs. Para-aural abscessation may occur and the source of any discharging fistulae can be investigated radiographically, using a metal probe or positive contrast sinography.

Radiography is insensitive for middle ear disease, although, chronic severe disease may result in increased opacity within the normally air-filled bulla and irregular thickening of the bulla wall due to periosteal new bone (Figure 12.43). Comparison of the two bullae on well positioned radiographs (as described above) is usually necessary to diagnose abnormalities with certainty as there is some variation in the appearance of the bullae between breeds; in particular the bullae of Cavalier King Charles Spaniels are normally small and thick-walled. Osteolysis of the bulla wall secondary to osteomyelitis is a rather unusual finding. Otoliths (mineral opacities in the bulla) have been described in three dogs, although in two they were an incidental finding (Ziemer *et al.*, 2003). They were visible as mineral

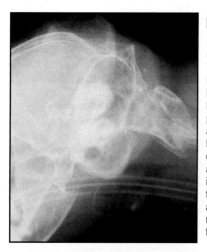

**12.43**
Middle ear disease in a 7-year-old Domestic Short-haired cat caused by a large aural polyp. The affected tympanic bulla shows loss of normal aeration and the bulla wall is thickened due to the presence of active periosteal new bone formation.

opacities on radiography and CT and were thought to represent mineralized necrotic material due to current or previous middle ear disease.

Inner ear disease is rarely diagnosed radiographically, although sclerosis of the petrous temporal bone may occur and be visible on a well positioned DV radiograph in which a confident comparison between the two sides can be made.

CT and MRI are both excellent tools for investigation of middle and inner ear disease. CT will show bone changes and the presence of soft tissue or fluid within the tympanic bulla (Figure 12.44), although an apparent increase in the thickness of the wall of a fluid-filled bulla can be a misleading artefact (Barthez *et al.*, 1996). MRI is much less sensitive for demonstrating bony changes, but is excellent for showing abnormal bulla material and peribullar inflammation. Bulla fluid has been found to be a common non-clinical finding on MRI in the Cavalier King Charles Spaniel and Boxer, and is probably due to partial occlusion of the Eustachian tube by excessive pharyngeal soft tissue in these breeds. In severe cases of inner ear disease there is loss of the normal fluid signal from the cochlea and semi-circular canals on MRI, although false negative findings are common.

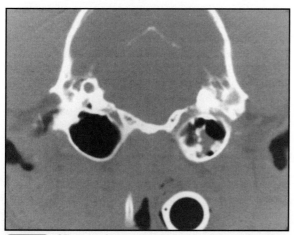

**12.44** CT scan of chronic middle ear disease in a dog (bone window). The wall of the affected bulla is diffusely thickened and the lumen contains both soft tissue and otoliths. The opposite bulla appears normal but both external ear canals are occluded by inflammatory soft tissue due to chronic otitis externa. (Courtesy of the Glasgow University Veterinary School.)

More recently, ultrasonography has been described for the detection of middle ear fluid, defying the conventional notion that bone is impermeable to ultrasound waves (Griffiths *et al.*, 2003). The normal air-filled bulla creates acoustic shadowing and reverberation artefacts but, if fluid-filled, the bulla lumen can be seen as an anechoic area.

## Salivary glands

### Neoplasia
Neoplasms of the salivary glands are uncommon and are likely to be adenocarcinomas. If confined to soft tissue no radiographic signs other than possible soft tissue swelling will be present, although an imaging search for metastases should be made. Severe retropharyngeal lymphadenopathy may be visible radiographically. Salivary gland malignancies may cause osteolysis of adjacent bone by direct extension. If necessary, sialography could be used to show disruption to the normal lobular architecture of the affected gland, but MRI is a much better technique for demonstrating the extent of salivary tissue neoplasms.

### Miscellaneous

***Salivary calculi:*** Small, discrete mineralized opacities in the region of a salivary gland or duct should give rise to the suspicion of sialolithiasis (salivary calculi), especially if a suspected sialocele is also present (Figure 12.45). Secondary duct rupture is a possibility. Sialography can be employed to confirm the location of the calculi.

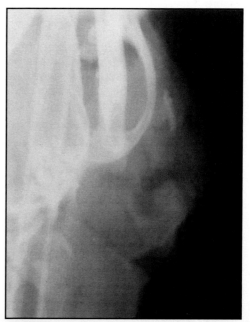

**12.45** Parotid sialoliths in an 8-year-old Cavalier King Charles Spaniel with a large salivary mucocele. A line of small, discrete, mineralized bodies are seen in the region of the parotid salivary duct. When removed surgically, they were found to be joined together as a serrated linear structure. (Reproduced from Jeffreys *et al.* (1996) with permission of the *Journal of Small Animal Practice*.)

*Sialoceles:* (Also known as salivary mucoceles and salivary cysts.) Saliva leaks from a damaged gland or duct and forms a subcutaneous fluid-filled area, which may become very large. Two types of sialocele occur:

- Sublingual sialoceles (ranulae)
- Intermandibular/cervical sialoceles.

Most sialoceles arise from an abnormality of the rostral part of the sublingual gland; submandibular salivary gland lesions are less common, although, they may occur simultaneously. Parotid and zygomatic lesions are rare; the latter may give rise to exophthalmos.

Unless a sialolith is present, survey radiography is unrewarding as it shows only soft tissue swelling. Sialography is usually required to confirm the gland or duct of origin, which is often not apparent on clinical examination. Radiological signs of abnormality include dilatation or rupture of the affected salivary duct, filling defects due to abnormal tissue or debris, gland abnormality and communication of the duct with the mucocele.

## References and further reading

Barthez PY, Koblik PD, Hornof WJ, Wisner ER and Seibert JA (1996) Apparent wall thickening in fluid filled versus air filled tympanic bulla in computed tomography. *Veterinary Radiology and Ultrasound* **37,** 95–98

Bischoff MG and Kneller SK (2004) Diagnostic imaging of the canine and feline ear. *Veterinary Clinics of North America: Small Animal Practice* **34,** 437–458

Dennis R (2000) Use of magnetic resonance imaging for the investigation of orbital disease in small animals. *Journal of Small Animal Practice* **41,** 145–155

Dennis R, Barnet KC and Sansom J (1993) A case of unilateral exophthalmos and strabismus due to craniomandibular osteopathy. *Journal of Small Animal Practice* **34,** 457–461

Dickie AM and Sullivan M (2001) The effect of obliquity on the radiographic appearance of the temporomandibular joint in dogs. *Veterinary Radiology and Ultrasound* **42,** 205-217

Featherstone H and Llabres Diaz F (2003) Maxillary bone epithelial cyst in a dog. *Journal of Small Animal Practice* **44,** 541–545

Garosi LS, Dennis R and Schwarz T (2003) Review of diagnostic imaging of ear diseases in the dog and cat. *Veterinary Radiology and Ultrasound* **44,** 137–146

Griffiths LG, Sullivan M, O'Neill T and Reid SWJ (2003) Ultrasonography versus radiography for detection of fluid in the canine tympanic bulla. *Veterinary Radiology and Ultrasound* **44,** 210–213

Hofer P, Meisen N, Bartholdi S and Kaser-Hotz B (1995) A new radiographic view of the feline tympanic bulla. *Veterinary Radiology and Ultrasound* **36,** 14–15

Jeffreys DA, Stasiw A and Demis R (1996) Parotid sialolithiasis in a dog. *Journal of Small Animal Practice* **37,** 296–297

O'Brien RT, Evans SM, Wortman JA and Hendrick MJ (1996) Radiographic findings in cats with intranasal neoplasia or chronic rhinitis: 29 cases (1982–1988). *Journal of the American Veterinary Medical Association* **208,** 385–389

Pastor KF, Boulay JP, Schelling SH and Carpenter JL (2000) Idiopathic hyperostosis of the calvaria in five young bullmastiffs. *Journal of the American Animal Hospital Association* **36,** 439–445

Sullivan M, Lee R, Jakovljevic S and Sharp NJH (1986) The radiological features of aspergillosis of the nasal cavity and frontal sinuses in the dog. *Journal of Small Animal Practice* **27,** 167–180

Sullivan M, Lee R and Skae C (1987) The radiological features of sixty cases of intra-nasal neoplasia in the dog. *Journal of Small Animal Practice* **28,** 575–586

Trower ND, Gregory SP, Renfrew H and Lamb CR (1998) Evaluation of the canine tympanic membrane by positive contrast ear canalography. *Veterinary Record* **142,** 78–81

Ziemer LS, Schwarz T and Sullivan M (2003) Otolithiasis in three dogs. *Veterinary Radiology and Ultrasound* **44,** 28–31

# 13

# Skull – nasal chambers and frontal sinuses

## Christopher R. Lamb

## Indications

Indications for radiography of the nasal cavity and frontal sinuses include:

- Nasal discharge, epistaxis, sneezing
- Head trauma
- Swelling, distortion, pain affecting maxillary or frontal regions
- Proptosis
- Epiphora.

## Radiography and normal anatomy

For information on the general radiographic technique see Chapter 12.

### Standard views

For standard lateral and ventrodorsal (VD) projections of skull see Chapter 12. The lateral view is unhelpful in many animals with nasal disease because superimposition of left and right nasal chambers tends to mask unilateral abnormalities; however, it is useful when looking for signs of disease affecting the nasal bones or cribriform plate. Similarly, a VD view is often unhelpful in animals with nasal disease due to superimposition of the mandibles over much of the nasal chambers.

A lateral radiograph centred over the nasopharynx should be considered in animals with clinical signs of nasal disease but no apparent abnormalities affecting the nasal cavity. Radiographs of the thorax are indicated in animals with signs of trauma or suspected rhinitis because of the possibility of concurrent thoracic conditions. Conversely, thoracic radiography is not usually helpful in dogs and cats with nasal neoplasia because metastasis to the lung from primary nasal neoplasms is rare.

### Special views

Radiography of the skull requires accurate patient positioning and attention to detail. General anaesthesia is required unless the patient is particularly depressed. Several specialized radiographic projections are useful for investigating dogs or cats with nasal signs:

- Dorsoventral (DV) intra-oral
- Ventral 20 degrees rostral-dorsocaudal oblique
- Rostrocaudal skyline
- Left or right 45 degrees ventral – right or left dorsal oblique.

### Dorsoventral intra-oral

DV intra-oral (Figure 13.1) is the single most useful radiograph for nasal disease because it provides a view of the nasal cavity without superimposed structures. This view also allows optimal comparison of the left and right sides, which aids recognition of asymmetrical or subtle lesions. A regular cassette is too thick to fit in the mouth of all but the largest dogs, hence it is necessary to use a thin film carrier, such as a soft cassette (Figure 13.2a). By placing the film carrier into the mouth corner first, it is possible to include the entire nasal cavity and the cribriform plate in most patients (Figure 13.2b).

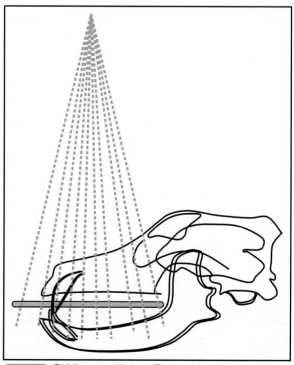

**13.1** DV (intra-oral) view. The patient is in sternal recumbency with the film in the mouth. The X-ray beam is vertical.

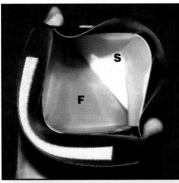

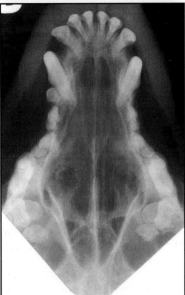

**13.2**
**(a)** Flexible film carrier held open to show the film (F) and screen (S).
**(b)** The DV (intra-oral) radiograph is the single most useful view for nasal disease because it provides a view of the nasal cavity without superimposed structures.

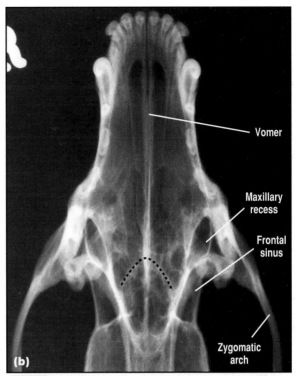

**13.3** (continued) V20° R-DCdO (open-mouth VD) view. **(b)** V20° R-DCdO (open-mouth VD) radiograph of a canine skull with anatomical landmarks indicated. The dotted line indicates the cribriform plate.

### Ventral 20 degree rostral-dorsocaudal oblique

A ventral 20 degree rostral-dorsocaudal oblique ('open-mouth VD'; V20°R-DCdO) view (Figure 13.3) is useful when it is not possible to include the most caudal

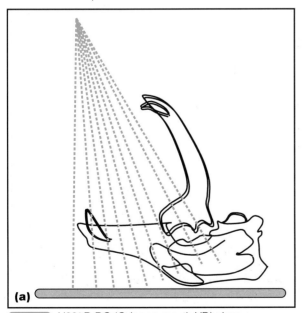

**13.3** V20° R-DCdO (open-mouth VD) view.
**(a)** The patient is placed in dorsal recumbency and the mouth opened. The X-ray beam is directed 20 degrees from vertical to show more of the caudal aspect of the nasal cavity. (continues) ▶

aspect of the nasal cavity on the DV intra-oral radiograph or when a thin film carrier is not available. The anaesthetized patient is placed in dorsal recumbency with the maxilla parallel to the cassette and the mouth held open using tapes, a gag or a perspex positioning frame. The X-ray tube head is tilted so that the primary beam strikes the mid-nasal cavity with minimal superimposition by the mandible. This view does not work well in brachycephalic dogs, hence an alternative has been described in which the dog is positioned in dorsal recumbency with the mouth closed and the X-ray beam angled from caudoventral to rostrodorsal by about 30 degrees. The relatively wide mandible of brachycephalic dogs causes less superimposition on the nasal cavity than in many other breeds.

### Rostrocaudal skyline

A rostrocaudal (RCd) skyline view (Figure 13.4) is useful for examination of the frontal sinuses, which may be the site of primary or secondary lesions in animals with nasal signs. This radiograph is usually performed using a vertical X-ray beam with the patient in dorsal recumbency and the hard palate vertical. Alternatively, a caudorostral (CdR) radiograph may be made with a horizontal X-ray beam, the patient in sternal recumbency, and the beam directed caudocranially towards a cassette propped up against the patient's external nares (Figure 13.5). This view has the advantage of making any fluid in the sinus visible as a horizontal fluid–air interface. For both the RCd and CdR views it is difficult to get suitable positioning in domed-headed dogs and short-nosed cats, such as Persians, because the frontal sinuses may be small or absent.

193

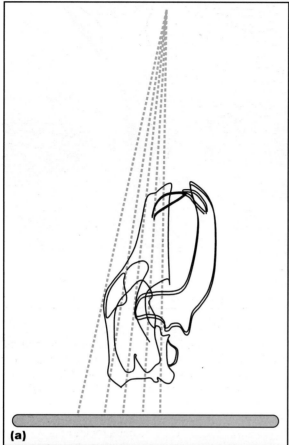

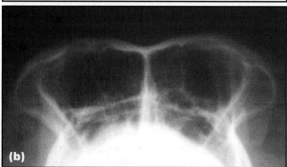

13.4  RCd (skyline). **(a)** The patient is placed in dorsal recumbency with the neck ventroflexed so that the hard palate is vertical. A vertical X-ray beam is centred on the external nares so that the diverging beam strikes the frontal sinuses. **(b)** Corresponding radiograph. Important for examination of the frontal sinuses, which may be the site of primary or secondary lesions in animals with nasal signs.

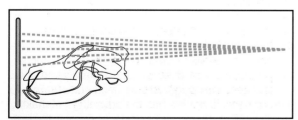

13.5  An alternative radiograph of the frontal sinuses may be made with a horizontal X-ray beam, the patient in sternal recumbency, and the beam directed towards a cassette propped up against the patient's external nares.

### Left or right 45 degrees ventral – right or left dorsal oblique

Left or right 45 degrees ventral – right or left dorsal oblique (Le45°V-RtDO or Rt45°V-LeDO) lateral radiographs made with the mouth open may be used to examine the upper dental arcades in animals with nasal conditions that may also involve the teeth, such as trauma or certain neoplasms (see Chapter 14).

### Normal anatomy

The anatomy of the nasal cavity is best depicted by the DV intra-oral view (Figure 13.6). On this view the nasal cavity is divided into left and right by the vomer, a long narrow bone that lies between the maxillae. The cartilaginous nasal septum is not visible radiographically because of superimposition by the vomer (Harvey, 1979). The nasal cavity is normally relatively lucent because of its air content but it also contains multiple fine folded bones (the turbinates) covered by mucosa. On the basis of the radiographic appearance of the turbinates, the nasal cavity may be divided into three zones:

- Rostral (canine to the third premolar) – numerous fine, slightly wavy, parallel lines represent the nasal conchae

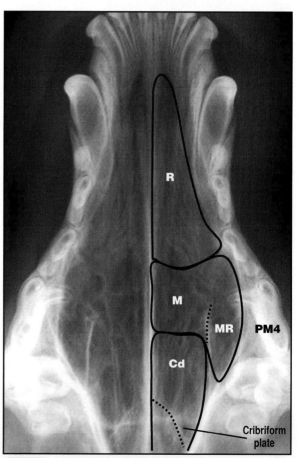

13.6  Anatomy of the nasal cavity showing the three zones: rostral (R), mid-zone (M) and caudal (Cd). Note the maxillary recess (MR), which is visible as a distinct oval lucency immediately medial to the fourth premolar and the cribriform plate (arrowed), from which the ethmoturbinates originate.

- Mid-zone (medial to the third and fourth premolars) – turbinates are rounded and more widely spaced, producing a bubbly appearance; the maxillary recess is visible as a distinct oval lucency immediately medial to the fourth premolar
- Caudal – has a series of linear paired lines that represent the ethmoturbinates, which originate from the cribriform plate.

The contribution of the turbinates to the radiographic appearance of the nasal cavity is best illustrated by a radiograph of a skull with the turbinates removed (Figure 13.7a). In this experiment, loss of turbinates results in a reduced number of fine lines and an overall increase in lucency. This appearance mimics the effect of destructive rhinitis (or rhinectomy). Alternatively, infusion of water into the nasal cavity leads to increased opacity and reduced visibility of turbinates (Figure 13.7b). This mimics the effect of swelling of the nasal mucosa, exudate or nasal haemorrhage. Loss of turbinate detail is usually interpreted as evidence of turbinate destruction, which implies a relatively aggressive disease.

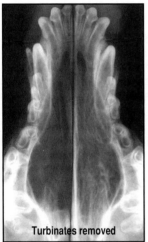

Turbinates removed

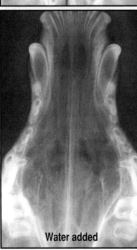

Water added

**13.7** Experiments to mimic the effect of nasal diseases. With the turbinates removed the nasal cavity is more lucent and lacks the numerous fine lines that are visible in the contralateral side. With the nasal cavity largely filled with water there is a diffuse increase in opacity. The turbinates are less clearly visible.

Variations in the appearance of the nasal cavity occur in dogs with different head shape. Dolichocephalic and mesaticephalic dogs are best suited to nasal radiography, but foreshortening of the nasal cavity in brachycephalic dogs and cats leads to greater superimposition of structures (Figure 13.8), which reduces clarity and makes interpretation more difficult.

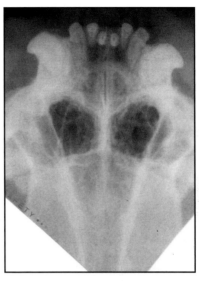

**13.8** DV (intra-oral) radiograph in a Bulldog. The internal anatomy of the nasal cavity is less well defined in brachycephalic dogs because the structures are foreshortened and thus superimposition by the soft tissues of the head occurs.

## Contrast studies

### Positive contrast rhinography

Positive contrast rhinography is a method for increasing the visibility of turbinates, nasal septum and the lining of the frontal sinus (Goring *et al.*, 1984a,b). The technique for contrast rhinography is as follows:

1. Infuse 30% w/v barium sulphate suspension through a feline urethral catheter into the dependent nasal cavity with the patient in lateral recumbency. The optimal volume of contrast medium is approximately 1 ml per 5 kg bodyweight.
2. Take lateral and DV (intra-oral) radiographs immediately.
3. If necessary, inject an additional small volume of contrast medium with the patient in dorsal recumbency to encourage flow of contrast medium into the frontal sinus; repeat radiography.

This technique may enable detection of otherwise occult nasal or nasopharyngeal masses, or abnormal communication between parts of the nasal cavity occurring as a result of invasive lesions or sinus formation.

### Dacryorhinocystography

Dacryorhinocystography is used to examine patency of the nasolacrimal duct in dogs and cats (Gelatt *et al.*, 1972). The technique for dacryorhinocystography is as follows:

1. Insert a fine catheter into the upper punctum.
2. Inject undiluted 300 mg I/ml water-soluble contrast medium slowly, while keeping digital pressure on the lower punctum to inhibit contrast leakage. Very small volumes of contrast medium are necessary: 0.2–0.3 ml for a cat or small dog; 0.3–0.5 ml for a medium to large dog.
3. Take lateral and V20°R-DCdO radiographs immediately.
4. Inject additional contrast medium and repeat radiographs if the duct is not adequately filled.

Dilatation of the nasolacrimal duct that deforms the adjacent bones may occur in association with chronic inflammation or a cyst in the lacrimal gland, a congenital condition known as dacryops (Grahn and Mason, 1995). Obstruction of the nasolacrimal duct may occur in association with exudates, foreign bodies (Figure 13.9), fractures, periodontal disease, rhinitis or nasal neoplasia. Extravasation of contrast medium into the nasal cavity indicates rupture of the duct.

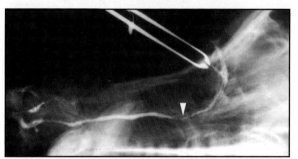

**13.9** Dacryorhinocystography. Injection of contrast medium into the upper punctum with the lower punctum occluded by an Allis forcep. The nasolacrimal duct is patent and contrast medium is leaking into the nasal cavity close to the external nares. There is an irregular filling defect (arrowhead) caused by a grass seed lodged in the nasolacrimal duct.

## Carotid arteriography

Carotid arteriography followed by selective embolization of nasal arteries has been used to treat persistent epistaxis in dogs (Weisse et al., 2004).

## Alternative imaging techniques

### Computed tomography

At institutions with computed tomography (CT), this modality has largely replaced radiography for examination of the nasal cavity in dogs and cats. A CT scan of the nasal cavity and frontal sinuses requires the patient to be perfectly still for approximately 5 minutes, hence it is usually done under a short anaesthetic. CT produces cross-sectional images, which eliminates the problem of superimposition that affects most skull radiographs, and enables a much more detailed assessment of the contents of the nasal cavity and adjacent structures than survey radiography (Figure 13.10). The extent of nasal lesions can be more reliably assessed with CT than with conventional radiography (Thrall et al., 1989; Saunders and van Bree, 2003), which makes CT particularly useful when planning surgical resection or external beam radiation therapy.

### Magnetic resonance imaging

In general, magnetic resonance imaging (MRI) is considered less useful than CT for examination of body parts containing air and bone in close proximity because neither of these normally has a signal, but nevertheless, MRI does provide an excellent depiction of nasal and extra-nasal structures (De Rycke et al., 2003). MRI is used to examine certain small animal patients with nasal disease if CT is not available or if a nasal lesion is

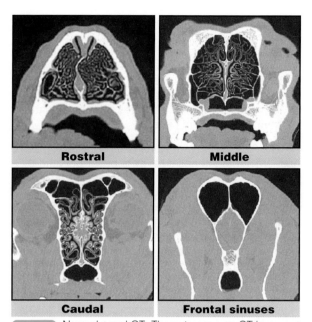

**13.10** Normal nasal CT. These transverse CT images of the rostral, middle and caudal parts of the nasal cavity and the frontal sinuses of a dog without signs of nasal disease illustrate the fine anatomical detail that is possible with this imaging modality.

suspected to involve other structures, such as the orbit or brain. Nasal neoplasms that invade the brain are particularly well depicted using MRI (see below).

## Ultrasonography

The extension of nasal neoplasms into the orbit may be detected ultrasonographically (Mason et al., 2001).

## Abnormal radiographic findings

### Trauma

Skull fractures are commonly observed in small animals. The choice of radiographic views will largely be dictated by physical findings, but will often include DV intra-oral, lateral and RCd skyline views to examine the nasal cavity (Figure 13.11a) and frontal sinuses (Figure 13.11b). Additional radiographs may be required to examine the mandible, zygomatic arches and temporomandibular joints (see Chapter 12).

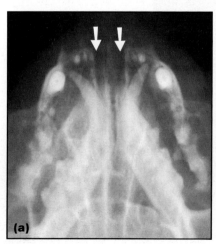

**13.11** Nasal trauma. **(a)** Separation of the incisive and maxillary symphysis (arrowed) in a DV radiograph of a cat that fell from a high window. (continued) ▶

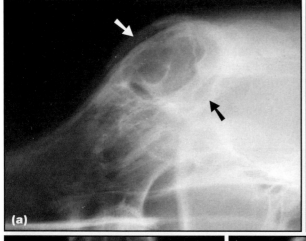

**13.11** (continued) Nasal trauma. **(b)** Multiple depressed frontal bone fractures (arrowed) in a dog that was hit by a car.

Frontal sinus mucocele refers to an accumulation of mucus in the frontal sinus that occurs after obstruction of the nasofrontal opening. The usual cause is trauma, leading to malunion. Radiographically, the affected sinus has an increased opacity because of retained secretions and is enlarged with thinning of the outer table of the frontal bone (Figure 13.12).

## Congenital and developmental conditions

### Cleft palate

A cleft palate is a congenital anomaly resulting from the failure of the sides of the palate to fuse, leaving a midline opening between the oral and nasal cavities. Although the diagnosis of cleft palate is usually possible on the basis of physical examination alone, radiography may be used to examine the affected bones (Figure 13.13) and assess the severity of any secondary rhinitis. Dogs with a cleft palate are prone to otitis media, which can also be assessed radiographically (and by CT or MRI).

### Immotile cilia syndrome

Animals with congenital abnormalities resulting in immotile cilia are prone to respiratory tract infections (Edwards *et al.*, 1989). Affected individuals or littermates may present at a few months of age with clinical and radiographic signs of relatively severe rhinitis and sinusitis (see below), and bronchopneumonia. The combination of immotile cilia, bronchiectasis and situs inversus is known as Kartagener's syndrome.

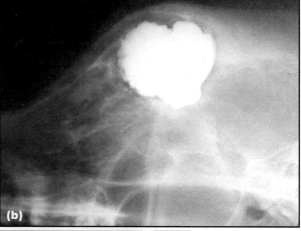

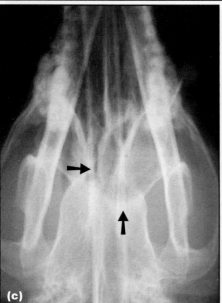

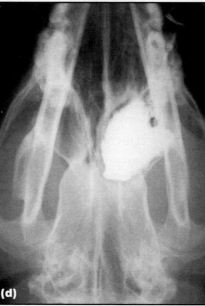

**13.12**

Frontal sinus mucocele. **(a, c)** Survey radiographs of a dog that had sustained fractures affecting the frontal bones several months previously. There is increased opacity and enlargement of the left frontal sinus (arrowed). **(b, d)** Contrast radiographs. A needle was inserted directly through the thin outer table of the frontal bone and contrast medium injected. Lack of flow of contrast medium into the nasal cavity indicates obstruction of the nasofrontal meatus and supports diagnosis of frontal sinus mucocele.

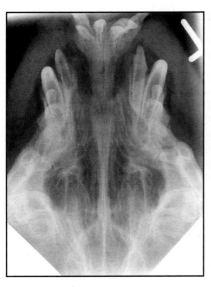

DV (intra-oral) radiograph of a young dog showing an unusual bilateral cleft affecting the incisive bones with resulting malposition of the incisors.

## Rhinitis and sinusitis

Rhinitis and sinusitis may be classified as:

- Allergic
- Hyperplastic
- Lymphocytic–plasmacytic
- Infectious
- Foreign body-associated
- Secondary to dental disease.

In the UK the most important nasal and sinus infection affecting dogs is aspergillosis, which causes a severe destructive rhinitis (Sharp *et al.,* 1991). This condition is less prevalent in other geographical areas and, depending on location, other fungi may colonize the nasal cavity. In cats, rhinitis may be caused by various respiratory infections including calicivirus, feline herpes virus-1, *Actinomyces, Bordetella bronchiseptica, Chlamydophila felis* and *Cryptococcus neoformans*. Rhinitis in cats has also been associated with systemic conditions, such as feline immunodeficiency virus (FIV) infection, and eosinophilic or lymphocytic–plasmacytic infiltration. Rhinitis (and any secondary sinusitis) may become chronic when inflammation is severe enough to cause structural changes in the nasal mucosa that compromise its immune function.

In recent studies, 55% of dogs and 30% of cats with rhinitis had radiographs that appeared to be normal (Russo *et al.*, 2000; Lamb *et al.*, 2003). Acute rhinitis causing minor mucosal swelling and serous discharge is unlikely to be recognized radiologically, but chronic rhinitis often produces radiographic signs. The different forms of chronic rhinitis can appear similar radiologically, hence the specific diagnosis will often depend on endoscopic, surgical or pathological results. The key radiographic signs of rhinitis in dogs with chronic nasal signs are:

- Lucent foci in nasal cavity
- Focal or multifocal loss of turbinate detail
- Localized soft tissue opacities.

Lucent foci occur when destructive forms of rhinitis (e.g. such as that caused by aspergillosis) destroy the turbinates and overlying mucosa but produce relatively little inflammatory tissue or exudates, hence the nasal cavity of an affected dog is relatively empty. When the abnormalities listed above occur together (Figure 13.14), a diagnosis of destructive rhinitis may be made with confidence.

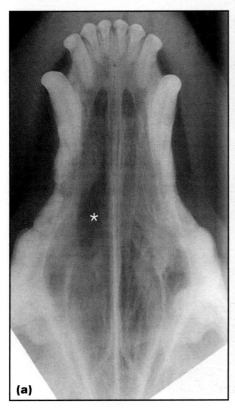

(a)

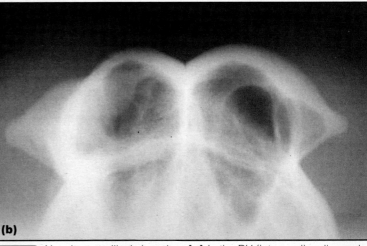

(b)

Nasal aspergillosis in a dog. **(a)** In the DV (intra-oral) radiograph there is increased opacity affecting the peripheral parts of the right nasal cavity and loss of turbinate detail, particularly medial to the third premolar where there is an oblong lucent zone (∗). The contralateral structures appear normal. **(b)** In the RCd (skyline) radiograph there is a relatively uniform thickening of the outer table of the right frontal bone, which has encroached on the lumen of the sinus. The zygomatic process now appears solid, whereas it normally contains the lateral aspect of the sinus (as on left). This combination of signs is typical of destructive rhinitis and chronic sinusitis.

Radiographic signs in cats with rhinitis are similar to those observed in dogs, but are more variable (Figure 13.15). Compared with dogs, more cats with chronic rhinitis have fluid and soft tissue opacity in the frontal sinuses because of exudative sinusitis.

A nasal foreign body is another possible cause of unilateral chronic rhinitis. The most common nasal foreign bodies are grass seeds and other plant fragments, which are invisible radiographically. Opaque foreign bodies, such as air gun pellets that lodge in the nasal cavity, are readily identified radiographically (Figure 13.16).

Rhinitis associated with nasal mites (*Pneumonyssus caninum*) is usually a subclinical infection (Gunnarsson *et al.*, 2001) and unlikely to produce any radiographic signs. In contrast, the tongue worm (*Linguatula serrata*) can cause a more severe haemorrhagic rhinitis that may be evident radiographically, although a definitive diagnosis will usually require endoscopy or rhinotomy. *Linguatula* is rare in the UK but prevalent in many other parts of the world.

## Neoplasia

Primary nasal neoplasms in the dog include a variety of cell types, including carcinoma (adenocarcinoma, mucoepidermoid carcinoma, squamous cell carcinoma) and sarcoma (chondrosarcoma, haemangiosarcoma, osteosarcoma). In cats with nasal and sinus neoplasia, the most frequent diagnoses are lymphoma, adenocarcinoma and squamous cell carcinoma. Most nasal neoplasms arise from the mucosa of the nasal cavity or frontal sinus and are malignant, spreading by local invasion and occasionally via lymphatics to the submandibular and retropharyngeal nodes. Benign nasal neoplasms are uncommon in dogs and cats.

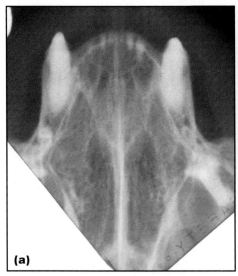
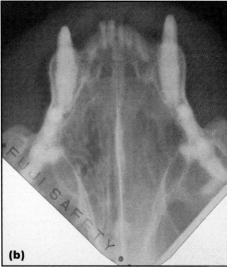
(a) (b)

**13.15** The variable appearance of rhinitis in cats. **(a)** DV (intra-oral) radiograph of a cat with rhinitis associated with a mixed bacterial infection, in which the intranasal structures were interpreted as within normal limits. **(b)** DV (intra-oral) radiograph of a cat with chronic necrotizing rhinitis, in which there is a generalized increase in opacity with loss of turbinate detail affecting the left nasal cavity. (Reproduced from Lamb *et al.*, 2003 with permission from the *Journal of Feline Medicine and Surgery*.)

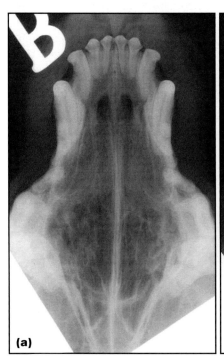
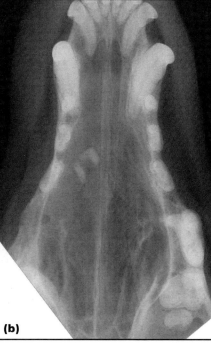
(a) (b)

**13.16** Nasal foreign bodies. **(a)** Normal-appearing DV (intra-oral) radiograph of a dog with persistent sneezing. Multiple pine needles were flushed from the nasal cavity. **(b)** Opaque nasal foreign body (piece of electrical insulation) lodged in the rostral part of the right nasal cavity. There is an increased opacity and loss of turbinate detail surrounding this object as a result of a locally severe rhinitis.

Cutaneous squamous cell carcinoma is a common neoplasm in cats, which frequently occurs on the nasal planum and the pinnae. Animals with this condition are not usually examined radiographically because of its superficial location.

The key radiographic signs of nasal neoplasia in dogs are:

- Lysis of bone around the margins of the nasal cavity
- A lesion affecting all parts of ipsilateral nasal cavity
- Generalized unilateral or bilateral soft tissue opacities

- Soft tissue and fluid opacity in ipsilateral frontal sinus
- Generalized loss of turbinate detail.

In contrast to destructive forms of rhinitis, nasal neoplasms tend to fill the nasal cavity with soft tissue (Russo *et al.*, 2000). This frequently results in a relatively uniform soft tissue opacity that may occupy the entire ipsilateral nasal cavity at the time of first presentation (Figure 13.17). More advanced neoplasms frequently extend beyond the normal boundaries of the nasal cavity, displacing the nasal septum, causing lysis of surrounding bones (Figure 13.18) and obstruction of the external nares (Figure 13.19).

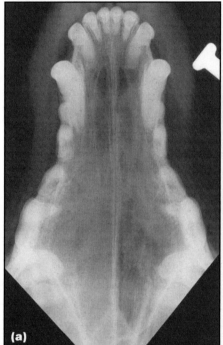

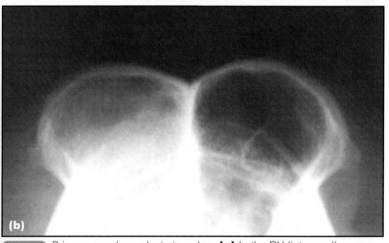

**13.17** Primary nasal neoplasia in a dog. **(a)** In the DV (intra-oral) radiograph there is increased opacity affecting the right nasal cavity and generalized loss of turbinate detail, resulting in a relatively homogenous appearance. The contralateral structures appear normal. **(b)** In the RCd (skyline) radiograph there is soft tissue and fluid opacity filling the ipsilateral frontal sinus.

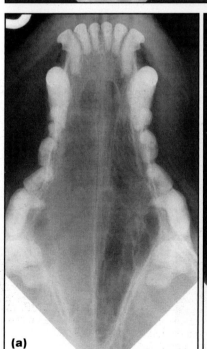
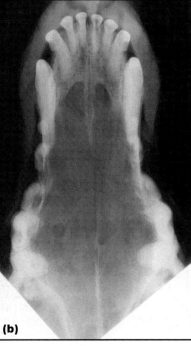

**13.18** Advanced nasal neoplasms. **(a)** Partial loss of the vomer and soft tissue mass bulging to the left in a dog with nasal carcinoma. **(b)** Bilateral increased opacity, generalized loss of turbinate detail, complete loss of the central portion of the vomer and multiple small lucent foci medial to the right fourth premolar compatible with lysis of the hard palate in a dog with advanced nasal carcinoma.

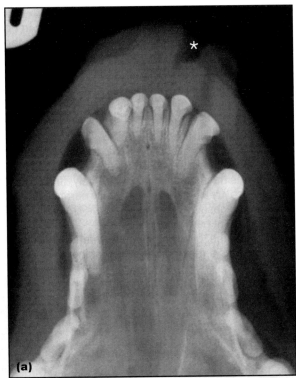

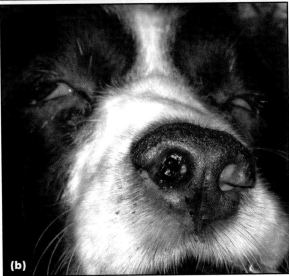

**13.19** Obstruction of external nares by nasal neoplasm. **(a)** DV (intra-oral) radiograph of a dog with a nasal neoplasm in which there is obliteration of the right nostril. The left nostril remains visible because of the air it contains (✱). **(b)** Photograph of this patient showing an ulcerated mass occluding the right nostril.

The radiographic signs in cats with nasal neoplasia are similar to those reported in dogs (Lamb *et al.*, 2003) (Figures 13.20 and 13.21). One noteworthy difference is the lower proportion of cats with nasal neoplasia that have soft tissue and fluid opacity in the frontal sinus compared to dogs. This and the higher proportion of cats with rhinitis that also have soft tissue and fluid opacity in the ipsilateral frontal sinus combine to reduce the significance of this sign, and it is less useful as a means of distinguishing these conditions than it is in dogs.

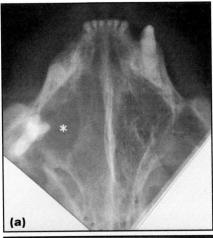

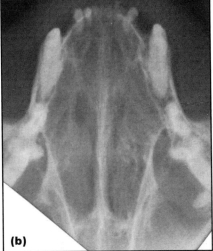

**13.20** Nasal neoplasia in the cat. **(a)** DV (intra-oral) radiograph of a cat with a granular cell tumour originating in the right nasal cavity. There is a relatively uniform increased opacity with loss of turbinate detail affecting the right nasal cavity and a focal lucent area (✱) as a result of bone destruction. **(b)** DV (intra-oral) radiograph of a cat with nasal lymphoma. There is a generalized increased opacity and obscured turbinates, more marked in the left nasal cavity. (Reproduced from Lamb *et al.*, 2003 with permission from the *Journal of Feline Medicine and Surgery*.)

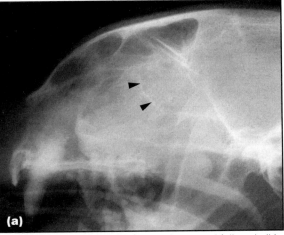

**13.21** **(a)** Lateral radiograph of a normal feline skull in which the cribriform plate is visible (arrowheads). (continues) ▶

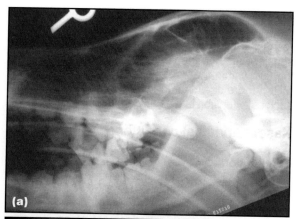

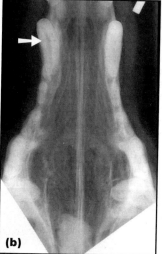

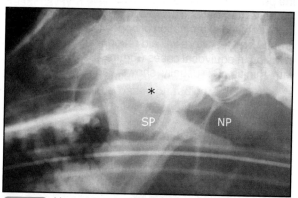

## Neoplasia

Malignant neoplasms may also be observed affecting the nasopharynx. The most common type in the cat is lymphoma (Allen *et al.*, 1999). Affected individuals usually have clinical signs that suggest a nasal lesion but radiographs centred on the nasal cavity may be normal. Under these circumstances it is important to consider the possibility that the lesion is nasopharyngeal and obtain a lateral radiograph to examine this area (Figure 13.27).

**13.25** Nasopharyngeal foreign body (pebble) in **(a)** lateral and **(b)** DV (intra-oral) radiographs of a stone-carrying dog. This object was removed orally using forceps. The enlarged pulp cavity affecting the right upper canine (arrowed) is the result of a tooth fracture that also occurred because of stone carrying.

**13.27** Nasopharyngeal neoplasm in a dog. Lateral radiograph of a dog with nasal signs showing a sessile soft tissue mass (★) on the dorsal aspect of the nasopharynx (NP). SP = Soft palate.

## Nasopharyngeal polyps

Nasopharyngeal polyps are non-neoplastic, inflammatory growths in cats that arise from the middle ear or the Eustachian tube and extend into the pharynx (Kudnig, 2002). Clinical signs reflect obstruction of the nasopharynx or the effects of otitis media and otitis interna. This lesion may be recognized in lateral radiographs as a rounded intra-luminal soft tissue structure in the nasopharynx that may displace the soft palate ventrally (Figure 13.26). Polyps may be treated effectively by surgery and carry a better prognosis than neoplasms.

## Stenosis

Nasopharyngeal stenosis is an uncommon condition that occurs in cats as a sequel to inflammation associated with upper respiratory tract infection. In this condition, a thin membrane of fibrous granulation tissue partially obstructs the nasopharynx, causing signs such as stertor and mouth-breathing. The membrane may be faintly visible on survey radiographs, although it is more clearly demonstrated by contrast rhinography or endoscopy (Figure 13.28). A recent report described treatment of this condition by fluoroscopically guided balloon dilatation (Boswood *et al.*, 2003).

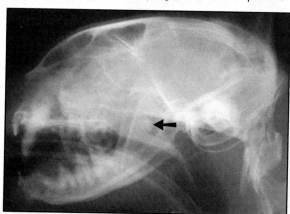

**13.26** Lateral radiograph of a cat showing a rounded intra-luminal soft tissue mass in the nasopharynx (arrowed). This appearance is typical of nasopharyngeal polyp in the cat. Larger lesions may also cause ventral displacement of the soft palate.

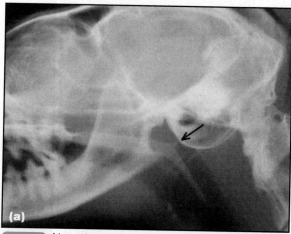

**13.28** Nasopharyngeal stenosis in a cat. **(a)** Lateral radiograph of the head showing a narrow strand-like soft tissue opacity across the nasopharynx (arrowed). At this site there is also a slight dorsal deviation of the soft palate. (Reproduced from Boswood *et al.*, 2003 with permission from *Veterinary Radiology and Ultrasound*.) (continues) ▶

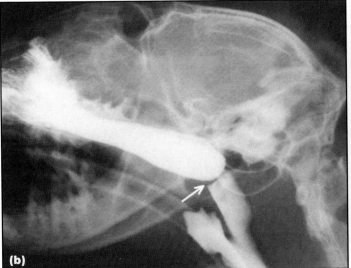

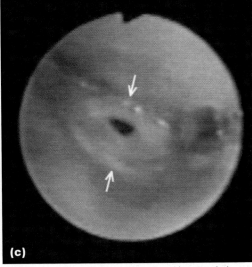

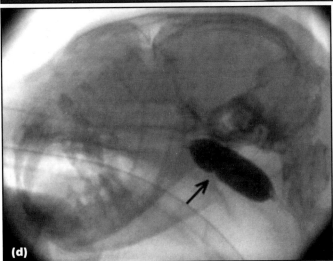

**13.28** (continued) Nasopharyngeal stenosis in a cat. **(b)** Positive contrast rhinography showing a partial obstruction to flow of contrast medium and a distinct septum in the nasopharynx (arrowed) at the same site as the strand-like soft tissue opacity in (a). **(c)** Retrograde endoscopic image of the nasopharynx (ventral at top) showing a pale, smooth membrane that spans the entire nasopharynx (arrowed) with only a single small orifice at its centre. (Note: variation in colour hue during reproduction of this image makes it erroneously appear that the cat was cyanotic.) **(d)** Lateral fluoroscopic image of the head during balloon dilatation to treat the stenosis. A waist in the balloon at the site of the septum (arrowed) was observed transiently before disappearing on full inflation of the balloon. (Reproduced from Boswood *et al.*, 2003 with permission from *Veterinary Radiology and Ultrasound*.)

## References and further reading

Allen HS, Broussard J and Noone K (1999) Nasopharyngeal diseases in cats: a retrospective study of 53 cases (1991–1998). *Journal of the American Animal Hospital Association* **35**, 457–461

Boswood A, Lamb CR, Brockman D, Witt A and Mantis P (2003) Balloon dilatation of nasopharyngeal stenosis in a cat. *Veterinary Radiology and Ultrasound* **44**, 53–55

De Rycke LM, Saunders JH, Gielen IM, van Bree HJ and Simoens PJ (2003) Magnetic resonance imaging, computed tomography, and cross-sectional views of the anatomy of normal nasal cavities and paranasal sinuses in mesaticephalic dogs. *American Journal of Veterinary Research* **64**, 1093–1098

Edwards DF, Kennedy JR, Patton CS, Toal RL, Daniel GB and Lothrop CD (1989) Familial immotile-cilia syndrome in English springer spaniel dogs. *American Journal of Medical Genetics* **33**, 290–298

Gelatt K, Cure T, Guffy M and Jessen C (1972) Dacryorhinocystography in the dog and cat. *Journal of Small Animal Practice* **13**, 381–397

Goring RL, Ticer JW, Gross TL and Ackerman N (1984a) Positive contrast rhinography. A technique for radiographic evaluation of the nasal cavity, nasal pharynx, and paranasal sinuses in the dog. *Veterinary Radiology* **25**, 98–105

Goring RL, Ticer JW, Ackerman N and Gross TL (1984b) Contrast rhinography in the radiographic evaluation of the nasal cavity, nasal pharynx, and paranasal sinuses in the dog. *Veterinary Radiology* **25**, 106–123

Grahn BH and Mason RA (1995) Epiphora associated with dacryops in a dog. *Journal of the American Animal Hospital Association* **31**, 15–19

Gunnarsson LK, Zakrisson G, Egenvall A, Christensson DA and Uggla A (2001) Prevalence of *Pneumonyssoides caninum* infection in dogs in Sweden. *Journal of the American Animal Hospital Association* **37**, 331–337

Harvey CE (1979) The nasal septum of the dog: is it visible radiographically? *Journal of the American Veterinary Radiology Society* **20**, 88–90

Kudnig ST (2002) Nasopharyngeal polyps in cats. *Clinical Techniques in Small Animal Practice* **17**, 174–177

Lamb CR, Richbell S and Mantis P (2003) Radiographic signs in cats with nasal disease. *Journal of Feline Medicine and Surgery* **5**, 227–235

Mason DR, Lamb CR and McLellan GJ (2001) Ultrasonographic findings in 50 dogs with retrobulbar disease. *Journal of the American Animal Hospital Association* **37**, 557–562

Russo M, Lamb CR and Jakovljevic S (2000) Distinguishing canine nasal neoplasia and rhinitis by radiography. *Veterinary Radiology and Ultrasound* **41**, 118–124

Saunders JH and van Bree H (2003) Comparison of radiography and computed tomography for the diagnosis of canine nasal aspergillosis. *Veterinary Radiology and Ultrasound* **44**, 414–419

Schwarz T, Sullivan M and Hartung K (2000) Radiographic detection of defects of the nasal boundaries. *Veterinary Radiology and Ultrasound* **41**, 226–230

Sharp NJH, Harvey CE and Sullivan M (1991) Canine nasal aspergillosis and penicilliosis. *Compendium on Continuing Education for the Practicing Veterinarian* **13**, 41–48

Thrall DE, Robertson ID, McLeod DA, Heidner GL, Hoopes PJ and Page RL (1989) A comparison of radiographic and computed tomographic findings in 31 dogs with malignant nasal tumors. *Veterinary Radiology and Ultrasound* **30**, 59–66

Weisse C, Nicholson ME, Rollings C, Hammer K, Hurst R and Solomon JA (2004) Use of percutaneous arterial embolization for treatment of intractable epistaxis in three dogs. *Journal of the American Veterinary Medical Association* **224**, 1307–1311

# 14

# Skull – teeth

## Gerhard Steenkamp

Dental radiography is essential for the practice of good veterinary dentistry. A thorough work-up of the oral cavity and even the nasal passages should always have some component of dental radiography associated with it. Ideally all first patients should undergo a full mouth radiographic examination in order to diagnose early lesions that are not apparent on intra-oral examination. With some practice the radiographic procedure may only add about 10–15 minutes to the overall time of the dental procedure.

This chapter should be read in conjunction with an appropriate veterinary dentistry text (see *BSAVA Manual of Canine and Feline Dentistry*) as it is beyond the scope of this text to guide the clinician through all the relevant dental terminology and oral pathology.

## Indications

There are many reasons to perform dental radiography and the following are some indications:

- Dental trauma
- Jaw fractures
- Retained deciduous dentition
- Anodontia (absence of teeth) and other dental developmental abnormalities
- Periodontal disease
- Endodontic disease
- Extraction of teeth
- Malocclusions
- Mandibular/maxillary masses
- Nasal discharge
- Discharging sinuses in the region of the mandible/maxilla
- Medico-legal reasons.

## Radiography and normal anatomy

Dental and standard X-ray machines may be used to take dental radiographs. Dental X-ray machines provide the operator with a very comfortable and easy option to use, which is usually situated in the dental operatory. The variations in using the two different types of X-ray machines are shown in Figure 14.1. Typical exposure factors for both units are shown in Figure 14.2.

For the safety of the patient and clinician, intra-oral radiographic examinations should always be performed with the patient under general anaesthesia.

| Variable | Dental unit | Standard unit |
|---|---|---|
| Kilovolts (kV) | Fixed 50–90 | Adjustable up to 150 |
| Milliamperes (mA) | Fixed 7–15 | Adjustable up to 500 |
| Time (s) | Adjustable | Adjustable |
| Film focal distance (FFD) | Fixed 20 cm | Adjustable up to 120 cm |
| Head adaptability | Rotation in many directions possible | More rigid, head not very adaptable to patient |
| Patient positioning | Lateral, sternal or dorsal | Patient has to be moved into various positions because the radiographic unit's head is not very adaptable |
| Radiographic unit position | Fixed in dental operatory | Not in dental operatory, excessive movement of patient results |
| Extra-oral radiographs | Limited due to size of collimator | Ideal |
| Intra-oral radiographs | Ideal | Good, with limitations as previously stated |

**14.1** Comparison of dental with standard X-ray machines for the taking of dental radiographs, using standard D-speed dental radiographic film.

| Species | Dental | | | Standard machine at FFD 105 cm | |
|---|---|---|---|---|---|
| | *kV* | *mA* | *s* | *kV* | *mAs* |
| Cat or dog <10 kg | 75 | 15 | 0.1–0.3 | 60 | 25–40 |
| Dog 10–30 kg | 75 | 15 | 0.2–0.4 | 66 | 25–40 |
| Dog >30 kg | 75 | 15 | 0.3–0.5 | 70 | 32–50 |

**14.2** Typical exposure factors for dental radiographs, using two different types of radiographic machine and standard D-speed dental X-ray film. kV = Kilovolts; mA = Milliamperes; s = Seconds.

## Radiographic film

The most common form of dental radiography is performed by placing the radiographic film inside the oral cavity (intra-oral technique). The radiographic film should be small enough to fit inside the oral cavity without causing damage to any adjacent soft tissue structures. There are various sizes of dental radiographic film that can be used. Figure 14.3 summarizes these along with the uses of the film.

| Size | Description | Code | Uses |
|---|---|---|---|
| 0 (2.2 x 3.5 cm) | Periapical (paediatric) | DF 54 | Cats and small dogs: incisors, premolars and molars |
| 2 (3.1 x 4.1 cm) | Periapical | DF 58 | Cats and small dogs: canines, nasal (DV). Dogs >10 kg: incisors, premolars, molars and canines |
| 4 (5.7 x 7.6 cm) | Occlusal | DF 50 | Dogs >10 kg: canines, molars or nasal (DV) |

**14.3** Different sizes of dental radiographic film and their uses in veterinary dentistry.

Dental radiographic film differs from the standard radiographic film in that it is a non-screen double emulsion film, which comes individually packed and ready to use. These features result in superb radiographic detail but the film is unfortunately slow and increased exposure times are needed. Dental radiographic film comes in two speeds:

- D = Ultra (slower)
- E = Ekta (faster).

The D-speed film is used most commonly and all references to exposure factors in this Chapter refer to D-speed film. For E-speed film the proposed exposure time should be halved.

Each dental film consists of an impervious cover, which is white on the side that should be exposed, and dually coloured (white and green) on the side that should not be exposed. The backside of the film will often also bear the inscriptions 'Backside' or 'Other

side towards beam'. On opening the packet, by pulling the tag on the backside, there should be a lead foil closest to the back in order to prevent back scatter degrading the film. Therefore, should the incorrect side of the film be exposed, the image will be underexposed and blurred. In front of the lead foil, one or two films are situated between two layers of black paper.

Dental radiographic film is too small to use markers in order to identify the side of the mouth from which the image was taken. For identification purposes each dental film has a raised dot or contralaterally a dimple in one of the corners (Figure 14.4), which should always be placed so that the dot points towards the X-ray beam. When evaluating a developed film the dot will serve as a reference point for the direction of the X-ray beam and, therefore, determining which side of the mouth was radiographed is possible. When using a dental film extra-orally, it is important to note this down as the raised dot is now situated outside the oral cavity. Failure to label extra-oral radiographs accurately may lead to confusion with re-evaluation at a later stage.

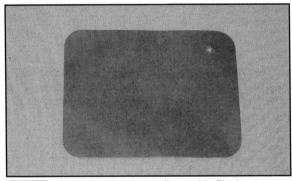

**14.4** An occlusal dental radiographic film lead backing, showing the convex dot that should always point towards the X-ray beam.

## Film positioning

The ideal film position would be parallel to the tooth's long axis and perpendicular to the X-ray beam. This position will give the most accurate image of the tooth. Due to the oral anatomy of dogs and cats this view is only possible when radiographing the mandibular molars and premolars, excluding the first premolar (Figure 14.5).

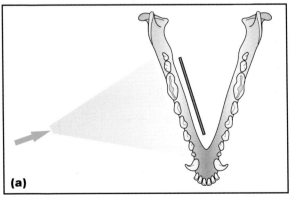

(a)

**14.5** An intra-oral parallel radiograph can only be made of the mandibular premolars and molars, excluding premolar one. **(a)** Placement of the dental film. (continues) ▶

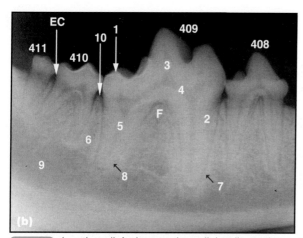

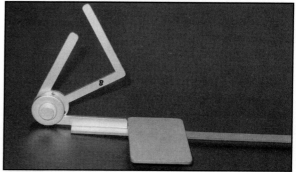

**14.7** A Pattol® device that helps the radiographer determine the bisecting angle. The incident beam should always be perpendicular to the bisecting angle (B).

**14.5** (continued) An intra-oral parallel radiograph can only be made of the mandibular premolars and molars, excluding premolar one. **(b)** Parallel radiograph of the mandibular first molar area showing the normal anatomical structures. 1 = Enamel; 2 = Dentine; 3 = Pulp horn; 4 = Pulp chamber; 5 = Root canal; 6 = Alveolar bone; 7 = Lamina dura (radiopaque); 8 = Periodontal ligament space (radiolucent); 9 = Mandibular canal; 10 = Alveolar bone height; 408 = Fourth mandibular premolar tooth; 409 = First mandibular molar tooth; 410 = Second mandibular molar tooth; 411 = Third mandibular molar tooth; EC = Enamel–cementum junction (approximately); F = Furcation area.

To obtain an accurate image of all the other teeth, a bisecting angle technique should be employed. The principle behind this technique is that there is an angle between the tooth and the film. With the incoming X-ray beam perpendicular to the tooth, an elongated image will be made (Figure 14.6a). In contrast, if the incoming X-ray beam is perpendicular to the film, a foreshortened image will be seen (Figure 14.6b). When the X-ray beam is perpendicular to an imaginary line, formed by halving the angle that is formed between the tooth and the dental film, a true-sized image will be formed (Figure 14.6c). The Pattol® (J. Morita Manufacturing Company, Japan) is a device that can help the radiographer determine this bisecting angle (Figure.14.7). By adjusting the legs for the film and the tooth, the bisecting angle leg is automatically adjusted.

## Extra-oral radiographic techniques

Standard radiographic film can be used for overview radiographs of the maxilla or mandible (see Chapter 12). Dental radiographic film is used extra-orally for the near lateral view of the maxillary fourth premolar tooth in cats. When a normal bisecting angle radiograph of this area is taken, superimposition of the zygomatic arch over the roots of the fourth premolar makes interpretation difficult (Figure 14.8). The cat is placed in lateral recumbency with the tooth to be examined closest to the film. With the head tilted dorsolaterly the zygomatic arch can be avoided (Figure 14.9).

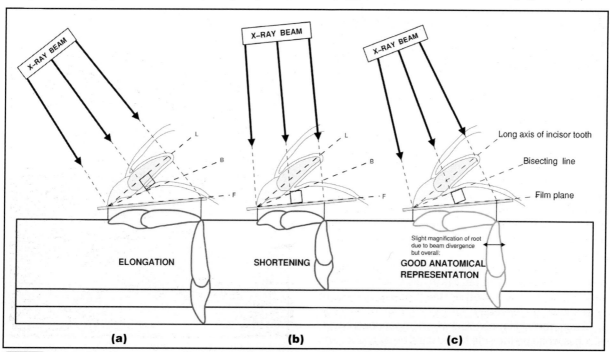

**14.6** **(a)** Incident beam perpendicular to tooth: elongation of image. **(b)** Incident beam perpendicular to film: foreshortening of image. **(c)** Incident beam perpendicular to the bisecting angle: life-size image. (© David Crossley and reproduced with permission.)

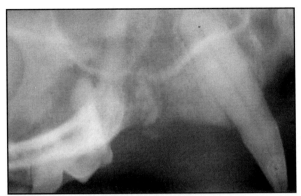

14.8 Superimposition of the zygomatic arch over the roots of the fourth premolar (208).

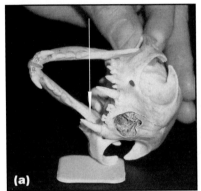

**14.9**

Near lateral technique. **(a)** Principle behind the technique, note that the roots are separated from the zygomatic arch. **(b)** Extra-oral dental radiograph of 208 of a dried skull.

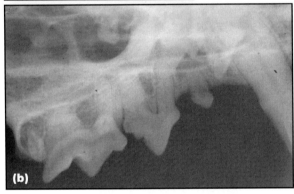

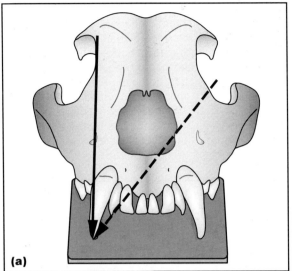

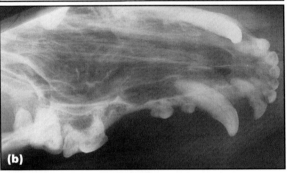

14.10 Intra-oral 45° oblique maxilla overview radiograph. **(a)** Placement of the dental film. **(b)** Radiograph clearly showing all the teeth, except for the incisors.

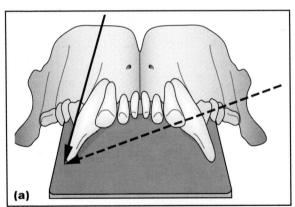

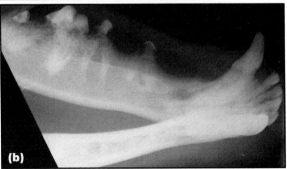

14.11 Intra-oral 30° oblique mandible overview radiograph. **(a)** Placement of the dental film. **(b)** Radiograph clearly showing all the teeth, except for the incisors.

## Intra-oral radiographic techniques

### Overview of a quadrant

In humans the panoramic view is a useful screening tool for a general evaluation for pathology of the jawbones and teeth (Mauriello *et al.*, 1995). For various reasons, a similar modality is not available for use in animals. In order for a practitioner to get an overview of the jawbones and teeth in dogs and cats, six views are commonly used. These include intra-oral 45° oblique views for each maxilla (Figure 14.10) and the approximately 30° oblique views for both mandibles (Figure 14.11). This approximates the bisecting angle technique used for teeth (see above) and gives a good overview of the jawbones and associated teeth, especially if the clinician wants to assess the extent of a large cystic or lytic lesion. These views can be exposed on to dental radiographic film in smaller patients, mammography film (excellent detail) in larger patients or on to standard film screen combinations in large-breed dogs. The last two of the six views are described below.

### Maxillary incisors and canines

With the patient in sternal or lateral recumbency, the film is placed between the mandibular and maxillary incisors. The bisecting angle between the incisors and film is determined and the X-ray beam directed perpendicular to this bisecting line (Figure 14.12).

In this view the maxillary canine root is often superimposed on the first or second maxillary premolar tooth. A bisecting angle technique from a lateral position is therefore often more valuable to assess the root of the canine tooth (Figure 14.13).

### Maxillary premolars and molars

With the patient in sternal or lateral recumbency, the film is placed palatally to the tooth or teeth to be visualized. The bisecting angle is calculated and the X-ray beam positioned perpendicular to it (Figure 14.14a). To separate the mesiobuccal and mesiopalatal roots of the maxillary fourth premolar tooth it is advised that at least two views of this tooth are taken, a lateral (Figure 14.14b) and an oblique lateral view, with the X-ray tube in a rostral oblique or caudal oblique direction (Figure 14.15).

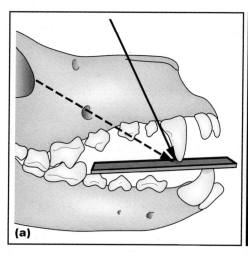
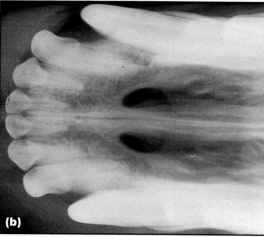

**14.12**
Bisecting angle technique for the maxillary incisors and canines. **(a)** Placement of the dental film. **(b)** Dental radiograph of maxillary incisors and canine teeth.

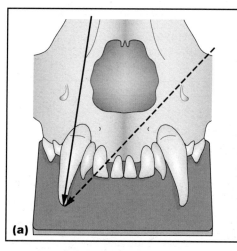
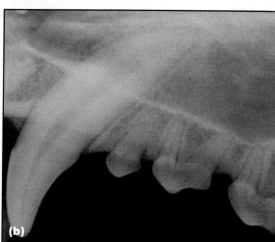

**14.13**
Lateral bisecting angle technique of the maxillary canine tooth. **(a)** Placement of the dental film. **(b)** Dental radiograph of the maxillary canine tooth.

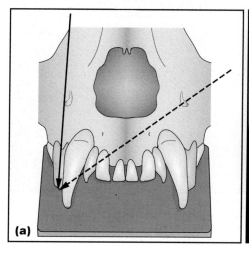
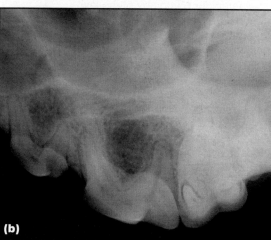

**14.14**
Bisecting angle technique for the maxillary premolars and molars. **(a)** Placement of the dental film. **(b)** Dental radiograph of the maxillary fourth premolar tooth. Note the superimposition of the mesiobuccal and mesiopalatal roots.

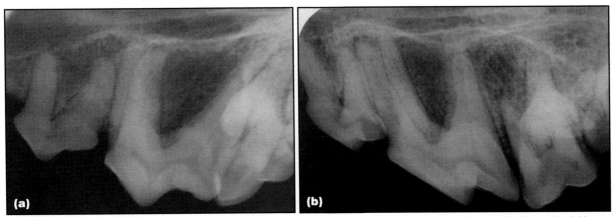

**14.15** In order to separate the two mesial roots for evaluation, one of two accessory bisecting angle views should be taken. **(a)** A rostral oblique dental radiograph. **(b)** A caudal oblique dental radiograph of the maxillary fourth premolar tooth. Both these views were taken on a dried skull. Note the separation of the mesial roots compared with Figure 14.14.

## Mandibular incisors and canines

With the patient in dorsal or lateral recumbency, the film is placed between the maxillary and mandibular incisors and canine teeth. If the frenulum of the tongue interferes with the film placement, the tongue can be depressed and the film positioned on the dorsum of the tongue (Figure 14.16).

## Mandibular first premolar tooth and canine

Due to the caudal extent of the symphysis, it is usually not possible for dental film to fit parallel to the first mandibular premolar. A bisecting angle technique is used for the first mandibular premolar. The film is positioned as above and the X-ray tube placed laterally. This view also gives additional information regarding the mandibular canine (Figure 14.17).

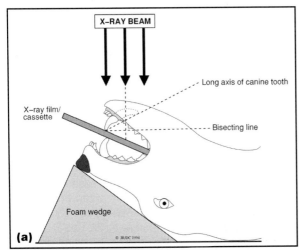
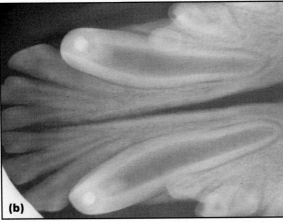

**14.16** Bisecting angle technique for the mandibular incisors and canines. **(a)** Placement of the dental film. (© David Crossley and reproduced with permission.) **(b)** Dental radiograph of mandibular incisors and canine teeth.

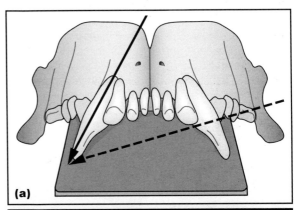
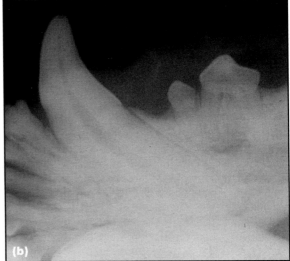

**14.17** Lateral bisecting angle technique of the mandibular first premolar tooth and canine. **(a)** Placement of the dental film. **(b)** Dental radiograph of the mandibular first premolar tooth and canine.

**Mandibular premolars (excluding first premolar) and molars**

This is the only place in the mouth of dogs and cats where a parallel technique can be used. The film is placed lingual to the mandible and ventrally it can displace the soft tissue structures to show the total height of the mandible (see Figure 14.5).

## Developing dental radiographic film

Dental radiographic film can be developed manually, automatically or may be self-developing. Self-developing film comes in two major forms: either the chemicals are attached to the film in a separate pocket; or the film packets may have a small opening on the side into which the chemicals are sprayed after exposure. The films are then processed according to the specific times as given by the manufacturers. Once developed, they are removed from their sachets and rinsed. The advantage is the fact that no darkroom or other developing equipment is required.

Manual processing is by far the most commonly used technique. Dental film can be processed in an ordinary darkroom, with regular manual developing chemicals, but the developing times will be quite long and it may take ten minutes or more to produce a good quality radiograph. Alternatively, a chair-side darkroom consisting of an enclosed box with a transparent orange (D-speed film) or red (E-speed film) lid can be used. These boxes have two rubber-protected holes where the operator can put their hands in. Inside the box there are usually three or four containers. Starting from left to right, these will be developer, stop bath, fixer and a water rinse (Figure 14.18). The stop bath is substituted with a water rinse in chair-side darkrooms where there are only 3 containers.

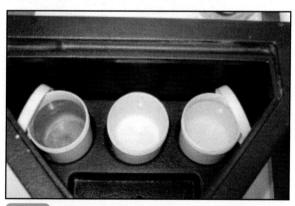

**14.18** Developing box and its three components.

The film is opened in the protection of the chair-side darkroom and a stainless steel film clip is attached to it, in order to carry it through the chemicals (Figure 14.19).

Dental radiography chemicals are usually rapid processing chemicals, and developing with a fresh solution will take about 20–30 seconds. After this the film is rinsed in water, or preferably in a stop bath, to prevent any further developing. It is then transferred to the fixer and can be viewed after approximately one minute of fixing. It is important to replace the film in the fixer solution after viewing, as at least 15 minutes is required for full fixation. After fixing, the film should be rinsed under running tap water for approximately 20

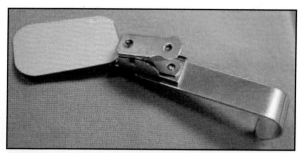

**14.19** Stainless steel dental film clips for use during the developing of films.

minutes. Any shortening of the fixing time or use of old chemicals will result in under or poor fixing, which will lead to discoloration of the film soon after the procedure.

Automatic film processors also use rapid chemicals, therefore these chemicals and machines may be used to process dental film. Should the practice choose not to invest in a dedicated dental automatic processor, an ordinary automatic processor can be used, taking the following into account. The main draw back of standard automatic processors is the fact that those using rollers have them spaced too wide apart and the dental film will be lost in the developing tank. Some practitioners attach the small dental film to a larger film using acetate tape. This will work, but many films may still be lost, or large areas of the film may not be processed because of the tape covering the surface. There are automatic developers that make use of a material sheet to feed the film through and these will work well with small dental films. Dedicated dental automatic processors have specific carrying mechanisms to transport the film through all the chemicals, producing a properly developed, fixed and dried image.

Digital dental radiography is becoming a commonly used diagnostic imaging technique in human dental practice, and many veterinary surgeons have also converted to this modality. The standard dental radiography machine is used but instead of film, a sensor is placed intra-orally and connected to a computer. Images are directly converted to digital images via the sensor and appear on the computer screen as such. This allows the operator to manipulate the images in many different ways depending on the software. Manipulation of the images is done to overcome slight over or underexposure, thereby reducing the amount of radiation the patient is exposed to from repeat radiographs.

## Normal radiographic anatomy

Figure 14.20 gives the dental formulae for the permanent and deciduous dentition of cats and dogs. The modified Triadan tooth identification system is shown in Figure 14.21.

| Species | Deciduous | Permanent |
|---------|-----------|-----------|
| Cat | 2 x (I 3/3 C 1/1 PM 3/2) = 26 | 2 x (I 3/3 C 1/1 PM 3/2 M 1/1) = 28 |
| Dog | 2 x (I 3/3 C 1/1 PM 2/2 M 1/1) = 28 | 2 x (I 3/3 C 1/1 PM 4/4 M2/3) = 42 |

**14.20** Dental formulae of deciduous and permanent dentition in the dog and the cat.

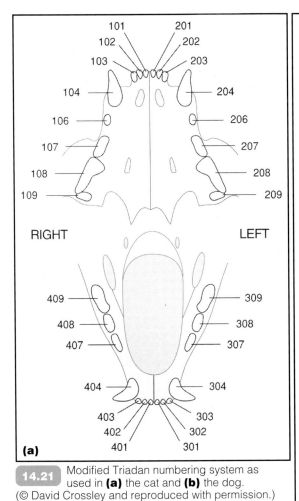

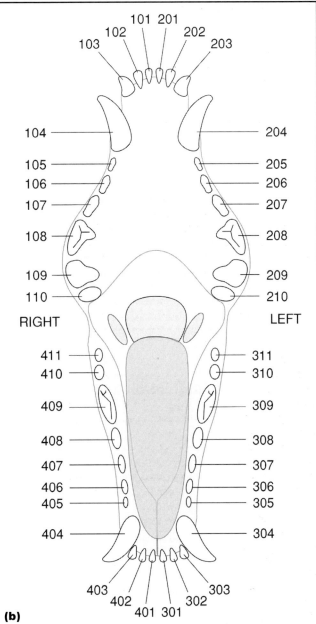

**14.21** Modified Triadan numbering system as used in **(a)** the cat and **(b)** the dog. (© David Crossley and reproduced with permission.)

Dental radiographs are much smaller than conventional radiographs and care should be taken when evaluating them. It is advisable to have a small light box or to make a cover for a normal size X-ray viewing box to reduce the peripheral glare. With most backlight removed the detail will be much clearer. Making use of magnification is also advisable to evaluate dental X-ray film thoroughly. The following normal anatomical structures should be assessed on all films (see Figure 14.5b):

- Enamel: very thin in carnivores, covering the crown
- Dentine: situated below the enamel of the crown and cementum of the root, amount increases with age
- Pulp cavity: the entire cavity of the tooth, housing all the neurovascular tissue. This cavity is lined by odontoblasts that form dentine throughout life. With age the pulp cavity decreases in size as dentine increases. The pulp cavity is divided into the:

  - Pulp chamber – that part of the pulp cavity that is situated in the crown
  - Pulp horn – part of the pulp chamber, extending into the cusps
  - Pulp (root) canal – that part of the pulp cavity that is situated in the root, extending to the apex
- Alveolar bone: the tooth-bearing bone of the jaws
- Lamina dura (radiopaque): the cortical bone of the alveolus
- Periodontal ligament space: the periodontal ligament is situated all around the root and is visible as a thin radiolucent line between the root and lamina dura
- Mandibular canal: this large canal starts mediocaudally at the mandibular foramen and extends rostrolaterally, exiting the mandible at one or more mental foramina situated in the premolar area, near the canine apex. It protects large neurovascular structures, and tooth roots

may often be seen to extend into it radiologically (especially the distal root of the first molar)
- Alveolar bone height: alveolar bone should always extend to just below the enamel-cementum junction, therefore always filling the furcation area of multi-rooted teeth.

## Contrast studies

Contrast studies are not in common use.

## Alternative imaging procedures

Computed tomography (CT) and magnetic resonance imaging (MRI) are very good modalities to assist the clinician in determining surgical borders for oral neoplasms (Kafka *et al.*, 2004; see Chapter 12). These modalities, especially CT, can be very informative regarding the extent of odontogenic neoplasms associated with the jawbones. CT or MRI is not commonly used as a diagnostic imaging modality for dentition only.

## Abnormal radiological findings

### Trauma

#### Dental trauma

***Dental fractures:*** Animals that have been involved in road traffic accidents, dogfights, have fallen from a height, have chewed hard objects, or suffered any other trauma to the head, should always be evaluated for tooth fractures. Crown fractures are most common and most obvious on visual inspection. Root fractures are rare, but can occur and should be ruled out (Figure 14.22).

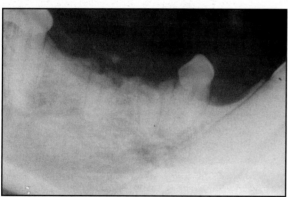

**14.22** Root fractures of 306 showing most of the roots still in the alveolus.

#### Tooth avulsions and luxations

- Tooth avulsion is the total removal of a tooth from its alveolus. This is most common in the canine teeth, especially the maxillary canines. The maxillary buccal bone plate is much thinner than the buccal bony plate protecting the mandibular canines. When a patient with tooth avulsion

presents and the tooth is not still visible, attached to the gingiva or presented for inspection by the owner, a radiograph should be taken to confirm an empty alveolus.
- Tooth luxation refers to the partial displacement of a tooth either into the alveolus (intrusion), out of the alveolus (extrusion), laterally or medially. Luxation is often associated with fracture of the alveolus. All of these features may only be visible once a radiograph of the affected area is taken and evaluated (Figure 14.23).

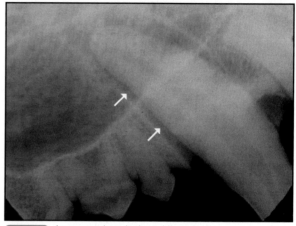

**14.23** Increased periodontal ligament space (arrowed) after reimplantation of a luxated 204.

***Tooth concussion:*** Discoloured teeth often point towards some traumatic insult; these teeth undergo pulpitis, leading to blood penetrating the dentinal tubules. Due to the pulpitis, the teeth often appear pink or grey–blue. The discoloration *per se* does not mean that the tooth has undergone irreversible pulpitis. In irreversible pulpitis, radiographic follow-up of these teeth will show a pulp canal that does not reduce in size compared with the contralateral tooth, or a periapical lucency may develop (see Endodontic disease, below).

#### Jaw fractures

Jaw fractures involving the dentate area (tooth-bearing part of jaw) should always be assessed with intra-oral radiography. Fractures through the alveolus of a tooth carry a poorer prognosis than those through alveolar bone only (Figure 14.24; see Chapter 12).

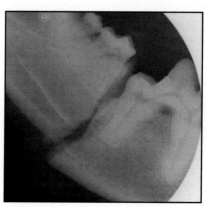

**14.24** Mandibular fracture, extending dorsally through the alveolus of 309 and 310.

## Congenital and developmental conditions

### Retained deciduous dentition

- Before retained deciduous teeth are removed it is always good practice to make sure the permanent counterpart is present. If a permanent tooth is not present, the anatomy of the deciduous tooth may be assessed and this tooth may be left *in situ* if it has no pathology present (Figure 14.25).

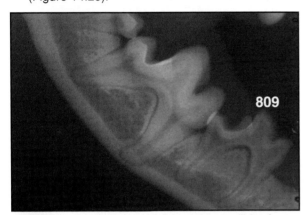

**14.25** Lateral radiograph of the right mandible of a Yorkshire Terrier. The deciduous molar (809) is still present but no permanent 408 is visible in the jawbone.

- Clinicians often find it difficult to establish which tooth is the deciduous and which tooth is permanent where they appear together in the mouth. Radiographs of the teeth in question will assist, as the roots of the permanent teeth are much larger than their deciduous counterparts.

### Anodontia and hypodontia

- The absence of a tooth or teeth may be due to the lack of development of all teeth (anodontia), previous extraction of a tooth or the lack of eruption of a tooth (hypodontia).
- Dental radiography will confirm the presence or absence of a tooth (see Figure 14.25).

### Tooth impactions

Teeth may fail to erupt for many different reasons, such as deformity of the tooth, obstruction by gingiva rich in collagen, bony obstruction (Figure 14.26), odontogenic cyst formation (Figure 14.27) or odontogenic neoplasms (see below).

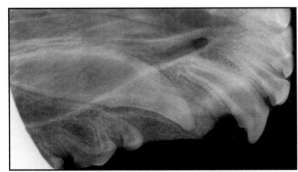

**14.26** Unerupted canine of a German Shepherd Dog due to a bony obstruction (possibly a retained deciduous tooth root).

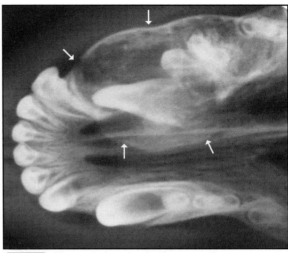

**14.27** Unerupted canine tooth, presenting as a dentigerous cyst (arrowed).

### Supernumerary tooth

The development of more than the required number of teeth (hyperdontia) may lead to the abnormal positioning of teeth (Figure 14.28). These extra teeth are referred to as supernumerary teeth and may have no clinical consequence for the patient, or they may lead to increased periodontal disease or traumatic malocclusion that can be painful.

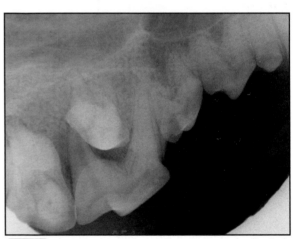

**14.28** A supernumerary maxillary premolar is situated palatal to the 208.

### Double-crowned teeth

Teeth with double crowns should always be evaluated radiographically. These teeth develop due to fusion of two separate teeth or the incomplete split of a tooth (gemination) (Figure 14.29). Clinically it is difficult, and sometimes impossible, to differentiate a double-crowned tooth from a supernumerary tooth. Double-crowned teeth will have just one root and this can only be determined radiographically. The author has seen this in German Shepherd Dogs where the presence of a supernumerary tooth is considered a fault (Figure 14.30). Many breeders will request extraction of the 'supernumerary' tooth, which most commonly is the first mandibular premolar tooth. The author discourages these extractions. Radiography is indicated to confirm whether the tooth is double-crowned or supernumerary.

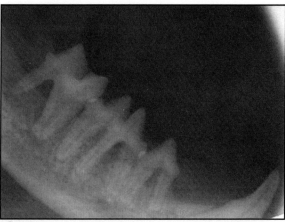

**14.29** Gemination of 308 in a cat. Note that in this case there is also a supernumerary root.

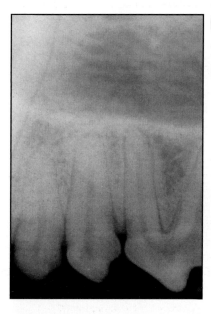

**14.30**
A supernumerary 105 in a German Shepherd Dog.

### Dilacerated tooth or root

Teeth that may have been damaged during odontogenesis can present with sharply angulated crowns or roots. Angulated roots may make the extraction of such a tooth very difficult and the clinician should be aware of this before extraction is attempted (Figure 14.31).

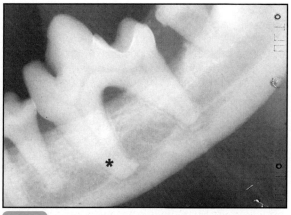

**14.31** Dilaceration of the mesial root (★) of 409.

### Supernumerary roots

- In dogs all the teeth rostral to and including the first premolar tooth, as well as the third mandibular molar, have only one root. The mandibular teeth caudal to the first premolar tooth are double-rooted teeth, except for the third molar.
- In cats this configuration is also followed; however, they have fewer teeth. All the teeth rostral to the premolars have only one root, as well as the single maxillary molar tooth situated palatal to the fourth premolar. The mandibular teeth caudal to the canine tooth are double-rooted teeth. The maxillary second and third premolars have two roots; the second maxillary tooth commonly has fused roots. The fourth maxillary premolar is the only tooth in the mouth of the cat that has three roots.
- There are numerous cases reported of excessive numbers of roots (supernumerary), especially of two-rooted premolar teeth with three roots (see Figure 14.29).

The clinician should be aware of these points before performing an incorrect extraction.

### Bulbous roots

An inconsistent but not uncommon finding is a small bulbous apex, especially of premolar teeth of both dogs and cats. This bulbous apex makes it impossible to remove the root by normal elevation. Should the clinician attempt this, the root invariably fractures. Preoperative radiographs of this condition should guide the clinician to more appropriate extraction techniques.

### Odontogenic cysts

Various odontogenic cysts may develop during odontogenesis, or from the remnants of odontogenesis (rests of Malassez or Ceres). Dentigerous cysts are the most common type of odontogenic cyst seen by the author, occurring mainly in the rostral mandible or maxilla (see Figure 14.27). Patients may present with a fluid-filled mass at the site of an unerupted tooth or an enlarged bony mass at the site of an unerupted tooth.

### Malocclusions

**Skeletal malocclusions:** These malocclusions are due to jaw length and/or width discrepancies. In certain breeds, especially the brachycephalic breeds, such as Boxers and Bulldogs, this inherited trait may be regarded as normal. A jaw of shorter length or narrower width than normal may cause mandibular canine penetration of the maxillary gingiva, palatine mucosa and bone, as well as the teeth. Bull Terriers, German Shepherd Dogs, Bearded Collies and Scottish Terriers are over-represented breeds with this condition. Radiography in these patients can assist in evaluating the full extent of the pathology present.

**Dental malocclusions:** Malocclusion of a single tooth or teeth in close proximity may be due to factors other than skeletal, such as delayed eruption of teeth for whatever reason. Apart from clinically evaluating the patient for these reasons, dental radiography may aid in the diagnosis of such problems.

## Infection and inflammation

### Periodontal disease

- Periodontal disease is an infectious/inflammatory process caused by plaque, which stimulates osteoclasts to destroy alveolar bone. The extent of bone loss around a tooth or teeth can be assessed by radiographic examination. Bone loss may be at a specific surface of a tooth root and may present clinically as a periodontal pocket. This type of bone loss is classified as vertical bone loss. If bone loss is radiographically evident across adjacent teeth it is classified as horizontal bone loss (Figure 14.32).

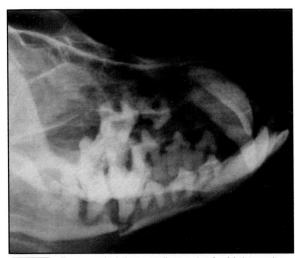

**14.33** Extra-oral oblique radiograph of a Maltese dog showing severe periodontal disease of 409, resulting in a pathological mandibular fracture.

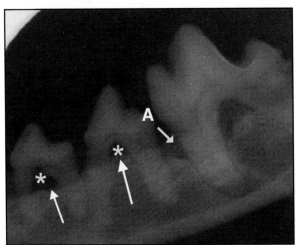

**14.32** Periodontal disease affecting all three teeth in this view. There is marked vertical bone loss present at the mesial and distal roots of 409, evident as an enlarged radiolucent area (A). There is no periodontal ligament visible in this area. Horizontal bone loss can be seen as the lowering of the alveolar bone height across all the teeth (arrowed). Complete bone loss is evident between the roots of teeth 407 and 408 (✱), whereas at 409 this bone loss is incomplete and does not extend all the way in between the two roots.

- Apart from alveolar bone height loss, the resorption may be subtler and the clinician may only see an increase in the width of the periodontal ligament space, with loss of the lamina dura.
- Periodontal disease may progress apically and enter the pulpal chamber through the root apex causing a pulpitis. This is called a perio-endo lesion.
- Severe periodontal disease may cause substantial bone loss, resulting in pathological bone fractures. This is especially seen in the toy breeds (Figure 14.33).

### Endodontic disease

- Complicated fractures of the teeth will leave the pulp exposed. In these cases pulpitis may progress through the apex of the tooth and cause disease in the periodontium (structures surrounding the tooth). This is called an endo-perio lesion (Figure 14.34).

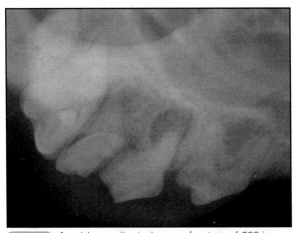

**14.34** An old complicated crown fracture of 208 in a dog. There is loss of the lamina dura and increased radiolucency around the apices of the rostral roots.

- In most cases a periapical lucency will develop, the nature of which cannot be determined radiographically (periapical cyst, granuloma or abscess). This pathological process may extend coronally via the periodontal ligament area and cause periodontal disease.

### Resorption

Tooth root resorption is a common finding in cats and also occurs in dogs (Figure 14.35). In cats odontoclastic resorptive lesions have been well documented and classified (Reiter and Mendoza, 2002) to assist the clinician in diagnosis.

Resorption will usually start at the cemento-enamel junction or on any surface of the root (internal or external) where osteoclasts are present. Radiographically there will be loss of the lamina dura, loss of the periodontal ligament space around the tooth as well as tooth substance loss. The resorbed tooth substance is often replaced by bone and ankylosis of the remaining tooth to the bone is formed. In these cases no periodontal ligament will be visible (Figure 14.36).

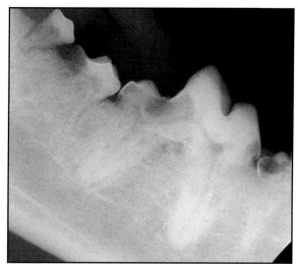

**14.35** Resorption lesions affecting 408, 409 and 410 in the mandible of this dog. Note the disappearance of the lamina dura and periodontal ligament space where ankylosis has occurred. 410 shows increased periodontal ligament space as with periodontal disease.

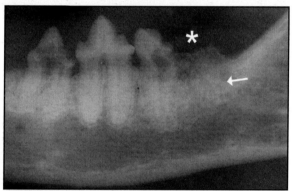

**14.36** Feline odontoclastic resorptive lesions in the right mandible of a cat, 407 and 409 are affected. The distal cusp of 409 (✱) is absent and the distal root has totally integrated with the alveolar bone (arrowed). No root is visible. The resorptive process of 407 is affecting the crown as well as the distal root. Here ankylosis is also evident, as there is no lamina dura or periodontal ligament space visible.

## Caries

- Caries can be distinguished from resorptive lesions in that they are common in dogs, especially the mandibular and maxillary molars of larger breeds. Furthermore the pathogenesis also differs markedly as caries is not an active resorptive process driven by osteoclasts, but a demineralization process of the crown, driven by bacteria and the fermentation of easily digestible carbohydrates.
- Early carious lesions should be distinguished from attrition or abrasion lesions with the aid of dental exploration and radiography. The extent of carious lesions must be thoroughly investigated, including the use of radiography.
- Typical lesions will cause loss of crown structure (enamel and dentine) and in more severe cases will extend into the root. Once the pulp is affected periapical pathology will develop (see above) (Figure 14.37).

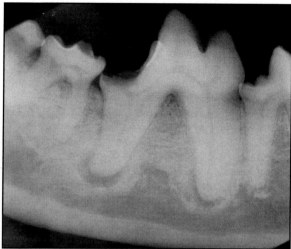

**14.37** Carious lesion of the distal cusp in 309. There is loss of crown material and apical lucency due to the caries invading the pulp cavity.

## Neoplasia

### Odontogenic neoplasms

- Any enlargement of the bones or soft tissues of the oral cavity should always be radiographically investigated. Odontogenic neoplasms develop during odontogenesis or from the remnants of odontogenesis (rests of Malassez or Ceres) and swelling will therefore be associated with the tooth-bearing areas of the jawbones.
- Odontogenic neoplasms may be:
  - Cystic (ameloblastomas)
  - Lytic (acanthomatous epulis; Figure 14.38)
  - Forming new bone (peripheral odontogenic fibromas)
  - Representing malformed teeth or multiple teeth (odontomas; Figure 14.39).

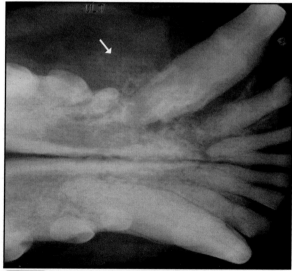

**14.38** Acanthomatous epulis of the left maxilla associated with 304. There is bone invasion represented by the moth-eaten appearance around 302, 303, 304 and 305. The periodontal ligament around these teeth has been destroyed. In this tumour metaplastic bone within the soft tissue component of the tumour is also visible (arrowed).

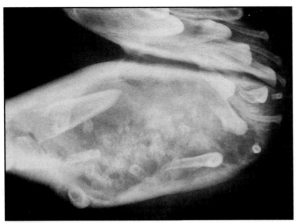

**14.39** Complex odontoma of the right rostral mandible in a small cross-breed dog.

## Non-odontogenic neoplasms

For information on non-odontogenic neoplasms see Chapter 12.

## Metabolic

For information on metabolic disorders see Chapter 12.

## Miscellaneous

### Dentally associated nasal discharge

Unilateral or bilateral nasal discharges may be either due to impacted teeth causing cystic swelling of the maxillary bones and penetration of the nasal passages (Figure 14.40), or due to infection extending from the teeth into the nasal passages (see Chapter 13).

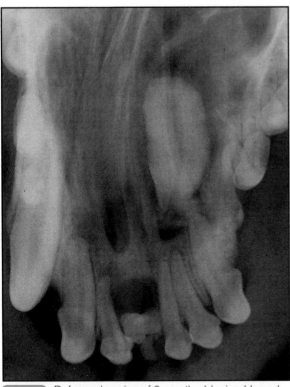

**14.40** Deformed canine of 8-month-old mixed-breed dog, which developed in the nasal passages, causing a purulent unilateral nasal discharge. A dentigerous cyst is also visible around the deformed 101 and 201.

## Discharging sinuses in the region of the maxilla or mandible

Carnassial or molar abscesses of the maxilla usually present as a firm swelling ventral to the eye. In severe cases these abscesses may burst and a draining sinus is formed. Apart from these abscesses there are other reasons for discharging sinuses in the maxillary or mandibular regions, and a thorough investigation of these areas should include a radiographic evaluation to rule out the presence of osteomyelitis, neoplasia or the presence of tooth root remnants (Figure 14.41).

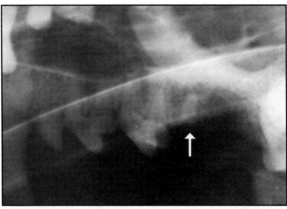

**14.41** Extra-oral oblique radiograph clearly showing a root remnant of one of the mesial roots after previous exodontia of the fourth maxillary premolar tooth.

### Medico-legal issues

Dental radiographs form part of the case record and will prove what pathology was present at the time of presentation.

## Further reading and references

Crossley D and Penman S (1995) *BSAVA Manual of Small Animal Dentistry, 2nd edn.* BSAVA Publications, Gloucester

DeForge DH and Colmery BH (2000) In: *An Atlas of Veterinary Dental Radiology.* Iowa State University Press, Ames

Eisner E (1998) Oral-dental radiographic examination. *Veterinary Clinics of North America: Small Animal Practice* **28**, 1063–1087

Gorrel C (1998) Radiographic evaluation. *Veterinary Clinics of North America: Small Animal Practice* **28**, 1089–1102

Harvey CE and Emily PP (1993) Oral examination and diagnostic techniques. In: *Small Animal Dentistry*, ed. CE Harvey and PP Emily, pp. 19–41. Mosby, St Louis

Kafka UCM, Carstens A, Steenkamp G and Symington H (2004) Diagnostic value of magnetic resonance imaging and computed tomography for oral masses in dogs. *Journal of the South African Veterinary Association* **75**, 169–172

Lommer MJ, Verstraete FJM and Terpak CH (2000) Dental radiographic technique in cats. *Compendium on Continuing Education for the Practicing Veterinarian* **22**, 107–117

Mauriello SM, Overman VP and Platin E (1995) Extraoral radiography In: *Radiographic Imaging for the Dental Team*, ed. SM Mauriello et al., pp. 278–295. JB Lippincott Company, Philadelphia

Mulligan TW, Aller MS and Williams CA (1998) *Atlas of Canine and Feline Dental Radiography.* Veterinary Learning Systems, Trenton, New Jersey

Reiter AM and Mendoza KA (2002) Feline odontoclastic resorptive lesions. An unsolved enigma in veterinary dentistry. *Veterinary Clinics of North America: Small Animal* **32**, 791–837

Verstraete FJM (1999) Routine full-mouth radiographs as a teaching tool in veterinary dentistry. *Journal of Veterinary Medical Education* **25**, 28–31

Verstraete FJM, Phillip PH and Terpak CH (1998a) Diagnostic value of full-mouth radiography in dogs. *American Journal of Veterinary Research* **59**, 686–691

Verstraete FJM, Phillip PH and Terpak CH (1998b) Diagnostic value of full-mouth radiography in cats. *American Journal of Veterinary Research* **59**, 692–695

# 15

# Spine – general

## Robert M. Kirberger

### Indications

The following are some of the indications for radiography of the spine:

- Mono, para- and quadriplegia
- Thoracic and pelvic limb paresis or paraparesis
- Ataxia
- Pain referable to a spinal lesion
- Stiffness
- Suspected vertebral deformities
- Sinus tracts in the lumbar region.

### Radiography and normal anatomy

#### General principles

- A complete clinical examination is required to rule out conditions that may mimic a spinal lesion (e.g. orthopaedic disease, such as bilateral cranial cruciate ligament rupture or conditions such as myasthenia gravis)
- A complete neurological examination is required to localize the lesion to one of the four major longitudinal divisions of the spinal cord. These are spinal cord segments C1–C5, C6–T2, T3–L3 and L4–Cd5. It is important to know that the spinal cord ends at about mid L6 and that spinal cord segments thus do not correspond with the vertebra of the same number. For example, spinal cord segment L6 is located at the caudal aspect of L4
- If a specific location or region of pathology is identified, the primary beam must be centred to this point
- Optimal quality radiographs are essential to identify subtle changes. This is ensured by:
  - collimating to the spine to reduce scattered radiation
  - using a grid to reduce the effect of scattered radiation on the radiograph
  - using high detail film–screen combinations
  - eliminating movement
- General anaesthesia is mandatory for radiation safety. It also prevents motion blur and allows for accurate positioning, as it relaxes the spine by reducing muscle spasm associated with

pain. If the plain films indicate a need for myelography this can be done under the same general anaesthetic
- Patients presented with suspected recent vertebral fractures should be handled with extreme care and with minimal movement. Horizontal beam ventrodorsal (VD) radiographs should preferably be taken to avoid having to rotate the patient.

### Standard views

#### Lateral view: neutral

*Positioning:* It is essential for accurate interpretation that the spine is parallel to the table top; foam supports should be positioned under the neck and lumbar spine to achieve this.

Rotation of the spine is prevented by using foam supports between the legs and, if necessary, below the sternum. For the cervical spine an additional foam wedge is placed below the nose to prevent rotation of the head, which in turn controls the position of the cranial cervical region (Figure 15.1). For examination of the lower cervical spine the thoracic limbs should be retracted, taking care not to cause rotation of the spine. This will decrease the tissue thickness in this region. Correctly positioned views will have superimposition of the following structures: wings of the atlas; transverse processes of C6; rib origins; lumbar transverse processes; and wings of the ilia.

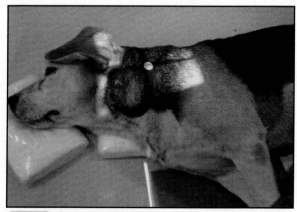

**15.1** Correct positioning and collimation for a lateral cervical radiograph.

*Centring points:* The beam should be centred on the area of suspected pathology. If no localizing signs are present, or if a complete vertebral survey is required, then the beam is centred at the following levels:

- Upper cervical (C2–3)
- Lower cervical (C5–6)
- Mid-thoracic (T8)
- Thoracolumbar junction (T13–L1)
- Mid-lumbar (L4–5)
- Lumbosacral (L7–S1).

Lower cervical radiographs need increased exposure factors to compensate for the increased thickness of tissues, compared with the upper cervical region. Fewer films may suffice for smaller animals. To demonstrate suspicious lesions more clearly an additional view can be made, centred and tightly collimated to the area of interest, which will significantly improve radiographic contrast and definition, particularly in larger dogs.

*Normal anatomy:* The vertebral formula for the dog and cat is C7–T13–L7–S3 and Cd6–23. Normal anatomy and radiographs are illustrated in Figures 15.2 to 15.5. The following structures and their variations are readily identifiable on radiographs:

- Vertebral bodies: the ventral vertebral body margins of L3 and L4 are often poorly defined with some loss of their normal concave appearance. This is due to the origin of the diaphragmatic crura and is more pronounced in older larger dogs. C7 and L7 are often shorter than the adjacent vertebral bodies. In immature animals open physes will be seen
- Transverse processes: C6 has a particularly large ventral lamina, which helps to identify this vertebra
- Intervertebral disc spaces: the T10–11 space is often narrowed due to the presence of the anticlinal vertebra (T11), and the L7–S1 space is often wider compared with the rest of the intervertebral spaces. The spaces will appear to narrow towards the edge of the film due to divergence of the primary beam
- Intervertebral foramina: the intervertebral foramina act as windows to the vertebral canal, and are best seen in the lumbar region where they often have the appearance of a horse's head. This is partially due to the presence of the accessory process, which appears to but into the foramen from its cranial end. The thoracic foramina are poorly seen due to superimposition of the dorsal ribs. In the cervical region, except between C2 and C3, the foramina are not seen clearly as they open ventrolaterally and are thus not aligned to the primary beam
- The dorsal (lamina) and ventral (vertebral floor) border of the vertebral foramen is seen as a thin sclerotic line. The vertebral canal gradually widens in the lower cervical region and in the L3–6 region to accommodate the cervical and lumbar intumescenses

- Articular facets: in the cervical region the articular facets are orientated dorsally to ventrally, and on lateral views the joint space is seen as an oblique radiolucent line running over the vertebral canal between the vertebra. In the lumbar region the facets are orientated laterally to medially above the vertebral canal, and on lateral views the edge of the joint space is seen as a curved radiolucent line on the caudal aspect
- Spinous processes: C2 should overlap C1
- Bony haemal arches may be seen ventral to Cd4–6 and small haemal processes may be seen caudal to this level.

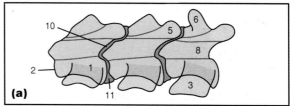

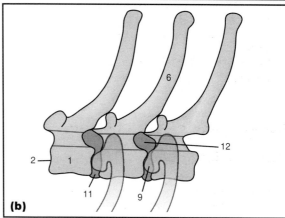

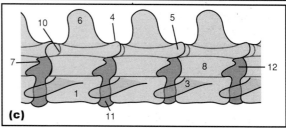

**15.2** Schematic representation of lateral vertebral views to illustrate normal structures. **(a)** Cervical. **(b)** Thoracic. **(c)** Lumbar. 1 = Vertebral body; 2 = Epiphysis/end plates; 3 = Transverse processes; 4 = Cranial articular facets; 5 = Caudal articular facets; 6 = Dorsal spinous process; 7 = Accessory process; 8 = Pedicle; 9 = Head of rib; 10 = Articular facet; 11 = Intervertebral disc; 12 = Intervertebral foramen.

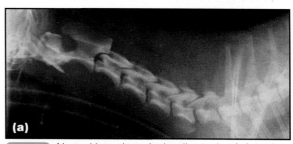

**15.3** Normal lateral cervical radiographs. **(a)** Adult small-breed dog. (continues) ▶

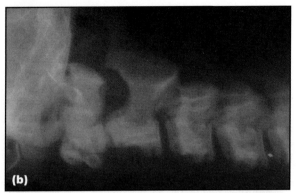

15.3  (continues) Normal lateral cervical radiographs. **(b)** Very immature large-breed dog, showing open physes.

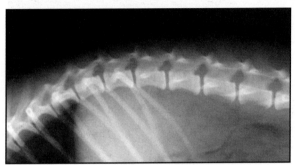

15.4  Normal lateral thoracolumbar radiograph of a small-breed dog.

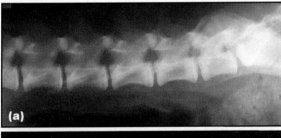

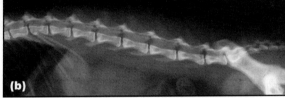

15.5  Normal lateral lumbar radiographs. **(a)** 7-month-old large-breed dog. **(b)** Adult cat. Note the sacrocaudal vertebral subluxation.

## Ventrodorsal view

***Positioning:*** The animal is placed on its back, preferably supported by a radiolucent trough or by firm pads placed on either side of the thorax. It is important to ensure that there is no rotation along the longitudinal axis of the spine. The pelvic limbs may be kept in a neutral position or be extended (Figure 15.6). Correctly positioned views will be symmetrical with the spinous process seen only as a central oval radiopaque structure. If the length of the spinous process becomes visible the spine is rotated. For the sacrum, the X-ray tube must be tilted 30 degrees caudally to ensure that the primary beam is perpendicular to the sacrum.

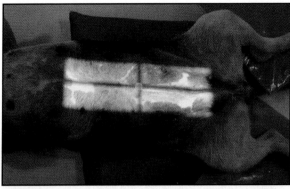

15.6  Correct positioning and collimation for a VD lumbar radiograph.

***Centring points:*** The centring points for the VD view are the same as those for the lateral view.

***Normal anatomy:*** The following structures and their variations are readily identifiable on radiographs (Figures 15.7 and 15.8; see also Lateral view comments above):

- The dens is seen cranial to the C2 vertebral body
- Mineralized laryngeal structures may be seen adjacent to the C2–3 region
- Transverse processes: C6 has particularly large laminae
- Intervertebral disc spaces: due to the natural curvature of the spine the disc spaces may vary in width, and evaluation of the disc space width should preferably be done on lateral views
- Intervertebral foramina are not seen, except in the cervical region where they may be partially visible
- The lateral borders of the vertebral foramen, representing the pedicles, are seen as thin sclerotic lines
- Articular facets: in the cervical region the articular facets are orientated dorsally to ventrally, and are seen as varying sized oval structures lateral to the invertebral disc spaces. In the lumbar region the facets are orientated laterally to medially, and the radiolucent joint spaces can be defined clearly
- Spinous processes are seen as central oval sclerotic lines.

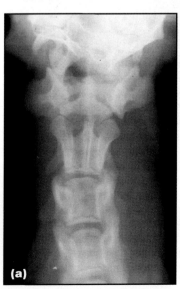

15.7  Normal VD cervical radiographs. **(a)** Very immature large-breed dog, showing open physes. (continues) ▶

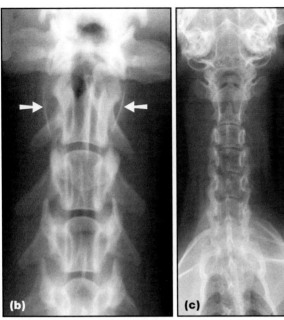

**15.7** (continued) Normal VD cervical radiographs. **(b)** Old large-breed dog with mineralized thyroid cartilages (arrowed). **(c)** Cat.

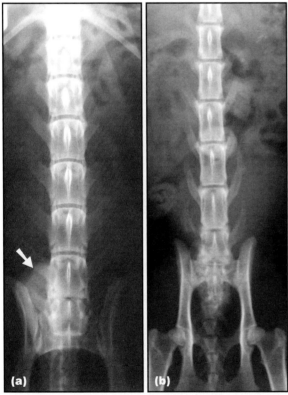

**15.8** Normal VD lumbar radiographs. **(a)** Large-breed dog. Soft tissue opacity adjacent to L6 is the prepuce (arrowed). **(b)** Adult cat. Note the sacrocaudal vertebral subluxation.

### Differences in canine and feline anatomy
Generally feline vertebrae are longer with a more sleek appearance than canine vertebrae.

There may also be more natural curvature to the spine in the cat.

## Special views

### Oblique cervical views
Plain film views (e.g. ventral 45° left-dorsal right (V45°Le-DRt) and ventral 45° right-dorsal left (V45°Rt-DLe)) highlight the intervertebral foramina and dens. In small-breed dogs with suspected cervical disc pathology, mineralized disc material that has herniated dorsolaterally may be seen in the intervertebral foramen (Figure 15.9).

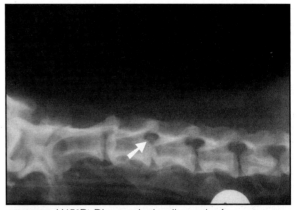

**15.9** V45°Rt-DLe cervical radiograph of an intervertebral foramen (arrowed). Herniated disc material is present in the C3–4 intervertebral foramen.

***Positioning:*** The animal is placed on its back, preferably supported by a radiolucent trough or by firm pads placed on either side of the thorax. The dog is then rotated 45 degrees to the left side; the exposure is repeated with the dog rotated 45 degrees to the right side.

***Centring points:*** As this view is primarily indicated in small breeds a single exposure centred to C4 will usually suffice.

***Normal anatomy:***

- The dens is seen as a slightly angulated structure just cranial to C2
- Intervertebral foramina are now seen. In views rotated to the left, the right foramina are seen and *vice versa*.

During myelographic studies oblique views centred to the region of interest are useful to determine the circumferential location of compressive lesions (Figure 15.10). Particular indications are:

- Dorsolateral cervical cord compression due to articular facet changes and synovial cysts
- Ventrolateral cervical cord compression by herniated disc material
- Dorsolateral or ventrolateral cord compression due to thoracolumbar disc herniation
- Lateral and VD films are normal (e.g. herniated disc material may be seen only on an oblique view) (Figure 15.11).

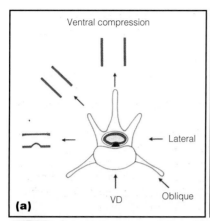 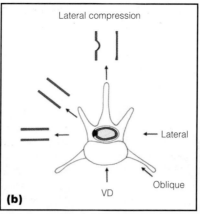 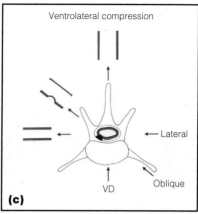

**15.10** Schematic representation of the myelographic visibility of extradural cord compression at various locations. **(a)** Ventral lesion. **(b)** Lateral lesion. **(c)** Ventrolateral lesion. (Reproduced from Kirberger (1994) with permission from the *Compendium on Continuing Education for the Practicing Veterinarian*.)

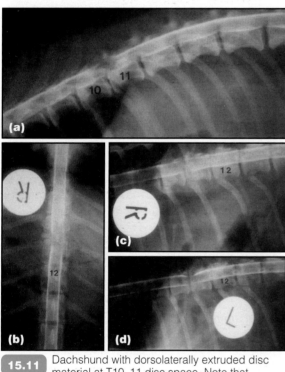

**15.11** Dachshund with dorsolaterally extruded disc material at T10–11 disc space. Note that significant compression is seen only on the left oblique view. **(a)** Lateral view. **(b)** VD view. **(c)** V45°Rt-DLe view. **(d)** V45°Le-DRt view.

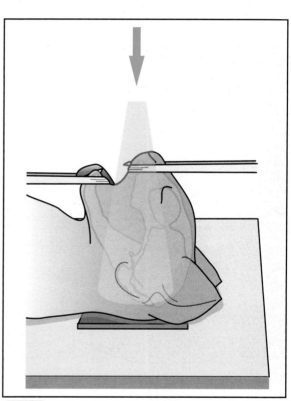

**15.12** Positioning for the RCd open-mouth view.

### Rostrocaudal open-mouth view

The rostrocaudal (RCd) open-mouth view is an additional view to evaluate the dens and associated structures. However, care must be taken with this view if atlanto-axial instability is suspected as excessive flexion may traumatize the cord further.

***Positioning:*** The patient is placed in dorsal recumbency and the head is flexed. The tongue is pulled forward between the mandibular canines, and the mandible secured with a loop of bandage so that the mouth is held in an open position. The palate should be tilted 5 degrees cranially.

***Centring points:*** The beam should be centred on the back of the soft palate. The endotracheal tube must be removed prior to radiographic exposure.

### Lateral view: stressed

Stressed lateral views may be used in the cervical or lumbosacral regions (see Chapter 18). Indications are:

- Flexed cervical views with plain film radiography to evaluate vertebral instability
- Flexed, hyperextended or traction views with myelography to evaluate the effect of vertebral movement on spinal cord compression lesions.

*Positioning:* To take a flexed cervical radiograph, a gauze bandage or thin rope is tied around the mandible caudal to the canine teeth and the free end passed between the thoracic limbs. The head is then pulled towards the front legs. Flexing of just the atlanto-occipital junction should be avoided; the head and whole cervical spine should be flexed.

Positioning for cervical traction views is as for the neutral cervical view, but with the head extended under traction. The thoracic limbs should be retracted with thin ropes and attached to the table. Using a gauze bandage or thin rope caudal to the canine teeth (or two ropes attached to each side of the dog's collar), traction should be applied by hanging one or more sandbags over the end of the X-ray table. This view is safer and achieves the same effect as the flexed cervical view. This is particularly true when compressive lesions are present ventrally in the vertebral canal where the view aids in differentiating hypertrophic annulus fibrosus from herniated disc material (Figure 15.13).

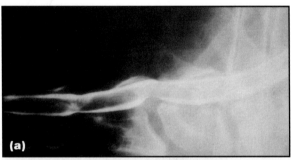
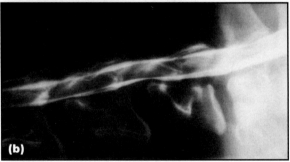

**15.13** Large-breed dog with extradural ventral cord compression at C6–7. **(a)** Neutral position. **(b)** Traction position. Note the wider intervertebral disc spaces and decrease in cord compression.

Hyperextended cervical radiographs may also be taken. There is no indication for this view with plain film radiography. It may be used during myelography to evaluate compressive lesions, particularly dorsal ligamentous hypertrophy.

## Physeal closure times
Interpreting radiographs of very young animals can be difficult due to the presence of physes and separate ossification centres, which should not be mistaken for pathology (see Figures 15.3b, 15.5a and 15.7a).

- The apex and body of the dens each has its own ossification centre, and both are ossified by the time the animal is 25 weeks old

- The atlas may still have a distinct separate ossification centre for its body in dogs less than 12 weeks of age
- The cranial vertebral physes close before the caudal physes, with the cranial physes virtually closed (cervical) or closed (thoracic and lumbar) by 38 weeks and all physes are usually closed by 1 year of age
- Sacral segments 2 and 3 are the last to fuse and may take up to a year to do so
- On lateral views the pelvic iliac crest is seen as a separate ossification centre from 4 months and may only fuse by 2.5 years, or later. The pelvic iliac crest is not seen on VD views.

The vertebral physes of the cat appear to close a bit earlier than those of the dog.

## Evaluation of a spinal radiograph
Each region of the vertebral column should be systematically evaluated. The major components of each vertebra and associated structures should be identified and compared with those adjacent to it. With the exception of the first two cervical vertebrae and at the junctions of the major levels of the vertebral column, most of the changes in vertebral conformation occur gradually. Complete assessment of the spine includes the systematic evaluation of the following:

- Vertebral alignment, in particular the vertebral canal floor which should have no abrupt change in level or angulation
- The length, shape and opacity of the vertebral bodies, transverse and spinous processes
- The presence of normal cortical and trabecular architecture. Specific evaluation of the sclerotic borders of the vertebral foramen (lamina and vertebral floor on lateral and pedicles on VD views) should be made as any vertebral lysis will often first be seen here
- The contour and opacity of the vertebral end plates
- Intervertebral disc space width and opacity. False disc space narrowing may occur due to an oblique projection of the vertebral end plates. This may occur towards the edge of the film or due to poor positioning (i.e. if the spine sags towards the cassette)
- Intervertebral foramen size, shape and opacity. Dural ossification may also be seen here
- Articular facets
- Paravertebral soft tissues.

Many radiological abnormalities may be present that are incidental findings (see Chapter 16) and many causes of spinal pathology may not be seen on plain films. The latter will only be identified with contrast studies or alternative imaging techniques. These include neoplasms and inflammatory, degenerative and vascular lesions (e.g. fibrocartilaginous infarcts) of the soft tissue components of the spine.

## Contrast studies

Myelography, the injection of a positive contrast medium into the subarachnoid space, can be performed via the cisterna magna or a lumbar route. The latter is regarded as safer for the patient but is more difficult to perform successfully. Provided the necessary care is taken in performing cisternal myelography this route is also safe. The reliability of the results can be improved by injecting the contrast medium at the standard site closest to the suspected lesion. Alternatively, either route can be used for the examination of the entire spinal cord but higher volumes of contrast medium will be required. However, with a cervical injection only the cranial edge of severe compressive lesions may be seen as there is not enough pressure built up to force contrast medium past the lesion, and contrast medium will preferentially flow into the cranial subarachnoid space. Lumbar myelography will, however, allow contrast medium to bypass lesions.

Indications for myelography include the following:

- Normal plain films, despite clinical evidence of spinal injury or disease
- Plain film changes that do not correlate with the site of pathology as indicated by the neurological examination
- Plain films that reveal multiple lesions which could be consistent with the neurological diagnosis
- A need to determine the degree and extent of cord pathology for surgical planning
- Diagnosis of certain conditions by exclusion of others, e.g. degenerative myelopathy or a fibrocartilaginous infarct, which may not produce myelographic changes.

Non-ionic low osmolar contrast media should be used and are relatively safe. Commonly used products are Iopamidol and Iohexol. These are available in concentrations varying from 180–370 mg iodine per millilitre, with the 240 and 300 mg concentrations commonly used by the author. The general dosage rate is 0.3 ml/kg for regional opacification and dosages of up to 0.45 ml/kg to evaluate the whole spine. Volumes of less than 2 ml for cats and small dogs result in unsatisfactory myelograms. The syringe may be hand-warmed to reduce the contrast medium viscosity. More recently, a non-ionic iso-osmolar dimeric contrast medium (Iotrolan) has become available and is said to be less nephrotoxic than the low osmolar contrast media.

A spinal needle must be used as it has a short bevel, which assists in preventing extradural contrast medium leakage. In small dogs a 22 gauge (4–5 cm long) needle is used, whereas in large dogs and very obese small dogs a needle up to 9 cm long may be required. The bevel must face in the direction of the lesion during the injection.

A general anaesthetic is given and the procedure is performed aseptically. Premedication with phenothiazine derivative tranquilizers should be avoided as they may reduce the seizure threshold. Hydration is maintained by means of appropriate intravenous fluids. After completing the myelogram the patient is immediately allowed to recover from anaesthesia or is taken directly to surgery. During the recovery period the patient is kept warm and under observation in case seizures occur. The head is rested on a foam plastic cushion to keep it higher than the rest of the body.

## Cervical myelography

### Positioning
The dog or cat is placed in lateral recumbency. The head and neck are supported on foam cushions to position the vertebral column and median plane of the head parallel to the table. An assistant holds the patient's head at right angles to the neck and the median plane of the nose and skull parallel to the table.

### Procedure
The spinal needle must penetrate the skin at a point in the exact median plane midway between the levels of the palpable external occipital protuberance of the skull and the edges of the wings of the atlas. The median plane is located by palpation with the index finger of the left hand; procedure described for right handed person:

1. The cord-like structure formed by the two rectus capitis dorsalis muscles should be felt for and the needle inserted in the middle of these, or in the palpable separation between the two muscles. If neither can be palpated, as in small patients, the midline must be determined with reference to the external occipital protuberance of the skull.
2. On skin penetration in small dogs and cats the stylet should be removed and the needle advanced slowly in the median plane (parallel to the table) in the direction of the angle of the jaw. When the tip of the needle enters the subarachnoid space of the cisterna magna, cerebrospinal fluid will immediately fill the transparent plastic hub of the spinal needle and begin to flow; this can be collected for analysis. Failure to stay in the median plane is likely to be complicated by perforation of venous sinuses in the spinal canal, in which case blood will escape from the needle. If this happens repeatedly the examination should be terminated or performed via the lumbar route. If resistance is encountered, which cannot be overcome with slight pressure, then the tip of the needle has probably come into contact with bone and the needle must be slightly withdrawn and redirected.

Or

2. In bigger dogs the same procedure is followed but the stylet is left in the needle until the resistance offered by the thick dorsal atlanto-occipital membrane is felt or after the ligament has been perforated. When this happens there is a slight but distinct 'pop' or decrease in resistance to the needle passage. As soon as

this happens, further advance of the needle must be halted and the stylet withdrawn. Cerebrospinal fluid should flow immediately. If it does not flow, the needle should be withdrawn slightly and then, if cerebrospinal fluid still does not flow, carefully inserted deeper until the fluid does flow. The needle should then be pushed in slightly further to ensure that its bevel does not become dislodged when the syringe is attached and to prevent extradural spillage.

3. Before the syringe containing contrast medium is attached to the spinal needle, the needle should be firmly gripped with the left hand index finger and thumb at its point of entrance through the skin and the palm of the hand supported on the draped neck. The syringe containing the contrast medium should be connected to the needle with the right hand. At this critical stage dislodging the tip of the needle or pushing it in deeper when applying pressure as the syringe is firmly inserted into the hub of the needle should be avoided. Alternatively, an extension tube may be used. The contrast medium is injected over one minute and the needle withdrawn.

If a cervical lesion is suspected the head can be lifted briefly before proceeding with taking radiographs. If a lesion is suspected in the thoracic or lumbar regions the patient may be inclined manually or even held vertically to assist the flow of contrast medium caudally. Contrast medium should reach the lumbosacral junction within two minutes if its flow is unimpeded. Only lateral radiographs are taken until a point of complete or partial obstruction to its flow is encountered, when a VD (upper cervical or thoracolumbar) or dorsoventral (DV; lower cervical) radiograph is taken. If no pathology is seen on the lateral views, VD and even oblique views must still be taken to look for lateralizing lesions. The endotracheal tube should be removed temporarily for the cervical radiographs as the wall of the tube has a similar appearance to the contrast medium columns, which can be confusing. If complete obstruction to flow is encountered the patient may be held in an inclined or vertical position for a few minutes before repeating the views to provide more contrast at the lesion location for improved resolution. Traction of the cervical spine may also help the flow of contrast medium beyond the lower cervical region if a compressive lesion is present.

**Normal cervical myelographic anatomy**
On lateral views (Figure 15.14):

- The subarachnoid contrast medium should be seen as a well marginated smooth line of varying thickness. Ventrally the soft tissues of the dorsal longitudinal ligament or annulus fibrosus may cause minor dorsal deviations of the ventral contrast column and this is most marked at C2–3. However, the dorsal contrast column will not be attenuated at this level. Dorsally a similar effect may be seen due to the flaval ligament

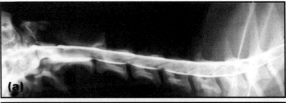
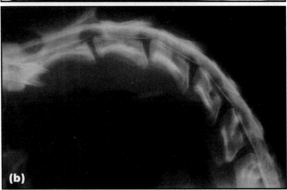
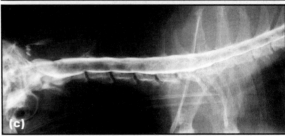

**15.14** Normal lateral cervical myelogram views. **(a)** Small-breed dog. **(b)** Large-breed dog with the neck in flexion. **(c)** Cat.

- The contrast medium columns may be quite wide cranially, particularly in the C1 and C2 regions, and then thin caudally
- Small dogs and cats have a relatively wide spinal cord in relation to the vertebral canal with resultant thin contrast medium columns. Large dog breeds have a relatively thinner cord with wide contrast medium columns
- At the lower cervical spinal curvature the spinal cord moves slightly dorsally, narrowing the contrast medium column on this side with concomitant widening of the ventral contrast medium column
- Thin fan-like radiolucent filling defect lines may be seen converging towards the intervertebral foramina; these are the nerve root filaments.

In addition to the above, on VD views (Figure 15.15):

- The basilar artery on the floor of C2 shows up as a serpent-like filling defect
- Optimal opacification depends on positioning as the contrast medium tends to gravitate to the most dependent region. If on lateral views a lesion is seen in the upper cervical region, VD radiographs must be made; if the lesion is in the lower cervical region, DV radiographs must be made to optimize the amount of contrast medium around the lesion.

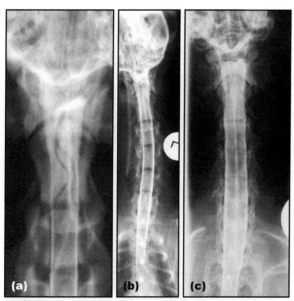

**15.15** Normal VD cervical myelogram views.
**(a)** Large-breed dog, illustrating filling defects over C2 caused by the basilar artery. **(b)** Small-breed dog. **(c)** Cat.

## Lumbar myelography

### Positioning

This procedure can be performed with the patient in sternal recumbency but the author prefers lateral re-cumbency. True lateral positioning of the spine by means of foam pads is essential to the success of the procedure and can be confirmed with fluoroscopy or a radiograph to look for superimposition of the ilial wings or lumbar transverse processes. Some clinicians like to flex the spine but this can hamper maintenance of a true lateral position.

### Procedure

A median approach is most commonly used. It is important not to insert the needle at a site of potential pathology.

1. The dorsal spinous process of L6 should be located just cranial to a line through the wings of the ilium (difficult in obese animals).
2. The spinal needle should be introduced flush against the cranial edge of L6 in a direction perpendicular to the long axis of the spine and parallel to the table top until solid resistance by bone is felt. The tip of the needle will now either rest on the floor of the vertebral canal or against the lamina of L5, in which case the needle must be slightly withdrawn and redirected remembering to stay strictly in the midline. A lateral radiograph may be taken to confirm the needle position.
3. When in the vertebral canal the needle bevel may be positioned in the dorsal subarachnoid space but this is technically difficult and usually the spinal cord is deliberately penetrated to reach the wider ventral subarachnoid space. This does not have any clinical effect on the patient.

Penetration of the cord often results in a jerk of the hindquarters, indicating correct needle placement. The needle is then retracted slightly and the stylet removed.

A paramedian approach may also be used, where the needle is inserted just lateral to the palpable L6 spinous process and directed cranioventromedially with the interarcuate space usually entered at a 45 degree angle.

4. Free flow of cerebrospinal fluid when the stylet is removed confirms the correct positioning of the tip of the needle. Lack of flow does not necessarily indicate wrong placement of the needle as severe compression or swelling of the cord will completely obstruct flow. If there is no flow 0.5 ml of contrast medium can be injected and a lateral radiograph taken to check for contrast medium in a normal subarachnoid location. If the needle tip is too deep an epidurogram will be seen (see Complications below). If severe compression is suspected the contrast medium can be injected rapidly (over 10 seconds) and radiographs taken immediately and again after 30 seconds. The first radiograph will show the caudal edge of the lesion to best advantage, while the slightly delayed exposure will demonstrate the cranial end. Rapid injection builds up sufficient pressure to force the contrast medium past the point of obstruction.

If attempting to enter the vertebral canal at L5–6 is unsuccessful, L6–7 and as a last resort L4–5 should be tried. The latter is not advised as there is an increased risk of intracord injection (see Complications below).

**Normal thoracic and lumbar myelographic anatomy**
On lateral and VD views (Figure 15.16) (see also Cervical myelogram):

- Small dogs and cats have a relatively wide spinal cord in relation to the vertebral canal with resultant thin contrast medium columns. Large dog breeds have a relatively thinner cord with wider contrast medium columns

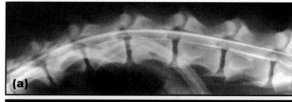
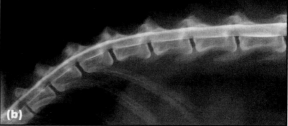

**15.16** Normal thoracolumbar myelogram views.
**(a)** Large-breed dog. **(b)** Cat.

- In the lumbar region there may be slight dorsal elevation of the ventral contrast medium column over the intervertebral disc spaces
- The thoracic cord is fairly narrow compared with the lumbar region where the lumbar intumescence widens the cord in the L4 region
- Contrast medium will tend to gravitate to the more dependent cervical and lumbar regions, particularly in larger dogs, possibly resulting in poor opacification of the caudal thoracic region. Thoracic subarachnoid filling can be improved by elevating the fore and hindquarters
- At the thoracolumbar spinal curvature the spinal cord moves ventrally, narrowing the contrast medium column on this side with concomitant dorsal widening of the contrast medium column, which may also extend more caudally
- In the dog the spinal cord ends at the L5–6 region but contrast medium opacification continues caudally within the dural end-sac, which has a variable length, up to the mid-sacral region. In the cat the cord ends a bit further caudally
- Within the dural end-sac linear radiolucencies may be seen, which represent the nerves of the cauda equine.

## Complications of myelography

### Clinical

- Seizures may occur when the patient regains consciousness and within the first 2 hours following anaesthetic recovery; they are more likely to occur with cervical myelography. Seizures can be controlled with intravenous diazepam.
- Aggravation of clinical signs may occur within the first day if stress radiographs of the neck were taken. In most cases the signs are reversible within 72 hours.
- Apnoea can occur if the injection is given too rapidly via the cisternal route.
- Distended lumbar canalograms (see below) may cause severe paresis or paralysis, depending on the amount of central canal distension.
- Death may occur with needle penetration of the cervical spinal cord.

### Procedural and artefactual

- The most common pitfall is partial or total extradural contrast medium injection during lumbar myelography. The contrast medium tends to escape via the intervertebral foramina, resulting in increased extradural opacification of this area on VD and lateral views. On the lateral views the extradural contrast medium has an undulating appearance and may mimic herniated disc material (Figure 15.17).
- Some of the above contrast medium may also be injected into venous sinuses or be absorbed into lymphatics, and may be seen ventral to the vertebrae during drainage.

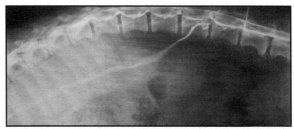

**15.17** Lumbar myelogram with extradural spillage and venous sinus drainage to the caudal vena cava via a vertebral vein.

- Multiple small radiolucent circular to oval filling defects within the subarachnoid space are gas bubbles inadvertently administered with the injection (Figure 15.18).

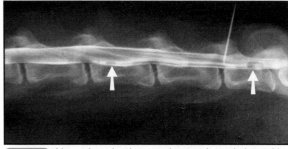

**15.18** Normal cat lumbar myelogram lateral view with radiolucent filling defects due to gas bubbles (arrowed).

- Subdural contrast medium injection or leakage results in an undulating scalloped appearance of the inner margin and may end in a knife-shaped point. Subdural contrast medium injection is seen up to five times more often with cisternal puncture (compared to lumbar puncture) as the dura is firmly attached to the dorsal atlanto-occipital membrane. Thus, there is no extradural space here and inadequate needle penetration of this region will result in the subdural artefact, more commonly seen affecting the dorsal contrast medium column. The contrast medium often appears more radiopaque than that seen with subarachnoid injections. This is possibly due to lack of dilution with cerebrospinal fluid.
- A canalogram occurs if contrast medium inadvertently enters the central canal during the procedure, but may also occur if there is a pathological communication between the subarachnoid space and the central canal. Iatrogenic canalograms are more likely to occur with lumbar myelography and needle puncture at L4–5 (Figure 15.19). Here the cord is wider (lumbar intumescence) with a subsequently narrowed subarachnoid space. The bevel of the needle may then be partly within the cord and some contrast medium may run along the needle shaft to enter the central canal. A 1–2 mm wide canalogram is unlikely to be clinically significant. However, if a lumbar pressure injection is made, the central canal may widen resulting in pressure necrosis of adjacent neural tissue with worsening of clinical signs. If L5–6 or

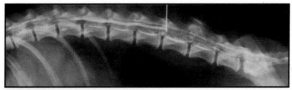

**15.19** Lumbar myelogram with needle placement at L4–5 and not positioned deep enough. Note the widened contrast medium-filled central canal from L1–L4 and continuing cranially as a 1 mm wide line.

L6–7 needle punctures are unsuccessful, and the L4–5 space has to be used, radiographs should be made after injecting a small volume of contrast medium to first check for a possible canalogram before proceeding with the rest of the injection.

## Myelographic lesion classification

For myelographic lesion classification see Figure 15.20.

- Extradural cord compression results in deviation and attenuation of one contrast medium column on one view with widening of the cord on the orthogonal projection (Figure 15.20b). The latter view will show attenuation of the contrast medium columns from within. Rarely an annular lesion may constrict the cord from all sides.
- Intradural extramedullary cord compression results in a split of the contrast medium column, with a 'golf tee sign' that is more visible on the cranial or the caudal margin, depending on the site of injection. The orthogonal view will show widening of the cord (Figure 15.20c).

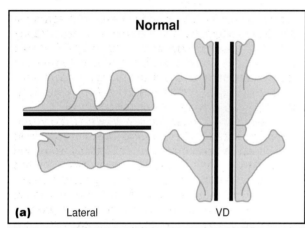

**Normal**

**(a)** Lateral    VD

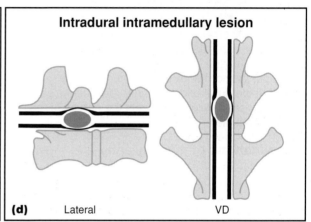

**Intradural intramedullary lesion**

**(d)** Lateral    VD

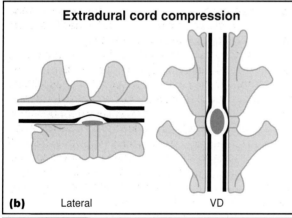

**Extradural cord compression**

**(b)** Lateral    VD

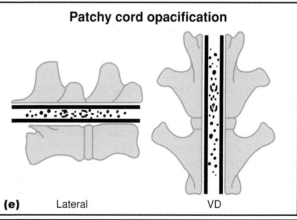

**Patchy cord opacification**

**(e)** Lateral    VD

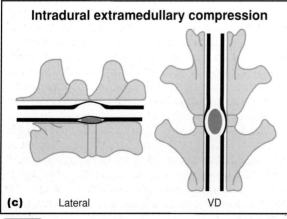

**Intradural extramedullary compression**

**(c)** Lateral    VD

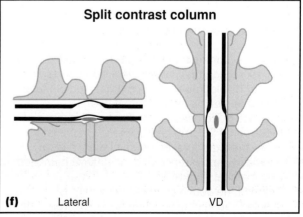

**Split contrast column**

**(f)** Lateral    VD

**15.20** Schematic classification of myelographically detectable vertebral canal pathology.

- Intramedullary cord enlargement results in widening of the cord and attenuation from within of contrast medium columns on all views (Figure 15.20d).
- Patchy opacification of the cord is associated with myelomalacia (Figure 15.20e).
- Split contrast medium columns (Figure 15.20f) may occur under the following circumstances:
  - intradural extramedullary lesions (as described above)
  - a compressive lesion, usually herniated disc material, located in a narrow area centrally on the floor of the vertebral canal
  - a compressive lesion, usually herniated disc material, located ventrolaterally.

The above may be distinguished by making orthogonal and oblique views.

## Special techniques for the lumbosacral region

For information on special techniques for the lumbosacral region see Chapter 18.

## Alternative imaging techniques

### Magnetic resonance imaging

Magnetic resonance imaging (MRI) produces excellent soft tissue detail and reasonable detail of bone and cartilage. The various imaging planes are readily acquired. There is no radiation danger and artefacts are minimal. However, the main limiting factors are its expense, prolonged anaesthesia when compared to helical computed tomography (CT), poorer resolution in cats and small dogs, and ferromagnetic substances in the patient that may cause severe artefacts.

The patient is usually placed in dorsal recumbency with the area of interest closest to a suitable coil. General anaesthesia is required and if inhalation anaesthesia is used the equipment must be non-ferrous. Procedures may take up to 30 minutes or more. Typically sagittal and parasagittal images are made first, the latter are particularly important to show up dorso- or ventrolateral cord compressions and intervertebral foraminal lesions that may not have been seen on myelography. The field of view is set to the region of interest and can be up to 40 cm long. Transverse images are then acquired. To save imaging and anaesthesia time these are often only done at the affected sites seen on sagittal images. Dorsal images of the whole region of interest may also be made. Slice thickness may vary from 2.5–3.5 mm and may be contiguous, overlapping or with a gap of up to 0.5 mm.

### Computed tomography

CT is very sensitive for subtle bone lysis, new bone formation or soft tissue mineralization. Visibility of pathology can be enhanced by CT myelography in a similar manner to routine myelography. Transverse images of the vertebral canal are produced. These can be reformatted to sagittal and dorsal images but with some loss of spatial and contrast resolution. Three-dimensional reconstruction can also be performed and is particularly useful for surgical planning.

Positioning is usually in dorsal recumbency with limbs strapped in flexion. Contiguous slices (up to 5 mm thick) are made of the affected region, with thinner slices in areas where better resolution is required, e.g. the intervertebral region. Different window levels and widths are used to enhance differentiation of various tissues (e.g. bone and soft tissue windows), allowing much greater definition of soft tissue opacities as compared with radiology. Tissue attenuation in a region of interest is expressed in Hounsfield units (HU), which usually range from −1000 HU for air to +1000 HU for bone. The normal spinal cord has intermediate attenuation, similar to that of the kidney. Degenerated extruded disc material will be hyperattenuated and can be readily seen.

### Myelography, MRI or CT?

Additional imaging is required in cases with equivocal plain film radiographs, and the choice of myelography *versus* advanced tomographic imaging by CT or MRI has to be made. The choice will often depend on matters not related to the specifics of each imaging modality but rather the familiarity of the clinician with the procedure, cost implications and availability of equipment.

Myelography is often the first choice as the veterinary surgeon can perform the procedure themself. With some practice myelography can be readily performed and is a very useful procedure. If executed properly it provides a lot of information, including circumferential location of pathology, a reason often cited for performing CT or MRI. An additional advantage is that a cerebrospinal fluid sample can be obtained for analysis. However, it is an invasive procedure, exposes the patient and workers to radiation, involves general anaesthesia and may result in complications (see above).

Advanced imaging with CT or MRI is non-invasive and gives multiplanar images of the structures being evaluated, resulting in cross-sectional images with no superimposition of structures, such as ribs or ilial wings. The craniocaudal and circumferential extent of pathology can be accurately determined and nerve roots can be followed caudally on contiguous transverse slices. If helical CT is used a vertebral column examination can be completed in less than 5 minutes. Examinations using standard third or fourth generation scanners may take up to 30 minutes. Bony changes are seen very well with CT but soft tissue differentiation is not as good as in MR images. In particular this applies to the spinal cord, although surrounding fat provides some contrast and also allows individual cauda equina nerve roots to be seen. Contrast may be improved by concurrent myelography (0.3 ml/kg of a 200 mg/ml solution diluted 1:5 to avoid beam hardening artefacts) but this then invalidates the advantage of the non-invasiveness of CT with the same disadvantages as cited for myelography.

MRI commonly uses T1-weighted (T1-W) and T2-weighted (T2-W) spin echo sequences. Numerous additional sequences, such as fat suppression and fast spin echo techniques may be available. Altering the spin or gradient of the echo sequence changes the contrast of various tissues, allowing characterization of their makeup. This then allows better evaluation of extradural, intradural extramedullary and intradural intramedullary lesions that may only be visible as filling defects on myelography. At the same time subtle intramedullary changes can be evaluated, which cannot be seen with myelography. Excellent anatomical detail is obtained with T1-W images but T2-W images give better tissue contrast, allowing distinction of discs, ligaments, grey and white cord matter, cerebrospinal fluid and fat. Distinction of the latter can be enhanced by using fat suppression sequences. Additional information can be obtained on T1-W images by administering a gadolinium-based paramagnetic contrast medium at 0.2–0.4 mmol/kg intravenously. Damaged capillaries will outline the vascular portion of a lesion, distinguishing it from any surrounding oedema, and may also show up pathology that was not visible on any other imaging sequence. A similar effect may be obtained with CT myelography.

With MRI cystic fluid is typically hypointense on T1-W and hyperintense on T2-W images, but intensity may vary depending on the fluid composition. Cervical articular facet synovial cysts and hydromyelia can thus be characterized. The nucleus pulposus in normal dogs is hyperintense on T2-W images due to its water content. Loss of this intense signal implies dehydration or herniation of the disc. Hyperintense extradural fat is readily seen and its displacement or obliteration is a good indication of a mass exerting cord pressure (also applies to CT). At the same time subtle changes in cord shape may also be appreciated. Hyperintense intra-parenchymal cord lesions on T2-W images may represent oedema, gliosis or even a dilated central canal. Neoplastic bone invasion and discospondylitis are easily appreciated with MRI and are seen much earlier than on radiographs. There is loss of the hypointense cortical bone signal, disruption of the more hyperintense bone marrow signal and in some cases neoplastic tissue can be seen in bone.

Besides the availability of equipment and clinician expertise, the choice of which imaging modality to use first also depends on the case presentation. The history, breed and clinical signs play an important role. A Dachshund with a T3–L4 myelopathy is likely to have a disc herniation and a well executed lumbar myelogram will provide all the information required to successfully treat the patient. A dog with clinical signs of discospondylitis and with normal survey radiographs should proceed directly to MRI as this is more sensitive for detection of early changes. In cervical vertebral malformation–malarticulation syndrome ('Wobbler syndrome') the age at presentation and breed may be important in deciding what modality to use. For example, the middle-aged Dobermann is likely to have a lower cervical disc problem with or without bony changes. Myelography is adequate in the vast majority of these cases. In a 1-year-old Great Dane there is a much greater likelihood of multiple lesions, involving the articular facets and pedicles. Although cervical myelography will provide most of the information required for this case, MRI will usually give additional information, such as the location of pathology induced by extradural pressure, which will

influence the choice of surgical decompression sites. Thus, in these cases MRI may be the initial imaging modality of choice. In a Cavalier King Charles Spaniel presented with persistent scratching of one side of the shoulder or neck region, syringohydromyelia is the most likely diagnosis and this is best seen with MRI as it is an intramedullary lesion. In some cases, e.g. lumbosacral pathology, the choice may be more difficult, and if there are marked bony changes on plain films CT may be a better option than MRI.

Irrespective of the imaging modality used, the imaging findings must still be correlated to clinical findings and neurological status. Many osseous or other changes may be incidental findings. Increasing numbers of abnormalities are seen with improved diagnostic modalities and their significance has to be correlated with the clinical presentation.

## Scintigraphy

Scintigraphy is useful in cases with normal plain film radiographs but where early bone changes are suspected, e.g. discospondylitis or occult spinal metastasis. The bone-seeking radiopharmaceutical will localize in regions of active bone turnover, resulting in a 'hot spot' indicating the lesion location. Dogs with extensive degenerative vertebral changes, such as spondylosis or spondyloarthrosis (which may be incidental findings), are not always good candidates for scintigraphy. Extensive isotope uptake will take place at these locations.

## Ultrasonography

Diagnostic ultrasonography may be used to evaluate vertebral contour changes and to guide fine-needle aspiration in degenerative, neoplastic or infectious conditions. It is particularly useful for evaluating the ventral vertebral bodies and associated discs from L3 to S1, using a transabdominal approach.

## References and further reading

Coulson A and Lewis N (2002) *An Atlas of Interpretive Radiographic Anatomy of the Dog & Cat* pp. 202–257. Blackwell Science, Oxford

Dennis R, Kirberger RM, Wrigley RH and Barr FJ (2001) Appendicular skeleton. In: *Handbook of Small Animal Radiological Differential Diagnosis* pp.42–45. WB Saunders, London

Kirberger RM (1994) Recent developments in canine lumbar myelography. *Compendium on Continuing Education for the Practicing Veterinarian* **16**, 647–854

Kirberger RM and Wrigley RH (1993) Myelography in the dog: review of patients with contrast medium in the central canal. *Veterinary Radiology and Ultrasound* **33**, 255–261

Penderis J, Sullivan M, Schwarz T and Griffiths IR (1999) Subdural injection of contrast medium as a complication of myelography. *Journal of Small Animal Practice* **40**, 173–176

Roberts RE and Selcer BA (1993) Myelography and epidurography. *Veterinary Clinics of North America: Small Animal Practice* **23**, 307–328

Sande R (1992) Radiography, myelography, computed tomography and magnetic resonance imaging of the spine. *Veterinary Clinics of North America: Small Animal Practice* **22**, 811–831

Scrivani PV (2000) Myelographic artefacts. *Veterinary Clinics of North America: Small Animal Practice* **30**, 303–314

Widmer WR and Blevins WE (1991) Veterinary myelography: a review of contrast media, adverse effects and technique. *Journal of the American Animal Hospital Association* **27**, 163–177

# 16

# Spine – conditions not related to intervertebral disc disease

## Fintan J. McEvoy

For information on general indications, radiographic technique, normal anatomy, evaluation of the spinal radiograph, contrast studies and alternative imaging techniques see Chapter 15. Intervertebral disc disease and 'Wobbler syndrome' are discussed in Chapter 17, and cauda equina syndrome in Chapter 18.

## Indications

Radiography for suspected spinal disease not related to intervertebral disc disease is appropriate in cases where:

- Clinical signs are referable to the spine or there is a breed disposition for congenital abnormalities
- There is a history of severe trauma, e.g. road traffic accident
- There is a suspicion of spinal disease from other imaging studies.

## Normal survey or contrast studies

On occasions no radiological abnormalities are seen in animals that have spinal disease. Such situations include:

- A number of breed-related congenital or hereditary diseases, typically presenting between 6 weeks and 8 months of life:
  - Progressive axonopathy (Boxers)
  - Inherited hypertrophic neuropathy in the Tibetan Mastiff
  - Neuroaxonal dystrophy in the Rottweiler and Papillon
  - Spinal muscular atrophy in the German Shepherd Dog, Rottweiler and English Pointer
  - Hereditary ataxia in the Fox Terrier and Jack Russell Terrier
  - Progressive neuropathy in the Cairn Terrier
- Inflammatory conditions:
  - Granulomatous meningoencephalomyelitis (GME)
  - Feline infectious peritonitis associated with meningitis
  - *Toxoplasma gondii* infection
  - *Neospora caninum* infection
  - Polyradiculoneuritis
- Dilatation of the central canal, syringomyelia and hydromyelia
- Intervertebral joint laxity: may require stress radiography as part of a directed search for the condition

- Fibrocartilage embolus or intramedullary haemorrhage
- Ischaemic neuromyopathy due to aortic thromboembolism
- Degenerative myelopathy.

## Abnormal radiological findings

### Trauma

#### Fractures

Fractures of the spine can be either pathological, where normal stresses result in fracture due to prior bone pathology, or traumatic as a result of abnormal stresses placed on normal bone. In assessing spinal fractures the following issues are important:

- Underlying bone disease
- Resulting instability
- Occult spinal trauma.

*Pathological fractures:* Focal bone lesions, particularly neoplasia, and diffuse disease (such as osteopenia, secondary to hyperparathyroidism) can result in fractures. It is important to recognize radiological evidence of these predisposing diseases, such as generalized osteopenia, focal bone lysis (Figure 16.1) or bone proliferation that is inconsistent with the age of the fracture (see also Chapters 3 and 4).

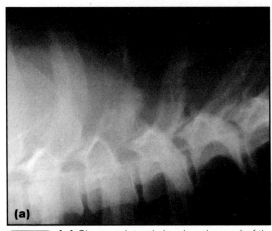

**16.1** **(a)** Close-up lateral view (myelogram) of the thoracic spine in an 8-year-old Labrador Retriever with osteosarcoma involving T6. Lysis of the dorsal spinous process is evident. Contrast medium can be seen within the subarachnoid space, which is narrowed and absent dorsally in this region. (continues) ▶

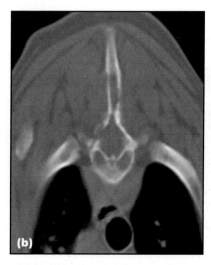

**16.1**
(continued)
**(b)** A transverse CT image from the same vertebra confirms the extensive lysis of the dorsal spinous process and further demonstrates marked bone lysis involving the lamina and body of the vertebra.

*Traumatic fractures:* Fractures of the spine, particularly of the articular facets and of the dens, result in vertebral instability. Close examination of the articular facets and of the alignment of adjacent vertebral bodies is important. Vertebral alignment should also be assessed by inspection of the dorsal spinous processes on ventrodorsal (VD) views and the vertebral canal on lateral views. Fractures of the vertebral bodies are best seen on lateral views, where recent traumatic fractures will appear as distinct radiolucent lines or as a deformity of the vertebral body (Figure 16.2). Fracture of the dens invariably leads to atlanto-

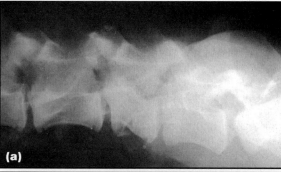

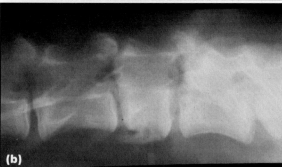

**16.2**  Lateral lumbar views of a dog with a fracture of L6. **(a)** Initial film showing a foreshortened vertebral body and fracture fragments with sharp edges compatible with a recent traumatic fracture. The vertebral canal does not appear significantly narrowed. **(b)** Similar view taken nine weeks later still shows a shortened vertebral body, no visible fracture fragments and a well organized callus on the ventral aspect of the vertebral body, indicating a healed fracture.

axial instability and spinal cord trauma. Non-fracture based atlantoaxial instabilities are described later in this chapter.

Compression fractures can occur in response to forces directed along the long axis of the spine. These are seen radiologically as a shortening of the vertebral body involved. Vertebrae in young animals have a high cancellous bone content rendering them more susceptible to compression fracture than the vertebrae of older animals, which have a higher cortical bone content. Bone fragments resulting from compression fractures may be forced into the spinal canal causing cord bruising or penetration. Spinal instability results if the facet joints are involved.

In dogs and cats, unlike certain other domestic species, the vertebral end plate is derived from a single ossification centre. Separations of the vertebral physes with or without associated fractures may be seen (Figure 16.3).

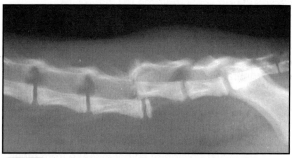

**16.3**  Lateral lumbar spine in a 5-month-old cat showing physeal separation and facet joint luxation after a traumatic incident.

When spinal cord compression results from spinal trauma, the rate at which compression occurs is a critical factor in determining the extent of cord trauma. Fracture callus is slow growing, and providing the cord survives the initial (rapid rate) insult, callus formation is unlikely to cause significant cord trauma during recovery.

**Vertebral luxations and subluxations**
Subluxations and luxations may persist after a traumatic incident and can, therefore, be easily detected (Figure 16.4). However, displacements may only be transient, resulting in no or little radiological evidence of displacement. Evidence, if present, may be quite

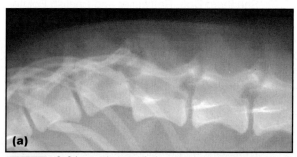

**16.4**  **(a)** Lateral view of the lumbar spine in an 11-month-old dog that sustained injuries in a road traffic accident. There is a severe subluxation of the spine involving L1 and L2. Fracture fragments are seen in the facet joint region. The marked step in the vertebral canal at this site and the acute nature of the injury suggests that significant spinal cord damage is likely. (continues)  ▶

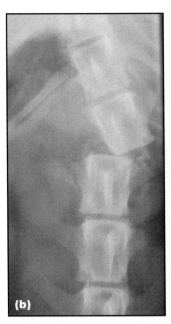

**16.4** (continued) **(b)** VD view of the lumbar spine in an 11-month-old dog that sustained injuries in a road traffic accident. There is a severe subluxation of the spine involving L1 and L2. Fracture fragments are seen in the facet joint region. The marked step in the vertebral canal at this site and the acute nature of the injury suggests that significant spinal cord damage is likely.

subtle and yet of great clinical significance due to cord bruising. The only remaining trace of a severe temporary luxation may be a mild degree of subluxation or small avulsion fragments. Thus, the extent of radiologically visible pathology gives little indication of the severity of cord trauma that can be present. Traumatic fracture luxations commonly occur at the thoracolumbar junction, which is a site of high intervertebral mobility.

## Congenital and developmental conditions

### Numerical abnormalities
Situations where there is an abnormal number of thoracic, lumbar or sacral vertebrae are not uncommon. These abnormalities are rarely clinically significant but can lead to confusion as to the location of lesions and ultimately to surgical intervention directed at the wrong vertebra or intervertebral space.

### Transitional vertebrae
Vertebrae that share characteristics with those from another location in the spine are considered transitional. Thus, cranial lumbar vertebrae that have associated ribs (which may be rudimentary), or sacral vertebrae that have discrete transverse processes or are incompletely fused are examples. Transitional vertebrae at sites other than the lumbosacral junction are often considered incidental findings. Lumbosacral transitional vertebrae, however, can be significant and may be associated with cauda equina syndrome and osteoarthrosis of the hips. The latter may result from an asymmetrical transitional vertebra, leading to asymmetry of the sacroiliac joints and abnormal loading of these joints. The extent and nature of the stress bearing articulation between the ilium and the transitional lumbosacral vertebra is best assessed on VD views. Radiological changes seen with lumbosacral transitional vertebrae include:

- Articulation of one or both transverse processes of the last lumbar vertebra with the ilium

- The presence of one or two transverse processes on S1
- Separation of the spinous process of S1 from the remainder of the sacrum
- Intervertebral disc spaces within the sacrum (typically between S1 and S2)
- Separation of the cranial articular process of S1 from the wing of the sacrum.

In cases where there is a separation between S1 and S2, there may be fusion of S3 with the first caudal vertebra and this fusion of three vertebrae should not be confused with a normal sacrum. Differentiation between a lumbarized sacral segment and a sacralized lumbar segment can be difficult. Assessment of the degree of asymmetry and the nature of the spinal attachment to the ilium is probably more important than clearly identifying the 'origin' of a particular transverse vertebra. Transitional lumbosacral vertebral anomalies are thought to be inherited, especially in the German Shepherd Dog (see Chapter 18).

### Block vertebrae
Vertebrae that are fused at birth due to failure of normal embryological segmentation are termed 'block vertebrae'. Any portion of adjacent vertebrae may be involved, total fusion or partial fusion of the vertebral body is typically recognized (Figure 16.5). Clinical signs related to adjacent intervertebral disc disease do occur rarely and are related to angulation of the vertebral canal and excessive moments of force at the articulation with adjacent normal vertebrae.

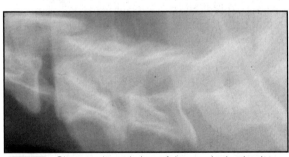

**16.5** Close-up lateral view of the cervical spine in a skeletally mature dog with an incidental block vertebra. C3 and C4 are fused at the level of the vertebral bodies. The vertebral canal appears wide and no clinical signs were present.

### Hemivertebrae
Failure in formation of a part of the vertebral body gives rise to a hemivertebra. The missing portion is either within the ventral or dorsal aspect of the vertebral body, which then adopts a wedge shape. The suggested embryological aetiology is that there is a failure of development within one of the two chondrification centres or sclerotomes that are present early in foetal development as precursors to the single ossification centre of the vertebral body. The resulting malformed vertebral body will be wedge-shaped, having its broad base either dorsally, ventrally or laterally. These various orientations result in kyphosis, lordosis or scoliosis, respectively (Figure 16.6).

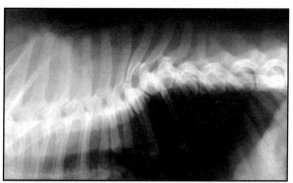

16.6 Lateral view of the thoracic spine in a skeletally mature dog with hemivertebrae. The bodies of T7–9 are wedge-shaped. There is an accompanying malformation of the articular facets and the dorsal spinous processes and also kyphosis. The vertebral canal appears a normal width.

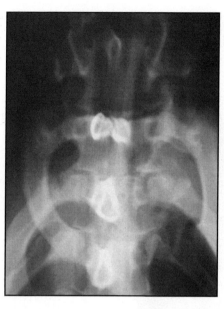

16.7 VD view of the cranial thoracic spine in a 5-year-old Beagle with spina bifida. The dorsal spinous process of T1 is paired. (© Y Ruel.)

Selective breeding for these vertebral abnormalities has been practised in certain breeds so that the condition is seen in the Boston Terrier, English and French Bulldogs and the Pug among others. When these abnormalities occur they are often multiple and grouped at single or multiple sites. Spinal cord abnormalities that accompany these vertebral abnormalities occur rarely. These vertebral abnormalities can be associated with clinical signs that are chronic and progressive (e.g. pain and pelvic limb weakness) and are usually manifest during the growth phase. Alternatively, hemivertebrae may not be associated with clinical signs. Diagnosis of clinically significant hemivertebrae requires that the clinical signs match the radiological location, and myelography may be indicated to demonstrate the site of spinal canal compromise.

### Butterfly vertebrae

A failure in development within both of the chondrification centres described above can also occur. This results in a vertebral body composed of two triangular units, with the apex of each opposing the other. The appearance on VD views resembles the wings of a butterfly. Clinical signs are rarely associated with this malformation and are determined by the exact geometry of the lesion, particularly the diameter of the vertebral canal in the affected region.

### Spina bifida

Failure of fusion of the dorsal part of the lamina, including the spinous process, can occur (Figure 16.7). Environmental and genetic causes are considered likely. The condition is reported in the English Bulldog, and in Manx cats, with sporadic accounts in other breeds. The condition may occur in a 'simple' form without associated cord abnormalities or neurological signs. Cord abnormalities, such as dysraphic defects ('split cord'), syringomyelia or hydromelia (see later) can, however, occur as part of the spina bifida syndrome. These changes are not seen on plain films, may be detectable using myelography, but are best seen using computed tomography (CT) or magnetic resonance imaging (MRI). Simple spina bifida can be

considered an incidental finding but one should be mindful of the potential for associated serious cord abnormalities. (For more information on spina bifida see BSAVA Manual of Canine and Feline Neurology.)

### Atlantoaxial instability

Atlantoaxial instability is typically, but not exclusively, seen in small breeds of dog. The dens of the axis (which arises embryologically from the body of the atlas) supports a number of ligamentous attachments that stabilize the atlantoaxial joint. Instability of this joint arises when the dens is absent, hypoplastic or fractured, or the ligaments themselves are absent or torn. Clinical signs are seen with dens or ligament pathology and are particularly severe with the latter as the abnormally mobile dens can abut against the cord and result in bruising. Signs, when present, are seen early in life and range from pain through varying degrees of ataxia to tetraplegia. Radiological signs include:

- Increased distance between the caudal aspect of the C1 lamina and the cranial extremity of dorsal spinous process of the axis (C2), which is exaggerated on flexion of the neck
- Absence, hypoplasia or fracture of the dens.

Care should be taken when trying to demonstrate these signs. A lateral view of the cranial cervical area with the neck in flexion is required. Practically, it is safer to obtain initial radiographs with the neck in slight flexion, to then inspect the radiographs, and if the lesion is not demonstrated convincingly, radiographs in moderate flexion can then be acquired (Figure 16.8). Oblique views (see Chapter 15) reduce overlap between the transverse processes of the atlas and the dens, allowing osseous dens pathology to be seen. RCd open-mouth views used to demonstrate the tympanic bullae (see Chapters 12 and 15) also show the dens free from significant overlap. The degree of occiptoatlantal and atlantoaxial flexion required to obtain this view is excessive in animals with suspected atlantoaxial instability and is therefore not recommended

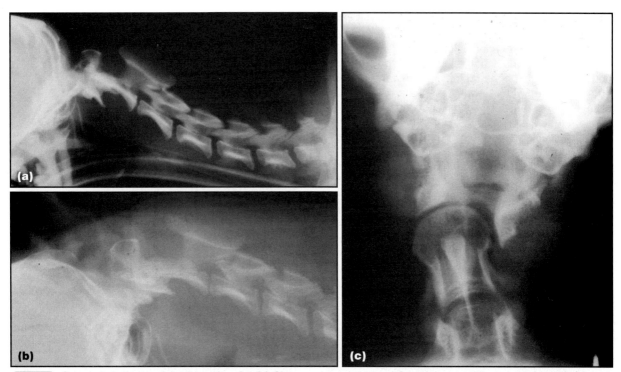

**16.8** Congenital atlantoaxial subluxation. **(a, b)** Close-up lateral views of C1–2 from two different dogs in different degrees of ventroflexion. The space between the neural arch of C1 and the dorsal spinous process of C2 is widened in each dog. **(c)** VD view of C1–2 in a 4-month-old Yorkshire Terrier with malaligned C1 and C2 due to an absent dens.

in this situation. The degree of instability and subluxation demonstrated is not related to clinical significance or to the likely outcome of surgical correction. In making a prognosis it is better to rely on the results of the neurological assessment.

### Breed-related conditions
As outlined above, certain breeds are overrepresented in accounts of specific congenital abnormalities. Thus, the Manx cat and brachycephalic dog breeds are associated with spina bifida. The German Shepherd Dog is noted for transitional vertebral abnormalities of the lumbosacral area. Hemi- and butterfly vertebrae are seen in Pugs and Bulldogs and in other breeds that have been selectively bred for a screw tail. Sacral agenesis, absence of part or all of the sacrum, is seen in the Manx cat.

Spinal dysraphism (myelodysplasia) is seen as part of a syndrome in certain severe forms of spina bifida or as an entity in itself as an hereditary trait, co-dominant, with variable expression, in the Weimaraner. Affected dogs typically show an abnormal 'bunny hopping' hindlimb gait as early as 6 weeks of life. Advanced imaging techniques, such as MRI, are required for a complete imaging diagnosis, but some of the components of these conditions may be evident on myelography. Dysraphism can be seen together with abnormalities of vesicourethral and urethral function.

### Arthrosis and degenerative conditions
For information on diseases of the intervertebral discs, see Chapter 17.

### Articular facet disease
The articular facets (zygapophyseal joints) act to provide stability and permit transmission of forces through the vertebrae. Their orientation relative to one another differs from being roughly horizontal up to the level of T10, to being more vertically orientated caudal to this. Thus, the joint spaces in the dog are best appreciated on lateral views cranial to T10 and on the VD view more caudally. Failure in development of the articular facets joints (facet aplasia) has been reported and may result in secondary spinal cord compression (Penderis *et al.*, 2005). Osteoarthrosis is seen radiologically as osteophyte formation with effacement of the normally clear joint margins. It is seen particularly in the lumbar area in large breeds of dog from middle age onwards. This is thought to represent a degenerative joint disease process and as the clinical significance of these changes is difficult to test, their significance remains uncertain.

Cystic lesions may arise from facet synovium. These are called synovial cysts and may occur at multiple facet joints in the cervical spine of young giant-breed dogs, or as solitary cysts in the thoracolumbar area of older large-breed dogs.

### Spondylosis
Spondylosis, also known as spondylosis deformans, is a degenerative disease of the spine characterized by the presence of one or more osteophytes, showing different degrees of development, occurring at the level of vertebral body end plates. The condition is seen mainly in medium and large-breed dogs. It is particularly prevalent in the Boxer, where it has shown moderate heritability. In severe cases the condition

causes loss of range of movement in the affected area, predisposing the animal to back pain. Radiologically these lesions are recognized on the lateral views.

The process arises at the junction of the vertebral body and the end plate (epiphyses). It can progress from a mild form with osteophytes situated on the edge of the epiphysis but not extending beyond the vertebral edge on the lateral view, to an intermediate form with osteophyte enlargement beyond the edge of the epiphysis, but not connecting with osteophytes on the opposite vertebra (Figure 16.9). The intermediate form in turn can progress to an advanced stage with bridging osteophytes situated on adjoining vertebrae. Any vertebrae may be affected but the caudal thoracic and cranial lumbar are the most common sites involved. Osteophyte formation can also involve the ventrolateral and lateral aspect of the vertebra, impinge upon the disc space or involve the intervertebral foramen. These non-ventral manifestations of vertebral spondylosis may be better seen in VD views.

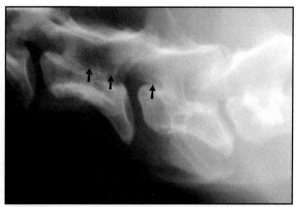

**16.10** Lateral cervical spine in a 12-year-old Flat Coated Retriever. A fine mineralized linear marking (arrowed) is seen running parallel and dorsal to the floor of the vertebral canal. This appearance is typical of dural ossification.

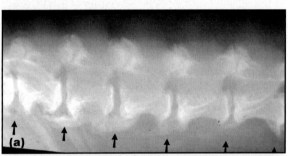

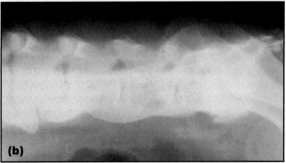

**16.9** Lateral lumbar spine from two different middle-aged dogs with spondylosis and osteoarthrosis. **(a)** Spondylosis (arrowed) extending beyond the vertebral edges and osteoarthrosis involving the articular facets. The latter is seen as a loss in clarity of the joint margin and distortion of the joints by new bone. **(b)** A more advanced stage of spondylosis with vertebral bridging involving multiple vertebral bodies.

### Spinal dural ossification (ossifying pachymeningitis)

Spinal dural ossification (ossifying pachymeningitis) has been described mainly in large-breed dogs, occurring late in life. Radiologically, it is seen as faint interrupted linear mineralized lines dorsally and ventrally within the vertebral canal. This may progress to marked mineralization, extending over large segments of the cord (Figure 16.10). CT and necropsy studies have confirmed the intradural nature of the mineralization. The finding is not associated with clinical signs. By identifying the location of the dura, the presence of ossification can help demonstrate extradural compression.

### Diffuse idiopathic skeletal hyperostosis

Adjacent vertebrae are stabilized by means of interconnecting ligaments that connect the tips of the spinous processes (interspinous ligament), the laminae (ligamentum flavum) and dorsal and ventral aspects of the vertebral bodies (dorsal and ventral longitudinal ligaments). Diffuse idiopathic skeletal hyperostosis (DISH) is a spinal enthesopathy that can also affect the appendicular skeleton. The condition has been reported in the dog and when the spine is involved, appears as an undulating wave-like or 'flowing' linear pattern of ossification involving these ligaments. Appendicular changes include ossification of other ligaments and tendons and subcutaneous calcification. Intra-articular structures are spared.

### Impingement of the dorsal spinous processes

Mutual compression of the spinous processes of closely approximated adjacent lumbar vertebrae is sometimes referred to as Baastrup's sign. In humans it is reported to occur as part of the degenerative disease processes in the spine, and can be associated with sclerosis and fracture of the spinous process and development of a neoarticulation between involved vertebrae with extension of the resulting synovial cavity to the intraspinal space. While radiological evidence of impingement has long been recognized in horses its clinical significance is questioned. Impingement of the dorsal spinous processes and the formation of neoarticulations have been reported in the dog. In addition, impingement can occur between any touching parts of adjacent vertebrae or between the vertebrae and the ilium.

### Infection

Infectious conditions are an important group in both the dog and cat. Vertebrae may become infected haematogenously or by local inoculation arising from bite wounds and migrating foreign bodies.

## Discospondylitis

Discospondylitis is an infection of the disc and adjacent vertebral end plates, usually developing via the haematogenous route and typically seen in large and giant breeds of dog. Bacteraemia may be associated with urinary tract, dental, valvular or other sites of focal infection. The clinical signs in discospondylitis appear to result from vertebral pain, intervertebral instability and extradural cord compression, which may be seen in severe cases. Multiple sites may be involved. It is thus important to radiograph the whole spine to determine the extent of the condition and to act as a control for follow-up films in the evaluation of response to treatment.

The onset of clinical signs may precede radiographic changes by as much as 3 to 4 weeks, while clinical recovery in response to appropriate treatment can occur despite the presence in the short term, of a worsening in radiological signs. Ultrasound-guided collection of material for culture from the lumbar area has been reported for the disease. Organisms cultured include *Brucella canis* but *Staphylococcus* spp. are most commonly encountered. *Aspergillus* spp. have been isolated from lesions in some affected dogs, particularly from German Shepherd Dogs, which may be predisposed to mycotic infection by immunosuppression. The progression of radiological signs is as follows:

1. In the early stages there may be a subtle widening of the intervertebral disc space without any opacity changes. Collapse rather than a widening of the disc space can occur rarely prior to osseous changes.
2. This is followed by a loss of opacity in the vertebral end plate or plates adjacent to the disc involved.
3. This progresses in later stages into marked lysis of the vertebral end plates, bone sclerosis within the affected adjacent vertebral bodies, focal or multifocal bone changes and narrowing of the intervertebral disc (Figure 16.11).
4. Proliferation of bone around the site can eventually lead to fusion of the vertebral bodies.

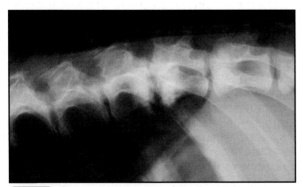

**16.11** Close-up lateral view of the thoracolumbar spine in a dog with advanced discospondylitis. There is a mixed proliferative and lytic process involving the T11–T12 end plates. There is loss of normal intervertebral disc material, resulting in collapse of the disc space.

## Spondylitis

Spondylitis is an infection localized to the vertebral body. Both parasitic and bacterial agents are encountered. In the case of bacterial infections, initial inoculation may result from migrating foreign bodies, bite wounds (particularly in cats) or by haematogenous spread. The route of migrating foreign bodies is not the same in all cases but some patterns are observed. There are convincing accounts of inhaled foreign bodies (typically grass or other seed awns that are barbed and so can move in one direction only) penetrating the airways after inhalation and migrating to various sites, resulting in pleural disease, fistulas and eventually vertebral body infections. It is proposed that the ventral borders of the bodies of L2–4 are preferentially involved when infection is via this route. This is due to their relationship with the origin of the diaphragmatic crura (Figure 16.12).

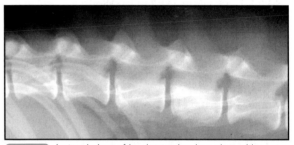

**16.12** Lateral view of lumbar spine in a dog with spondylitis. There is new bone formation at the ventral aspect of L2 and L3. Bone sclerosis is evident within the affected vertebral bodies. The spondylitis is likely to be secondary to a migrating foreign body.

Migrating larvae of the oesophageal worm *Spirocerca lupi* can stimulate vertebral inflammatory changes. The parasite during its life cycle must migrate ventrally from the aorta into the oesophageal wall, where it induces a parasitic granuloma in which adult worms reside. Some larvae take aberrant paths and migrate dorsally to reach the thoracic spine. Multiple thoracic vertebrae from T5–13 may be affected. Radiological changes range from a subtle loss of the normal ventral vertebral concavity due to the laying down of dense, solid periosteal new bone to a ventrally protruding periosteal reaction (Figure 16.13). If the reaction bridges the intervertebral space it can be difficult to distinguish

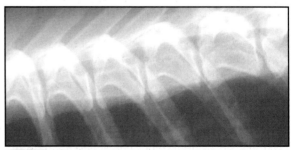

**16.13** Close-up lateral view of caudal thoracic spine showing spondylitis secondary to *Spirocerca lupi* infection. Note the lack of ventral concavity of the middle vertebral bodies due to a solid periosteal reaction. (Courtesy of R Kirberger.)

from spondylosis. The spondylitis seen with spirocercosis is usually associated with an oesophageal mass and typically only involves the central part of the vertebral body, while spondylosis arises in the region of the vertebral end plate.

### Physitis
Infection localized to the vertebral physes has been reported due to *Staphylococcus intermedius*. This occurs rarely and is seen in young dogs. The route of infection is haematogenous and presumably the physeal region in the vertebrae is predisposed as a result of blood flow characteristics in the region. A single report demonstrated this rare finding in a dog with a congenital portosystemic shunt (Walker *et al.*, 1999).

## Neoplasia
Neoplastic disease of the vertebrae may be primary, metastatic or locally infiltrative. To some extent each category has suggestive radiological signs, which are considered separately below. Radiological signs in general will be determined by the nature of the bone response (lytic or productive) to the neoplasm, the presence of pathological fractures and, on myelography, the degree of extradural compression present.

### Primary neoplasia
Primary neoplasia in the vertebral column may appear radiologically as a lytic, proliferative or mixed bone response. Due to the slow growing nature of such mass lesions, initial signs may relate to spinal pain rather than neurological deficits.

Malignant neoplasms encountered in the spine include osteosarcoma, chondrosarcoma and myeloma. Primary osteosarcoma can involve any part of the vertebrae. Lesions are typically confined to one vertebra but local metastasis to adjacent vertebrae can occur in advanced stages. Permeative bone destruction and disorganized bone proliferation extending into adjacent soft tissues are features of osteosarcoma. There is no apparent predilection site.

Neoplasia containing cartilage, of which chondrosarcoma and chordoma are examples, is also reported rarely in the spine. Chordomas arise from remnants of the notocord and occur in the vertebral body or in extraskeletal sites, including the spinal cord. These neoplasms will be seen radiologically if they cause destruction of adjacent normal bone, compression of the spinal cord (evident myelographically) or if they contain zones of mineralization. Multiple myeloma is seen as multiple lytic 'punched out' areas of bone with little or no bone response evident on the radiograph, or detectable on bone scintigraphy (Figure 16.14). Differentiation of multiple myeloma from certain forms of lymphoma is not possible on the basis of radiology alone.

Multiple cartilaginous exostoses (osteochondromatosis) appear as large smoothly marginated bone masses that are continuous with the underlying bone and may be cystic. Within the vertebrae they are typically associated with the dorsal spinous process. Other parts of the vertebrae can be involved as can the appendicular skeleton (see Chapter 3). These masses can occasionally result in spinal cord compression.

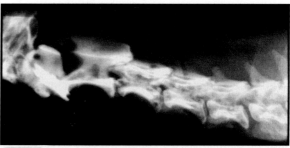

**16.14** Lateral cervical spine of a skeletally mature dog with multiple myeloma. Multiple focal lucencies with sharp margins are seen throughout the cervical spine. There is no evidence of new bone production in response to the lesions. (© Y Ruel.)

They are not neoplastic but transformation to chondrosarcoma or osteosarcoma can occur later in life. A focal, isolated cartilaginous non-osseous form called solitary cartilaginous exostosis is seen occasionally in large breeds of dog at the dorsal aspects of C1 and C2, or less frequently the tissues between the dorsal spinous processes of other vertebrae are involved. Radiologically the lesion appears as a mineralized zone closely associated with the underlying vertebra where modelling changes can be seen. Histologically the condition differs from multiple cartilaginous exostosis and calcinosis circumscripta (see below). The lesion does not contain bone and its classification is problematic (Bhatti *et al.*, 2001).

### Metastatic neoplasia
Metastasis can arise from a variety of distant primary neoplasms including mammary, prostate and thyroid carcinomas. While metastatic neoplasia can affect only one vertebra, multiple vertebrae are more commonly involved, often with lesions at various stages of development. Prostatic neoplasia can metastasize to the caudal lumbar vertebrae via the haematogenous route. During periods of attempted forced expiration against a closed glottis (Valsalva manoeuvre) raised intra-abdominal pressure causes blood from the hindlimbs and prostate to be redirected from the caudal vena cava to the vertebral venous sinuses. The new bone formed in response to metastases from prostatic carcinoma is 'fluffy' or 'brush-like' in appearance, involving the ventral borders of the vertebral bodies. Metastatic lesions arising from more distant sites may be mainly proliferative, lytic or mixed in nature. Their location and appearance do not give information on the site or cell type of the primary neoplasia involved.

### Infiltrative neoplasia
Soft tissue neoplasms (e.g. fibrosarcomas) adjacent to the vertebral bodies can extend locally to involve the vertebrae (Figure 16.15). Special care must be taken in evaluating radiographs to appreciate the presence of subtle paravertebral soft tissue changes. Paravertebral masses can be difficult to detect in the cervical area. Displacement of fascial plains and dystrophic mineralization, if present, are important radiological indicators. Soft tissue processes ventral to the thoracic spine are easily seen as they are outlined by a gas-filled lung but

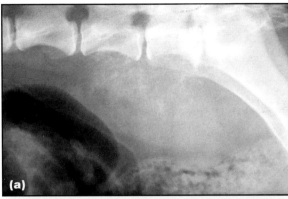

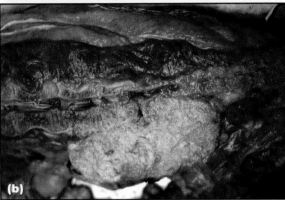

**16.15** Close-up lateral view of lumbar spine of an 8-year-old German Shepherd Dog. **(a)** There is a sublumbar mass arising from the medial iliac lymph nodes. This has resulted in a mass effect displacing the descending colon ventrally. The mass has a non-uniform opacity containing numerous linear mineral markings. The mineral component of the mass somewhat obscures the ventral surfaces of the underlying vertebrae. **(b)** Post-mortem examination confirmed the mineralized nature of the mass with local extension into L7 and S1. The histological diagnosis was fibrosarcoma.

can be missed if they are midline and merge with the mediastinal space. In the latter case this will amount to a dorsal mediastinal widening, which is best seen on a VD/dorsoventral (DV) view rather than on the lateral view. Ventral vertebral soft tissue changes are more readily identified in the lumbar area due to the presence in many animals of sublumbar retroperitonal fat, which provides adequate radiological contrast to permit detection. Neoplasms involving the medial iliac lymph nodes occasionally spread by infiltration to the adjacent lumbar vertebrae.

## Metabolic and storage diseases

The axial skeleton may be affected by systemic disease and show radiological changes over large segments or in its entirety.

### Renal secondary hyperparathyroidism

Chronic renal disease results in demineralization of the axial skeleton. This process can be present in considerable degree and remain undetectable radiologically until bone mineral content drops by at least 30%. The underlying mineral imbalance is caused in part as a result of the failing kidney's inability to excrete phosphate. High serum phosphorus levels and failing kidney function stimulate increased production of parathyroid hormone (PTH), which acts to restore a normal calcium (Ca): phosphate (P) ratio by mobilizing calcium from bone. Additionally, vitamin D synthesis by the failing kidney is reduced and this leads to impaired osteoid mineralization. Within the axial skeleton, the skull rather than the spine appears to be the preferential site of demineralization (see Chapter 12).

### Nutritional secondary hyperparathyroidism

Nutritional secondary hyperparathyroidism shares much of the pathogenesis of its renal counterpart except that the cause of Ca:P imbalance is nutritional. Foods with a low available calcium or vitamin D content stimulate PTH synthesis in order to restore circulating ionized calcium levels to normal. Renal function with respect to vitamin D synthesis is unaffected so that osteoid mineralization can proceed. The osteopenia is a result of a combination of lack of substrate for normal mineralization and increased mobilization of the calcium that has reached bone (see Chapter 3). It is typically seen in young dogs and cats and is best seen within the vertebrae. Radiological changes include reduced bone to soft tissue contrast. There is loss of the normal fine trabecular pattern as it is replaced by coarse trabecular bone. In severe cases folding pathological fractures within the vertebral bodies may be seen. When such fractures are present they are often multiple and at different stages of the healing process. In cats particularly, loss of bone stiffness results in excessive curvature of the spine.

### Osteogenesis imperfecta

Osteogenesis imperfecta is a rare heritable disease involving genes coding for type I collagen, a connective tissue component found throughout the body (including the vertebrae). Its radiological appearance is similar to the demineralizing conditions above and should be included in the differential diagnosis in young dogs with poor vertebral mineralization and pathological fractures in which secondary hyperparathyroidism has been excluded.

### Age-related osteopenia

A less marked cause of vertebral osteopenia can occur as an age-related change, particularly in cats.

### Hypervitaminosis A

Hypervitaminosis A is seen in cats fed exclusively on a raw liver diet. This results in bony exostoses involving the axial and appendicular skeleton. In the vertebrae new bone is typically, but not exclusively, deposited in the cervical area at ligamentous origin and insertion points. The ventral borders of the vertebrae are involved initially, but exostosis can extend to all parts of the vertebrae, resulting in severe cases in compression of the nerve roots and spinal cord (Figure 16.16). Similar proliferative bone changes may also occur on the appendicular skeleton (see Chapter 4). In addition the skeleton may show a diffuse increased opacity.

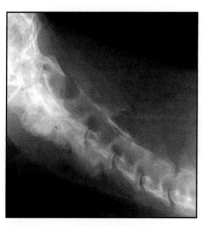

**16.16**

Lateral cervical spine in a 9-year-old cat with hypervitaminosis A. Proliferative well mineralized new bone formation is seen at the ventral aspects of C1–3.

## Mucopolysaccharidosis

Mucopolysaccharidoses are a group of rare lysosomal storage diseases where dermatan and heparan sulphate, which are metabolites of glycosaminoglycans (formerly know as mucopolysaccharides), accumulate intracellularly. This accumulation occurs because the enzyme catalysing their further breakdown is missing. As the metabolites accumulate they give rise to progressive functional and structural alteration throughout the body, including the spine. Multiple radiological changes including bone proliferation, changes in vertebral shape and vertebral fusion are seen (Figure 16.17).

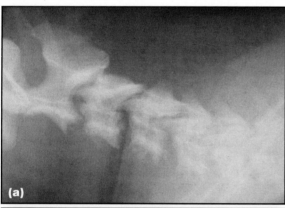

(a)

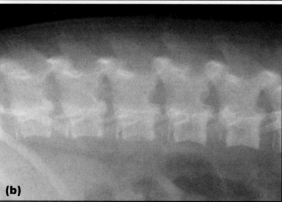

(b)

**16.17**  Mucopolysaccharidosis. Lateral views of segments of the **(a)** cervical and **(b)** lumbar spine in a 7-year-old cat. Note the incompletely ossified vertebral end plates, which have a 'folded' appearance, the shortening of the vertebral bodies and the irregular and widened intervertebral disc spaces.

## Congenital hypothyroidism

Congenital hypothyroidism is a rare condition described in many animal species, including dogs and cats. It causes generalized abnormalities, including delayed closure of vertebral physes and shortening of the vertebral bodies (see Chapter 3).

## Generalized osteosclerosis

Osteosclerosis can be used as a general term for bone hardening diseases, with or without accompanying changes in bone morphology. Osteopetrosis is a subdivision of this process, where there is no alteration in overall bone shape. Thus, radiologically there may be an increased bone opacity, primarily involving the medullary and cancellous bone, with normal morphology. Myeloproliferative diseases can result in osteosclerosis, manifest as replacement of the normally mainly fat-filled marrow cavity of long bones with either fibrous or osseous tissue. Radiological features include a generalized increase in bone opacity relative to soft tissues, cortical thickening, loss or filling of the medullary cavities with soft tissue or mineralized opacity (see Chapter 4). These conditions are encountered rarely in dogs and cats. Underlying disease processes can include feline leukaemia virus (FeLV) infection, extramedullary haematopoiesis, particularly in the end stages of pyruvate kinase deficiency, and medullary bone infarction. Osteopetrosis as part of the paraneoplastic process has also been suggested. The aetiopathogenesis of sclerosis in these conditions is poorly understood in domestic animals.

## Paravertebral soft tissue changes

Disease processes occurring adjacent to any of the vertebrae, seen as paravertebral soft tissue swelling or mineralization, can extend locally to involve the vertebrae. This applies particularly to infection and neoplasia.

## Calcinosis circumscripta

Calcinosis circumscripta (tumoral calcinosis) is seen as punctate deposits of amorphous mineralization, often close to joints and the spine (Figure 16.18) (see Chapter 3). There are occasional reports of this pro-

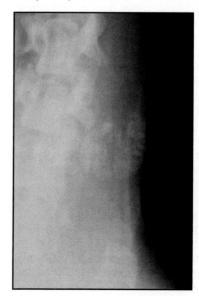

**16.18**

VD cervical spine view in a 13-month-old German Shepherd Dog. A roughly spherical zone of unstructured calcification, typical of calcinosis circumscripta, is present within the soft tissues of the neck adjacent to the vertebral column.

cess causing neurological signs due to spinal cord compression. Bone erosion local to the site of mineralization is possible. The aetiology is unknown but there appears to be a breed disposition in the German Shepherd Dog. Calcinosis circumscripta has been associated with chronic renal failure and footpad mineralization, although there are many reports of the condition in the absence of detectable renal disease.

## Non-osseous vertebral pathology

Diseases of the soft tissues within the vertebral canal resulting in cord compression are an important cause of neurological signs. Clinical signs will be most severe in cases where enlargement of the space-occupying lesion is rapid. If lesions are slow growing, there can be considerable displacement and compression of the spinal cord without severe clinical signs. Alternatively, the cord itself may become enlarged due to disease. These lesions are often not visible on plain films and myelography is required for their detection. Occasionally, in cases of chronic cord enlargement, pressure causes modelling of the vertebral canal resulting in subtle, though detectable, widening of the spinal canal: this can be evident on the plain films.

Soft tissue lesions within the spinal canal are typically classed as intramedullary, intradural–extramedullary and extradural. Masses at each location produce characteristic myelographic changes, which are described in Chapter 15. The distinction between the various locations is important as the differential diagnosis and treatment options will vary with the location of the mass.

### Extradural masses

Extradural lesions are common and important sources of spinal cord compression.

***Conditions associated with intervertebral discs:*** Intervertebral disc herniation and dorsal ligament hypertrophy are both examples of important compressive lesions and are considered in Chapter 17.

***Cystic lesions:*** There are two cystic lesions of note:

- Synovial cysts
- Arachnoid cysts.

*Synovial cysts:* Synovial cysts arise from the facet joints and are thus positioned dorsolaterally with respect to the cord. Demonstration of the lateralized compression that can result from these cysts typically requires the use of oblique views or preferably MRI.

*Arachnoid cysts:* Arachnoid cysts are dilatations or diverticula arising within the subarachnoid space. Since they communicate with the normal subarachnoid space, they fill with contrast medium during myelography and, depending on their size, cause variable degrees of obstruction to the passage of contrast medium in addition to cord compression. Arachnoid cysts can occur at any location along the spine but are typically seen in the dorsal region of the cervical and thoracolumbar spine (Figure 16.19).

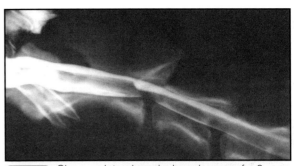

**16.19** Close-up lateral cervical myelogram of a 3-year-old Dobermann showing an arachnoid cyst. Note the enlargement of the contrast media-filled subarachnoid space dorsally at the level of C2 and C3, and the marked reduction in cord diameter. (© Y Ruel.)

***Abscess and haematoma:*** Benign swelling due to an abscess or haematoma can arise within the spine just as in any location throughout the body. These lesions, although benign and possibly trivial at other locations, are serious when they occur within the central nervous system. This is mainly because of the compression that results as they expand within the bony confines of the cranium or vertebral canal.

Bleeding from vessels that are extradural or within the subarachnoid space can occur as a result of trauma. Common causes include motor vehicle accidents, iatrogenically induced bleeding during myelography or as a postoperative complication of spinal surgery. The resulting haematoma can give rise to spinal cord compression. Spontaneous bleeding within the spinal canal, without known trauma, can occur in animals with coagulopathies. Von Willebrand's disease (deficiency in clotting factor VIII activity) in the Dobermann has been reported as presenting with various degrees of neurological deficit attributable to extradural haemorrhage.

***Juvenile polyarteritis syndrome:*** Juvenile polyarteritis syndrome, which leads to haemorrhage and progressive ataxia, has been reported in the Welsh Springer Spaniel. Bleeding can be seen as focal intradural or extradural swelling, or as a concentric narrowing or obliteration of the contrast medium column without displacement of the cord if the haemorrhage is diffuse and epidural. Cord compression can be seen if sufficient contrast medium is present to outline the concentrically narrowed cord. This may require a lumbar injection technique, with exposures made, if possible, during the final stages of the injection.

***Neoplasia:*** Neoplasic lesions can occur at any level in the spine. Plain film changes are rare. Slow growing masses, however, can cause remodelling of the surrounding neural arch. Nerve root neoplasms in particular are associated with widening of the intervertebral foramen. These may be primary (e.g. neurofibroma or sarcoma (nerve root tumour), schwannoma) or secondary (e.g. lymphoma). Extradural metastatic lymphosarcoma is by far the most common neoplasm of the spine seen in the cat. Affected cats may be FeLV or feline immunodeficiency virus (FIV) positive.

### Intradural–extramedullary masses

Neoplasia is the most commonly diagnosed disease at this location and is uncommon in both the dog and cat. Typically meningioma and neurofibromas are seen (Figure 16.20). Nephroblastomas typically occur in young dogs at the L1–4 region as intradural–extramedullary masses, and rarely, as extradural or intradural–intramedullary masses.

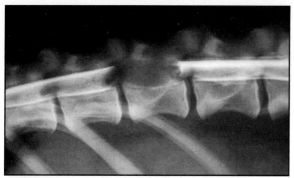

**16.20**  Lateral thoracolumbar myelogram from a dog with a meningioma. This intradural extramedullary neoplasm caused a filling defect in the contrast medium, extending the length of L1. The cord is compressed by the mass so that the myelographic appearance at the cranial aspect of the lesion is one of cord swelling (outward displacement of the contrast medium columns). Caudally and dorsally, however, the contrast medium to lesion interface is highly suggestive of an intradural mass (i.e. the contrast medium column stops abruptly and is widened with an irregular border). This irregular border represents the caudal limits of the intradural mass.

### Intramedullary disease

Swelling within the spinal cord can arise from neoplasia of any of the various cell types normally found in the spinal cord, as a result of infiltration by other cell types, from vascular disease and from disturbances in the flow of cerebrospinal fluid (CSF) through the central canal. Medullary neoplasia is rare in both dogs and cats (Figure 16.21). These lesions may be primary neoplasms of the spinal cord, such as astrocytomas and ependymomas, while lymphosarcoma is the most important metastatic neoplasm.

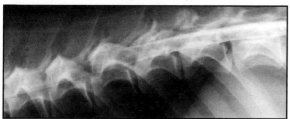

**16.21**  Lateral caudal thoracic myelogram after lumbar puncture in a middle-aged dog with an intramedullary neoplasm. There is diffuse cord swelling within the thoracic region. The long transition zone between swollen and normal cord can be seen on this image at the level of T11 and T12. Note the narrow contrast medium columns positioned at the outer limits of the vertebral canal, indicating a uniform cord swelling. These features are common to cord swelling of any origin. (© Y Ruel.)

*Hydromyelia and syringomyelia:* The term hydromyelia refers to a fluid-filled central canal lined by normal ependymal cells. This is differentiated from syringomyelia where the lining of a fluid-filled central canal is compromised so that fluid leaks into the parenchyma of the cord, or fluid is present in cavities within the cord that are not lined by ependymal cells and do not communicate with the central canal. Clinically and radiological differentiation between the two conditions can be problematic and the term 'syringohydromyelia' is used as an all-encompassing alternative.

Cord swellings associated with dilatation of the central canal are more and more recognized, due to the increased awareness of the condition and availability of MRI. The central canal runs the length of the spinal cord. Dilatation can occur over variable lengths of the canal and may be congenital or acquired. Acquired dilatation can result from accidental injection of contrast medium during a myelographic procedure, either via a lumbar puncture or as a result of an inappropriate cisternal puncture. The significance of inadvertent central canal injection relates to the degree of central canal dilatation induced. An opacified central canal of less than 1 mm diameter in the dog will typically be clinically insignificant. Greater accumulations and inadvertent injection via the cisternal route are likely to result in a worsening of neurological signs post-myelography. The appearance of contrast medium in a normal diameter or dilated (>1 mm) central canal can be also seen at sites of cord trauma distant to the site of injection, e.g. at sites of severe intervertebral disc prolapse.

*Chiari malformations in Cavalier King Charles Spaniels:* The primary anatomical abnormality is partial 'herniation' or overcrowding of the cerebellum through the foramen magnum. This, it is proposed, gives rise to disturbances in circulation of CSF and eventually over a prolonged period to central canal dilatation. The syndrome includes characteristic clinical signs. Imaging diagnosis is optimal using MRI (Figure 16.22). Typically, no radiological abnormality will be

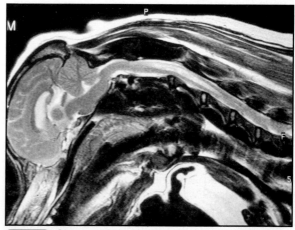

**16.22**  Chiari malformation in a Cavalier King Charles Spaniel: sagittal T2-weighted MRI, showing overcrowding of the cerebellum with resulting 'herniation' through the foramen magnum. CSF is hyperintense and can be seen in a dilated central canal (C2–4 region), indicating hydromyelia. (© P Mantis.)

seen in cases of central canal dilatation on plain radiography, but the slow expansion of the cord, particularly within C2, may lead to a detectable widening or dorsal convexity of the vertebral canal. Myelography may show a uniform narrowing of the contrast medium columns on multiple views of the area involved due to widening of the spinal cord. If the dilatation is severe and the cord is pressed against the wall of the spinal canal, then accidental injection of contrast medium into the CSF-filled cavity is possible if not likely, with the result that the dilated central canal is clearly imaged (Figure 16.23).

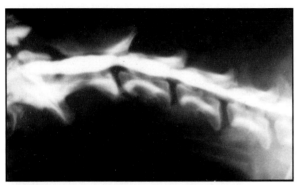

**16.23** Cervical myelogram from a Boxer showing severe hydromyelia. Note the small gap between the outer margins of the contrast medium column within the central canal and the wall of the vertebral canal, indicating marked compression and atrophy of cord material. The contrast medium was inadvertently placed in the central canal rather than the subarachnoid space during a cervical puncture. (© P Mantis.)

***Circulatory abnormalities:*** Infarcts and haemorrhage are well described in the spinal cord and can give rise to focal cord swellings. Infarcts can occur as a result of thrombi or emboli within either the venous or arterial parts of the spinal vasculature. Much of the intrinsic blood supply to the spinal cord can be considered end arterial, segmental in nature with vessels supplying lateralized segments of tissue. Emboli, when they do occur, can be associated with marked lateralization of clinical signs. They can arise from a number of sources, including heart valves in endocarditis, but may also be fibrocartilaginous in nature. In the latter case the material found appears identical to that of the nucleus pulposus of the intervertebral disc. The mechanism(s) by which this material can gain access to the spinal arterial system, and possibly even more perplexing into the venous system, is the subject of much speculation and investigation and to some extent remains unresolved. In diagnosis, clinical signs mentioned above, can be highly suggestive, particularly in young dogs up to 6 years of age. There is no well documented breed disposition. Radiological changes, if present, are non-specific and are a function of cord swelling, i.e. normal plain radiographs with signs of focal intramedullary swelling on myelography. Subtle extradural signs on myelography at the disc space in the area of infarction (centrally displaced contrast medium columns) can occur and may be related to the underlying embolic event.

## Myelomalacia

Myelomalacia typically refers to a haemorrhagic infarction of the spinal cord. It can be seen either as a focal or diffuse process. Radiological signs may be a non-specific cord swelling demonstrated on myelography. However, many dogs with myelomalacia show the more suggestive signs of contrast media infiltration, either focal or diffuse, into the cord (Figure 16.24). Care must be taken to ensure that the contrast medium is actually within the cord rather than epidurally and that other causes of contrast media within the cord, e.g. iatrogenic injection, hydromyelia and syringomyelia and inadvertent placement of contrast medium in the central canal have been eliminated. It is suggested that the greater the length of cord involved the worse the prognosis. The condition can be described as progressive if involvement of progressively higher or lower spinal segments is seen on sequential neurological or imaging examinations.

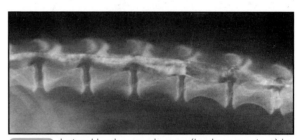

**16.24** Lateral lumbar myelogram (lumbar puncture) in a 5-year-old Dachshund. There is a marked accumulation of contrast material within the spinal cord indicative of myelomalacia. In addition, a trace of contrast medium is seen as an incidental finding within the epidural space. (Reproduced from Lu D *et al.* (2002) with permission from *Veterinary Radiology and Ultrasound*).

## References and further reading

Bailey CS and Morgan JP (1992) Congenital spinal malformations. *Veterinary Clinics of North America: Small Animal Practice* **22**, 985–1015
Beaver DP, Ellison GW, Lewis DD, Goring RL, Kubilis PS and Barchard C (2000) Risk factors affecting the outcome of surgery for atlantoaxial subluxation in dogs: 46 cases (1978–1998). *Journal of the American Veterinary Medical Association* **216**, 1104–1109
Bhatti S, Van Ham L, Putcuyps I, De Bosschere H, Polis I and Van Goethem B (2001) Atlantoaxial cartilaginous exostosis causing spinal cord compression in a mature Bernese Mountain Dog. *Journal of Small Animal Practice* **42**, 79–81
Campbell BG, Wootton JA, Krook L, DeMarco J and Minor RR (1997) Clinical signs and diagnosis of osteogenesis imperfecta in three dogs. *Journal of the American Veterinary Medical Association* **211**, 183–187
Caswell JL and Nykamp SG (2003) Intradural vasculitis and hemorrhage in full sibling Welsh Springer Spaniels. *Canadian Veterinary Journal* **44**, 137–139
Court EA, Watson AD and Peaston AE (1997) Retrospective study of 60 cases of feline lymphosarcoma. *Australian Veterinary Journal* **75**, 424–427
Dennis R (1987) Radiographic examination of the canine spine. *Veterinary Record* **121**, 31–35
Dickinson PJ, Sturges BK, Berry WL, Vernau KM, Koblik PD and Lecouteur RA (2001) Extradural spinal synovial cysts in nine dogs. *Journal of Small Animal Practice* **42**, 502–509
Done SH, Drew RA, Robins GM and Lane JG (1975) Hemivertebra in the dog: clinical and pathological observations. *Veterinary Record* **96**, 313–317
Dvir E, Kirberger RM and Malleczek D (2001) Radiographic and computed tomography changes and clinical presentation of spirocercosis in the dog. *Veterinary Radiology and Ultrasound* **42**, 119–129

Frendin J, Funkquist B, Hansson K, Lonnemark M and Carlsten J (1999) Diagnostic imaging of foreign body reactions in dogs with diffuse back pain. *Journal of Small Animal Practice* **40,** 278–285

Galloway AM, Curtis NC, Sommerlad SF and Watt PR (1999) Correlative imaging findings in seven dogs and one cat with spinal arachnoid cysts. *Veterinary Radiology and Ultrasound* **40,** 445–452

Gnirs K, Ruel Y, Blot S, Begon D, Rault D, Delisle F, Boulouha L, Colle MA, Carozzo C and Moissonnier P (2003) Spinal subarachnoid cysts in 13 dogs. *Veterinary Radiology and Ultrasound* **44,** 402–408

Johnston DE and Summers BA (1971) Osteomyelitis of the lumbar vertebrae in dogs caused by grass-seed foreign bodies. *Australian Veterinary Journal* **47,** 289–294

Jones BR, Gruffydd-Jones TJ, Sparkes AH and Lucke VM (1992) Preliminary studies on congenital hypothyroidism in a family of Abyssinian cats. *Veterinary Record* **131,** 145–148

Kirberger RM (1989) Congenital malformation and variation of the lumbar vertebrae in a dog. *Journal of the South African Veterinary Association* **60,** 111–112

Kirberger RM (1993) Myelography in the dog: Review of patients with contrast medium in the central canal. *Veterinary Radiology and Ultrasound* **34,** 253–258

Knaus I, Breit S, Kunzel W and Mayrhofer E (2004) Appearance and incidence of sacroiliac joint disease in ventrodorsal radiographs of the canine pelvis. *Veterinary Radiology and Ultrasound* **45,** 1–9

Macri NP, Van Alstine W and Coolman RA (1997) Canine spinal nephroblastoma. *Journal of the American Animal Hospital Association* **33,** 302–306

Lu D, Lamb CR and Targett MP (2002) Results of myelography in seven dogs with myelomalacia. *Veterinary Radiology and Ultrasound* **43,** 326–330

Morgan JP, Miyabayashi T and Choy S (1986) Cervical spine motion: radiographic study. *American Journal of Veterinary Research.* **47,** 2165–2169

Penderis J, Schwartz T, McConnel JF, Garosi LS, Thompson CE and Dennis R (2005) Dysplasia of the caudal vertebral articular facets in four dogs: results of radiographic, myelographic and magnetic resonance imaging investigations. *Veterinary Record* **156,** 601–605

Sanders SG, Bagley RS, Silver GM, Moore M and Tucker RL (2004) Outcomes and complications associated with ventral screws, pins, and polymethyl methacrylate for atlantoaxial instability in 12 dogs. *Journal of the American Animal Hospital Association.* **40,** 204–210

Shamir MH, Tavor N and Aizenberg T (2001) Radiographic findings during recovery from discospondylitis. *Veterinary Radiology and Ultrasound* **42,** 496–503

Shores A (1992) Spinal trauma. Pathophysiology and management of traumatic spinal injuries. *Veterinary Clinics of North America: Small Animal Practice* **22,** 859–888

Dombrowski Silverstein DC, Carmichael KP, Wang P, O'Malley TM, Haskins ME and Giger U (2004) Mucopolysaccharidosis type VII in a German Shepherd Dog. *Journal of the American Veterinary Medical Association* **224,** 553–557

Thomas WB (2000) Discospondylitis and other vertebral infections. *Veterinary Clinics of North America: Small Animal Practice.* **30,** 169–182

Thomas WB, Sorjonen DC and Simpson ST (1991) Surgical management of atlantoaxial subluxation in 23 dogs. *Veterinary Surgery* **20,** 409–412

Tomlinson J (1996) Surgical conditions of the cervical spine. *Seminars in Veterinary Medicine and Surgery (Small Animal)* **11,** 225–234

Walker MC, Platt SR, Graham JP and Clemmons RM (1999) Vertebral physitis with epiphyseal sequestration and a portosystemic shunt in a Pekingese dog. *Journal of Small Animal Practice* **40,** 525–528

Watson AG, de Lahunta A and Evans HE (1988) Morphology and embryological interpretation of a congenital occipito-atlanto-axial malformation in a dog. *Teratology* **38,** 451–459

# Spine – intervertebral disc disease and 'Wobbler syndrome'

## Jeremy V. Davies

For indications, radiographic technique, contrast studies and alternative imaging techniques, see Chapter 15. Caudal lumbar intervertebral disc disease is discussed in Chapter 18 under cauda equine syndrome.

## Intervertebral disc disease

### Terminology

The terminology 'disc disease' presupposes that the condition in question is a degenerative or other process that culminates in disc failure. However, acute disc ruptures do occur and may not be accompanied by the more universal disc degeneration that is seen in chondrodystrophic breeds in particular.

A consideration of the basic structure of intervertebral discs invites the terminology that accompanies the different disc lesions encountered in clinical practice. The annulus is the fibrous outer portion that encloses the elastic nucleus pulposus. The normal nucleus is gelatinous in composition and has a high water content which with magnetic resonance imaging (MRI) is demonstrated clearly on T2-weighted images (Figure 17.1a). With age, or premature degeneration in susceptible breeds, the nucleus loses water content (Figure 17.1b) and as a result loses elasticity. This in turn may lead to a deformation that does not 'recoil' to normal shape; such a disc can then remain deformed with the annulus bulging. Biomechanical factors dictate that any such bulge usually extends into the vertebral canal, hence, disc protrusion. It is also possible for the fibres of the annulus to tear, allowing a protrusion into the vertebral canal. This might best be called disc herniation. The extreme form of this is where the annulus tears, allowing the escape of nuclear material into the vertebral canal. When this event is acute, and often the result of vigorous activity, the escaping material may be an admixture of nuclear material, fibrous strands of annulus and blood products, hence, disc extrusion. The ultimate conclusion of this degenerative process is calcification.

Previously disc lesions have been classified as Hansen types 1 and 2. Type 1 disc lesions are seen in chondrodystrophic breeds, such as the Dachshund, where chondroid degeneration leads to calcification. Acute onset signs are typical. In contrast, type 2 disc lesions are seen in non-chondrodystrophic breeds and calcification is less frequently a feature. Chronic development of signs is more typical. More recently a 'type 3 – Miyabayashi' disc lesion has become unofficially

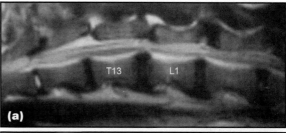
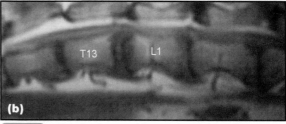

**17.1** MRI of a 4-year-old cross bred dog with a herniated disc. **(a)** T2-weighted image shows a normal hydrated disc nucleus with a high signal (white) on the left of the image and other nuclei at various stages of dehydration and degeneration. The T13–L1 disc at the centre of the image has herniated into the vertebral canal. The nucleus of this disc has a mottled MR signal. **(b)** T1-weighted image more clearly shows the herniation of nuclear material into the vertebral canal.

accepted (T Miyabayashi, personal communication). This involves the slow protrusion or extrusion of disc material that subsequently mineralizes. As with other types of disc lesion, accompanying chronic bony proliferation of the vertebral bodies (spondylosis) and facets (spondyloarthrosis) may develop. This is a slowly developing process that may not be accompanied by severe motor deficits (Figure 17.2).

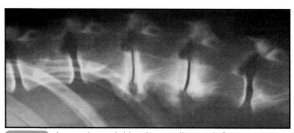

**17.2** Lateral cranial lumbar radiograph from an 11-year-old Springer Spaniel with collapse of the L1–2 and L2–3 disc spaces with mature ventral and abaxial spondylosis. Calcific material is seen within the vertebral canal at L1–2. This may be a composite shadow from calcified herniated material ('type 3 – Miyabayashi') and an extension of the spondylosis.

A further variation is the low volume high velocity disc lesion. This may cause significant contusion and cord swelling with little or no macroscopic disc material visible in the canal. The forces involved may even disrupt the meninges and penetrate the cord parenchyma (Figure 17.3).

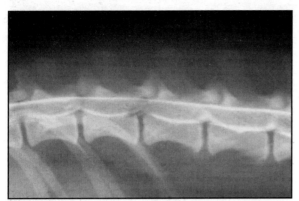

**17.3** Lateral lumbar radiograph after a lumbar myelogram in a 2-year-old Cavalier King Charles Spaniel. There is some epidural contrast medium spillage. There is loss of myelographic and epidural contrast over the L1–2 disc. Slight thinning of the dorsal column at this level confirms a low volume compression.

The currently preferred terminology in diagnostic imaging is disc herniation and for consistency this term will be used throughout this Chapter in common with the other sections of the manual.

## Degenerative disc disease

It is convenient to consider the radiological changes that may be present by dividing them according to the anatomical location:

- Plain film findings
  - Intervertebral disc space
  - Intervertebral disc
  - Vertebral canal
  - Intervertebral foramen
  - Vertebral body
  - Facet joints
  - Vacuum phenomenon
- Myelographic findings
  - Thecal sac
  - Cord swelling
  - Ascending myelomalacia.

A number of anatomical features dictate the likely location of clinically significant disc lesions:

- There is no disc at C1–2
- The intercapital ligament that lies between rib heads 2 to 10/11 reinforces the dorsal annulus making herniation less likely, although occasional cranial thoracic disc herniations have been reported
- Those parts of the spine that are the fulcrum of movement contain the most vulnerable discs, i.e. the cervical and thoracolumbar junction segments. The latter region is in contrast to the lower lumbar spine of humans that is most vulnerable

- The dorsal longitudinal ligament is stronger in the cervical than the thoracolumbar region. This may reduce the incidence of cervical herniation. The spinal cord in the cervical vertebral canal is afforded relatively more space. This will, in turn, allow more space occupation before clinical signs develop. This relative space can be quantified as the cervical spinal cord-to-canal ratio. Small-breed dogs have a higher cord-to-canal ratio and so small extradural compressions are likely to be more significant the smaller the breed
- The ventral part of the annulus is much thicker and stronger than the dorsal part, reducing the likelihood of ventral and lateral herniation. Frequently ventral spondylosis is noted in the thoracic region. Whilst this may be considered a response to 'instability', the thoracic segments supported by the rib cage and sternum are inherently stable. It is possible, therefore, that ventral osteoproliferation is an indication of the route of escape of herniated disc material in this region.

### Plain film findings

*Intervertebral disc space:* Providing the X-ray beam penetrates the disc space precisely perpendicular to its orientation the shape and size can be assessed. Minor deviations in beam centring and positioning will compromise the perpendicularity, giving a false impression of disc space narrowing. It is possible to compare the shape and size of adjacent disc spaces, providing that only those spaces in the central part of the exposed area are scrutinized. Common practice would suggest a plain film view extending throughout the area of interest, e.g. mid-thoracic to mid-lumbar spine, with subsequent beams much more tightly collimated and centred to a small number of vertebrae under scrutiny.

Loss of disc space size implies that some annulus or nuclear material has been displaced. The line of least resistance is toward the vertebral canal. Lateral and ventral herniation is infrequent. Changes in shape may also be detected (Figure 17.4). Most often this will manifest as a triangulation or 'wedging' of the disc space, narrowed dorsally. When subtle reductions in

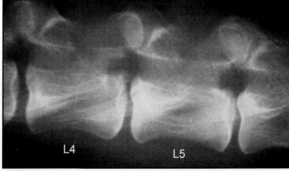

**17.4** Close-up lateral lumbar view in an 8-year-old German Shepherd Dog. The L4–5 disc is narrowed, more so dorsally than ventrally ('wedging') implying herniation of disc material. There is evidence of mineralization of the dorsal annulus. The superimposed lateral transverse processes opacify the nuclear part of the disc.

disc space size occur this may translate more obviously as a change in size and shape of the associated intervertebral foramen.

***Intervertebral disc:*** The intervertebral disc is, normally, radiolucent and is appreciated by extrapolation as the structure lying between the end plates of adjacent vertebrae. The degenerative processes that affect discs culminate in the calcification of the nucleus or annulus. Once there is sufficient calcium content to be appreciated radiologically the disc can be seen. This calcification may only be with the disc *in situ* and may actually identify normality as far as the shape and position of that disc. However, it confirms that the disc or discs are subject to degenerative changes and, therefore, have an increased potential to herniate. It is often the case that the only faintly calcified discs are more at risk from herniation than those that have completely calcified. These intermediate degrees of calcification may render the disc unable to regain shape following deformation. If a calcified disc herniates then calcific material may be visible within the intervertebral foramen or adjacent vertebral canal (Figure 17.5).

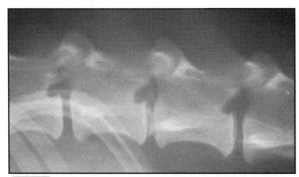

**17.5** Close-up lateral lumbar view in a 4-year-old Cocker Spaniel. The L1–2 disc has calcified and some of the calcified nuclear material has herniated into the vertebral canal and is seen clearly through the intervertebral foramen.

As many discs will not be calcified, contrast studies may be necessary to document the presence and degree of any herniation. Most often myelography is the contrast study of choice. The enhanced soft tissue separation of helical computed tomography (CT) will demonstrate some disc anatomy without contrast, and the structure and degree of hydration of a disc is readily demonstrated using MRI.

***Vertebral canal:*** The vertebral canal is largely encased in bone and so soft tissue changes therein will be virtually impossible to detect using plain radiography. If herniated disc material is sufficiently calcified it will be visible (Figures 17.6). Plain film radiography in cases of suspected disc disease often focuses on the lateral views. In a large proportion of disc herniation cases hemilaminectomy or pediculectomy may be the surgical procedure of choice, and so determining the side of any herniated material is imperative. This needs to be determined on ventrodorsal (VD)/dorsoventral (DV) or oblique views. If during routine lateral views heavily calcified material is suspected to have herniated, it is

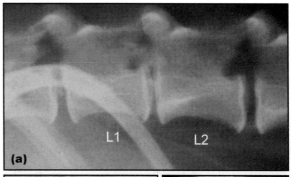

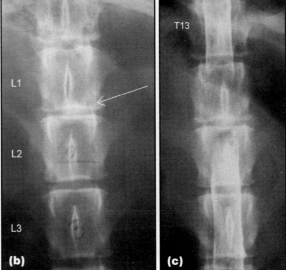

**17.6** 5-year-old Bichon Frise with a herniated L1–2 disc. **(a)** Lateral view with a large calcified mass of disc material easily seen in the intervertebral foramen. Also note the collapsed intervertebral disc space and reduced articular facet joint space. **(b)** On the VD view the large calcified mass of disc material (arrowed) can be seen lying to the left of the midline. A hemilaminectomy could be performed on the strength of this information. This image has been annotated on the original film for the benefit of the surgeon in the operating theatre, where it can be helpful to have annotations that are visible from a distance. **(c)** VD lumbar myelogram view of the same dog. It is less easy to interpret as far as determining the side for surgery, underlining the benefits of biplanar plain views when obvious calcific material is present.

worth attempting to demonstrate this on a VD view prior to myelography. Not every myelographic study is faultless in the identification of the side of herniation and in these cases the lack of a plain film VD view is regretted! Therefore, it is worth considering using biplanar survey views in all cases, or at least performing the VD views, if obviously calcific material is suspected to lie within the canal. Dural calcification (ossifying pachymeningitis) is an occasional incidental finding and where this is present adjacent to an intervertebral disc it will act as an indicator for extradural compression. This has been colloquially termed 'automyelography'.

***Intervertebral foramen:*** The intervertebral foramina, located on each side of a spinal segment, should be exactly superimposed on a well positioned radiograph. The shape varies slightly from breed to breed and from anatomical region to region. In the caudal thoracic and lumbar regions the foramen is often described as resembling a 'horse's head'. When small disc herniations occur and there is very minor loss of disc volume, it may be easier to detect changes in the shape or size of the foramen rather than the accompanying reduction in size of the disc space itself (Figure 17.7). Beam centring and positioning inaccuracy can distort the appreciation of the foramen but comparison with the two adjacent foramina should be reliable. As the foramen is an anatomical defect in bone, it may be possible to appreciate smaller and less calcified quantities of herniated disc material. The accessory process that overlies the foramen in the lumbar region must not be confused with pathological disc change.

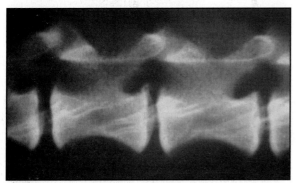

**17.7**   Close-up lateral view of the lumbar spine in a 4-year-old Beagle. The intervertebral foramen at the centre of the image is smaller and of a slightly different shape to those cranial and caudal to it.

In the thoracic region the ribs will be superimposed on the foramen. This is most noticeable in the barrel-chested breeds, such as the Bulldog, Pug and Pekingese. Even minor rotation or poor centring can then make these calcific shadows inviting as possible calcified disc material. In the cervical region VD oblique views will provide an *en face* view of the foramen on each side. This can reveal small amounts of calcified herniated disc material that might be overlooked even using myelography. This is most likely to be the case in chondrodystrophic breeds and should be considered as a possible routine part of the examination.

***Vertebral body:*** Changes associated with infection (discospondylitis and spondylitis) are addressed in Chapter 16. Well organized benign, chronic proliferative change ventral and abaxial to adjacent vertebral bodies is common. It is most often termed spondylosis, and is usually expected in middle and older aged individuals. It is especially prolific in Boxers sometimes being present as early as one year of age. Whilst this bony proliferation may reduce intervertebral movement, which is minimal, its clinical effects are usually of no direct clinical significance (Figure 17.8). However, it is an indicator of an intervertebral joint where dynamics may have been altered and, therefore, the disc may have been subjected to unnatural forces and have greater potential for herniation. It may also be a consequence of previous disc failure or fenestration. Likewise congenital anomalies, such as fused or block vertebrae, transitional

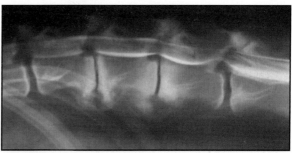

**17.8**   Lateral thoracolumbar view in a 7-year-old cross bred dog. Mature spondylosis changes are present at L1–2 and L2–3 with associated narrowed disc spaces, indicating previous disc herniation, but there is no attenuation of the myelogram. However, at L3–4 where there is no evidence of spondylosis there is a large disc herniation manifest by the dorsal displacement and attenuation of the ventral contrast medium column and attenuation of the dorsal contrast medium column at this point.

vertebrae and hemivertebrae, may direct abnormal loading in the intervertebral disc inviting failure. Radiologically all these changes should be noted as indicators of an increased potential for disc herniation.

***Articular facets:*** The facet joints are small synovial joints and are subject to the typical changes expected with osteoarthrosis (i.e. enlargement, soft tissue thickening, bony proliferation). On rare occasions such proliferative change may encroach on the dorsal parts of the vertebral canal and cause compression (Figure 17.9). Encroachment can only be assessed by myelography or tomographic imaging (MRI and high resolution CT). As the facet joints are abaxial to the canal, quite exuberant change on a lateral or VD view should not be assumed to compromise the vertebral canal.

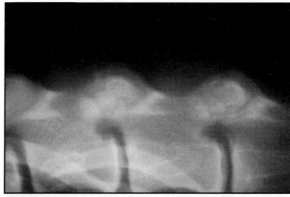

**17.9**   Close-up lateral view of T13–L1 region in an 8-year-old Labrador Retriever. Articular facet osteoarthrosis is seen at this level. This has caused loss of edge sharpness of the composite shadow of the two superimposed joints and some ventrally protruding bony material that may encroach the vertebral canal.

An assessment of the size of the facet joint space is sometimes possible and by comparing this with adjacent joints, loss of joint space can be an indicator of a shortening of the gap between vertebrae and consequent loss of disc volume.

***Vacuum phenomenon:*** The presence of linear lucent gas streaking within the disc is recognized commonly as evidence of disc degeneration in human patients. In humans vacuum phenomena are considered a reliable indicator of disc degeneration but are very rare in the presence of disc infection or neoplasia. The phenomenon is occasionally seen in dogs, where it is assumed (by extrapolation from human radiology) that it is an indicator of disc herniation. It is most often seen in veterinary radiography in stressed views, e.g. cervical traction views and extended lumbosacral views. The phenomenon may be overlooked on conventional radiographs but is more readily recognized on high-definition CT images. The source of the gas is widely debated (Figure 17.10).

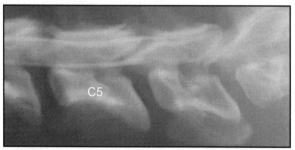

**17.10** Lateral cervical view after a myelogram followed by traction in an 11-year-old Springer Spaniel. The vacuum phenomenon can be seen as a linear gas shadow parallel to the caudal end plate of C5. In this case the affected disc was C6–7 where the compression has been ameliorated by traction and the vacuum phenomenon is probably merely a consequence of that traction.

## Myelographic findings

***Thecal sac:*** The contents of the neural canal can be extrapolated from the myelographic findings. Extradural compression from a herniated disc or cord swelling, resulting from cord insult, should be identifiable. On rare occasions it is established that ascending myelomalacia is underway following disc herniation as evidenced by seepage of contrast medium from the thecal sac into the parenchyma of the spinal cord.

Occasionally acute disc lesions may be accompanied by severe haemorrhage. This may produce a mixture of disc debris and organizing blood products that cause a circumferential compression over a wide area. Because of the physical nature of this material, especially the blood clots, an irregular filling defect may be created (Figure 17.11).

It is convenient, from a radiological point of view, to consider the meningeal structures as a composite thecal sac. It is within this sac that myelographic contrast

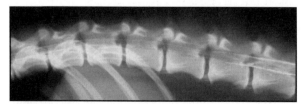

**17.11** Lateral thoracolumbar view after a myelogram of a 2-year-old cross bred dog. Note the circumferential attenuation of the myelogram from T11 to L4.

medium is delivered and dispersed. However, there are both anatomical and pathological limitations. Anatomically, the thecal sac is of varying length in different individuals. As many as 15% of thecal sacs may terminate cranial to the lumbosacral joint. This renders anatomy caudal to that point a 'blind spot' for myelography. Cord swelling may obstruct the flow of contrast medium, making accurate identification of the site and nature of any compression difficult. This phenomenon is particularly pertinent when contrast medium is distributed by gravity following a cisterna magna injection. Lumbar puncture administration does allow contrast medium to be 'forced' past an area of cord swelling but if this occupies several vertebral body lengths the actual causative lesion may not be identified.

The importance of identifying the side of a compressive lesion, especially when hemilaminectomy or pediculectomy is anticipated, cannot be overstated. A number of factors may thwart this objective. To minimize the likelihood of failure a number of precautions can be taken. If contrast medium is delivered under fluoroscopic control, the flow of contrast medium past a lesion can be monitored directly. The radiation safety and equipment constraints of this approach usually render it impractical. It has been found that exposure of the VD/DV view, immediately following the injection of contrast medium by lumbar puncture, is most likely to give best thecal filling and consequent identification of a compressive lesion. It behoves the operator to have all imaging facilities ready before injection as the time between injection and exposure can then be an absolute minimum.

Oblique views may also enhance the possibility of identifying the point of compression, particularly if extruded disc material is only located ventrolaterally or dorsolaterally, which may occasionally happen. It could be argued, therefore, that a standard protocol immediately following lumbar injection should be VD/DV, both oblique views and finally a lateral view in quick succession. The choice of DV rather than VD may be preferred by those who administer the lumbar puncture injection, with the dog in sternal rather than lateral recumbency. The slight magnification caused by the DV positioning is of no consequence but the time saved in re-positioning the dog in VD recumbency may make a difference to the identification of the compressive lesion (Figure 17.12).

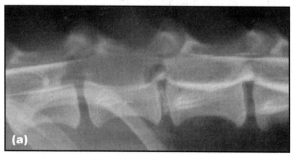

**17.12** Cranial lumbar views after a myelogram in a 4-year-old Cocker Spaniel. **(a)** On the lateral view there is comprehensive loss of thecal contrast medium from cranial L1 to mid L2, confirming the presence of either a compressive lesion or cord swelling at this level. *(continues)* ▶

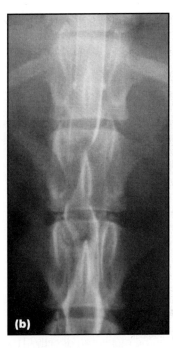

**17.12**
(continued) Cranial lumbar views after a myelogram in a 4-year-old Cocker Spaniel. **(b)** The VD view shows a large extradural compression on the left, mostly within the vertebral canal of L1. The granular calcification within the narrowed L1–2 disc space confirmed the degenerate status of the disc. This case demonstrates cranial migration of herniated disc material.

## Cord swelling

Any insult to the spinal cord, especially if acute and violent, may result in cord swelling. This will have greatest effect in the more tightly packed parts of the vertebral canal, e.g. the thoracolumbar junction. This is possibly the most common site to be investigated clinically. Cord swelling is likely to be circumferential, symmetrical and extend equally either side of the insult. By extrapolation, the point of injury can be assumed to be the midpoint of the swelling as revealed by myelography. This tenet is reasonable but not wholly reliable. It also will not offer information as to the side of any compression. Relatively mild swelling will obstruct the gravitational flow of contrast medium from a cisternal puncture. It is, therefore, necessary to carry out a lumbar puncture through which sufficient pressure can be exerted to force injected contrast medium past a swollen cord. The contrast medium that surrounds the swollen part of the cord rapidly dissipates and so exposures should be made during, or immediately following, injection to maximize the possibility of identifying the compressive lesion. For this reason the VD/DV view should be exposed first.

## Ascending myelomalacia

Incidences rising to 5% have been suggested for the irreversible ischaemic damage to the cord that can result from acute injury. If intrathecal contrast medium is introduced when the thecal–medullary barrier has been broken there will be seepage and mixing of the contrast medium with the parenchyma of the cord. This obviously carries a hopeless prognosis. The failure of the thecal barrier will not occur immediately, and so very early investigation following the acute injury may not detect the developing myelomalacia.

## Cervical disc disease

As with all parts of the spine, careful positioning for radiography is essential in order to evaluate the cervical disc spaces (see Chapter 15). Rotation and 'dipping' (spine not parallel to the table top) are the most common errors. Centring and obliquity also play a major role in the accurate assessment of the intervertebral foramina. Both effects may obscure or enhance the image.

### Small breeds of dog

Degenerative disc disease affecting the cervical discs is recognized in the same group of chondrodystrophic breeds that are affected by thoracolumbar disc herniation. There are some notable breed predilections. The Beagle is a breed where cervical disc problems may be more common than thoracolumbar herniations. Conversely, the Dachshund is more commonly affected by thoracolumbar herniation. Cocker Spaniels are also frequently affected. The Whippet is also affected but this may reflect its relationship to the Greyhound and Lurcher rather than its chondrodystrophic conformation. In the chondrodystrophic breeds there may be multiple disc degenerations though the presenting signs may be attributable to one only. It is therefore important to use myelography, CT or MRI to determine with certainty which disc is affected. The two commonly used surgical procedures are fenestration and ventral slot decompression. Quantification of the size of the lesion from those special studies will assist procedure selection.

The radiological signs (described above) for recognizing degenerative disc disease in chondrodystrophic breeds pertain to both cervical and thoracolumbar disc herniations. In the small breeds C2–3 and more cranially disposed intervertebral disc herniations predominate (Figure 17.13).

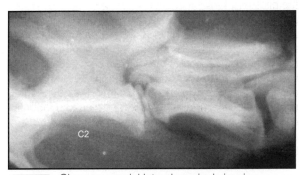

**17.13** Close-up cranial lateral cervical view in a 4-year-old Dachshund. The C2–3 disc is calcified and has fragmented, allowing some calcific material to herniate into the vertebral canal. The disc space is clearly narrower than C3–4.

### Large breeds of dog

Cervical disc protrusions (not including those that fall within the 'Wobbler' category, discussed below) in large dogs affect a variety of breeds sporadically. The Dalmatian, Greyhound and Lurcher may be overrepresented. In the larger breeds more caudally disposed discs, especially C5–6 and C6–7, are involved and this may make separation from 'Wobbler' dogs somewhat arbitrary. Because these breeds are not affected by disseminated degenerative disc change, calcification may not be a feature, and myelography, CT or MRI may be the only means of demonstrating a lesion (Figure 17.14).

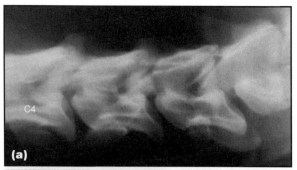

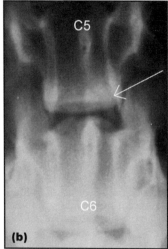

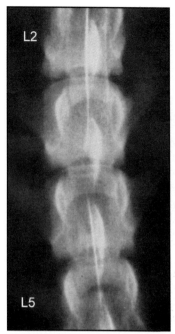

**17.14** Close-up caudal cervical views in a 10-year-old Dalmatian. **(a)** A large calcified shadow is visible just craniodorsal to the C5–6 disc space. This space is narrower than C6–7 but positioning does not allow an accurate size assessment. **(b)** The large herniation of calcified disc material is faintly seen to the left of the midline at C5–6, superimposing on the caudal aspect of C5 (arrowed).

**17.15** Close-up VD view after a myelogram in a 6-year-old Dachshund. Most of the contrast medium is in the central canal and has resulted in a non-diagnostic myelogram. Fortuitously the VD view of the central canalogram has isolated the level and side of the compression: left side, L3–4.

## Thoracolumbar disc disease

Thoracolumbar disc disease probably represents the most frequent spinal disease requiring the attention of the clinician. Most animals present as potential emergencies so, despite the increasing availability of CT and MRI, myelography is likely to remain the investigation of choice in the foreseeable future. Myelography has proved successful in confirming the location of a thoracolumbar disc herniation, although it is not always accurate in determining lateralization. The meticulous use of oblique views will increase accuracy significantly. Technique protocols to maximize identification of the location of herniated disc material have already been discussed.

The cord swelling expected in most of these cases will compromise the efficacy of myelography via the cisterna magna route, and so the operator needs to be familiar with the more challenging technique of lumbar puncture. Even in experienced hands complete failure is possible. More often annoying artefacts, including epidural injection that obscures the thecal contrast and central canal injection may thwart the procedure (Figure 17.15). However, it is rare that the particular disc involved is missed. If the clinician or radiologist misinterprets the side of the compression, the surgeon can always perform a bilateral hemilaminectomy. A compromise must be drawn between persistent efforts to 'get the perfect picture' by repeated lumbar injections and exploratory surgery at the correct level to decompress on one or, if necessary, both sides.

## Intravertebral disc herniation

For information on intravertebral disc herniation (Schmorl's node), see Chapter 18.

## 'Wobbler syndrome'

'Wobbler syndrome' is an enigmatic condition that poses many questions, not least of which is the nomenclature that surrounds it. Certainly to the layman 'Wobbler' seems universally accepted though the not uncommon variation 'Wobbler's syndrome' suggests some eponymous connection!

There are a number of synonyms for 'Wobbler syndrome':

- Cervical vertebral malformation malarticulation syndrome
- Cervical spondylopathy
- Cervical spondylolisthesis/subluxation
- Cervical stenosis
- Cervical vertebral instability
- Caudal cervical malformation
- Caudal cervical spondylomyelopathy
- Cervical stenotic myelopathy (more often used in equine neurology)
- Disc-associated 'Wobbler syndrome' (DAWS).

For the purposes of this Chapter the condition is referred to as caudal cervical malformation (CCM). The condition most often presents as a pelvic limb ataxia, with or without neck pain, progressing to include thoracic limb neurological deficits and ultimately quadriplegia (see *BSAVA Manual of Canine and Feline Neurology*). Large and giant-breeds predominate and the Dobermann is over represented. The Dobermann and Great Dane together account for about 80% of cases. Other large breeds (e.g. Rottweiler) may be similarly affected and the classic age of presentation is 4 to 10 years. Other manifestations that have been termed 'Wobbler syndrome' include juvenile Basset Hounds with a congenital bony deformity of the vertebral canal and juvenile giant-breeds (e.g. Great Dane, Irish Wolfhound, Borzoi) with cranial cervical malformation. Some reports suggest a male predominance but this is questionable.

253

The radiological features encountered in these different clinical manifestations should be considered when assessing plain and contrast radiographs from suspected cases.

- Vertebral changes:
  - Vertebral canal stenosis (sagittal narrowing, funnelling, dyssymmetry or medially deviating pedicles)
  - Vertebral body deformity often promoting disc failure
  - Facet joint enlargement and encroachment
- Soft tissue changes:
  - Ligamentous hypertrophy
  - Disc degeneration and protrusion, thickening and hypertrophy of the disc annulus
  - Synovial cysts
- Dynamic changes
  - 'Tilting' or 'tipping' of adjacent vertebrae relative to each other
  - Disc space collapse
  - Effect of traction
- Postoperative changes.

## Vertebral changes

### Vertebral canal stenosis

The bony canal of a patient with vertebral canal stenosis may be congenitally narrow in a number of ways. Viewing the vertebral canal within each vertebra gives an impression of a funnel-shaped structure that is dorsoventrally narrower cranially than caudally (sagittal diameter). This narrowing or funnelling is accentuated in those breeds with elongated vertebrae, for example the Great Dane and Basset Hound, where, if excessive, it causes cord compression. Lateral narrowing of the transverse diameter due to medially deviating pedicles, particularly caudally (either symmetrically or asymmetrically) has also been described in the Basset Hound, Great Dane and the Boerboel. On some VD views medial deviation of the pedicles can be suspected, and if canal compromise is confirmed myelographically the diagnosis is reliable. Until transverse tomographic imaging (CT or MRI) was available, confirmation of more exotic vertebral canal deformities, as reported in Basset Hounds, was a post-mortem exercise. As these are conformational defects they are likely to provoke signs in adolescent or young adult dogs (Figure 17.16).

### Vertebral body deformity

In the Dobermann, in particular, the centra of the caudal cervical vertebrae may lose their normal 'building brick' shape with the cranioventral margin obliquely incomplete (Figure 17.17). This deformity may be of variable severity and probably has two effects.

- It will diminish the caudal support of the intervertebral disc, inviting premature degeneration and failure.
- It may be linked with the apparent 'tilting', often seen in this breed that may be exaggerated on stressed flexed lateral views.

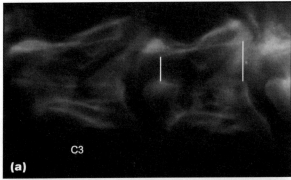

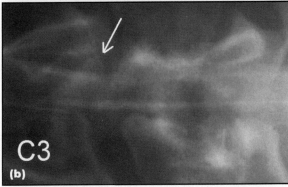

**17.16** Close-up caudal cervical views in a 2-year-old Great Dane. **(a)** The plain film shows funnel-shaped vertebral canals within the caudal cervical vertebrae with the cranial diameter being less than the caudal. **(b)** A myelogram confirmed the dorsoventral compromise of the vertebral canal at C3–4.

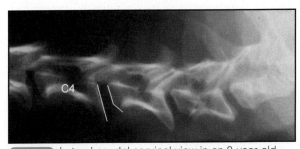

**17.17** Lateral caudal cervical view in an 8-year-old Dobermann. The white lines show the discrepancy between adjacent vertebral end plates, in particular the oblique cranioventral margin of the cranial vertebral end plate of C5.

This dynamic component compounds any degenerative process in the intervertebral disc. The likely sequence of events is: vertebral body deformity, increased movement at the intervertebral joint and ultimately premature degeneration of the intervertebral disc. There may be associated spondylosis.

### Articular facet enlargement

The facet joints are synovial joints and may respond to damage similarly to other more major synovial joints. The joint may distend and the capsule thicken. Periarticular osteophytes may develop and these can often be detected on plain radiographs. Any or all of these components may encroach the vertebral canal, causing DV or lateral cord compression (Figure 17.18).

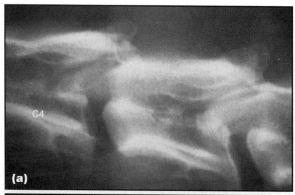

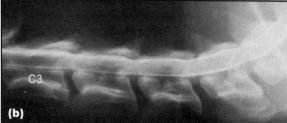

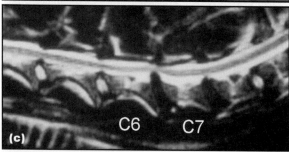

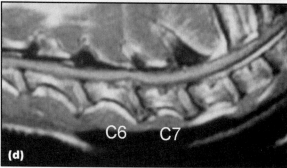

**17.18** Caudal cervical region in a 9-year-old Dalmatian. **(a)** Plain film shows facet joint enlargement, which may be associated with visible bony change but may be more of a soft tissue thickening. No new bone can be seen at the facet joints on this plain film. **(b)** The myelogram shows the dorsal encroachments of the vertebral canal by synovial hypertrophy of the facet joints and the ligamentum flavum. Oblique views may separate these differentials. **(c)** T2-weighted MRI shows disc herniation at C6–7. The disc is dehydrated and clearly degenerate. Dorsal encroachments are also noted at C4–5 and C5–6 and C7–T1. **(d)** T1-weighted image shows more clearly the mushroom-shaped disc herniation that consists of longitudinal ligament and annulus and some degenerate nuclear material.

## Soft tissue changes

In order to see soft tissue changes myelography, CT or MRI will be required, as even severely affected dogs may have quite normal plain film radiographs. The dorsally located ligamentum flavum or the ventrally located dorsal longitudinal ligament may thicken. This hypertrophy is presumably the result of a fibrotic response to chronic damage or loading. The resulting dorsal or ventral compression may contribute to the clinical signs exhibited by the affected dog. Nuclear material may partially escape but is usually constrained by the outer fibres of the annulus. Escape of nuclear material into the vertebral canal is unlikely.

The change that is probably of greatest consequence is the encroachment of the vertebral canal by disc elements. This is most likely to be a thickening or hypertrophy of the fibrous disc annulus with dorsal displacement but not extrusion of the disc nucleus. This is the likely active lesion in the Dobermann and, in view of the possible dynamic components of the disease in this breed, might be seen as a natural response to instability.

Extradural synovial cysts, arising from the facet joints, have been described in a small number of young giant-breed dogs including the Great Dane. These dogs are usually affected by multiple cysts. This is in contrast to the solitary cysts recognized in the thoracolumbar region of middle-aged large-breed dogs. It is questionable whether this should fall within the definition of CCM; it is clearly, though, a valid differential. The clinical signs arising from cervical spinal cord compression will mimic those seen in typical 'Wobblers' and the breeds or types involved overlap those that are recognized as being susceptible to other forms of CCM. The cysts can cause dorsolateral cord compression, which may be seen on oblique myelographic views but their precise imaging characteristics have only come to light since the availability of MRI. On MRI the compressive lesions can be clearly seen to contain fluid and are not confluent with the thecal sac as they are extradural structures.

## Dynamic changes

The 'tilting' or 'tipping' of vertebrae may be a hypothetical concept, only reproduced by particular stressed radiographic views, and may not be a realistic situation in the living standing animal. However, the correlation of this feature with ligamentous and annulus hypertrophy does support strongly the hypothesis that instability may be an aetiological factor. It should be mentioned that the modern Dobermann has a neck and forelimb conformation that concentrates forces in the caudal cervical spine. The development of ventral spondylotic change is further evidence to support some degree of instability. The spondylosis is presumed to be a natural ankylosing response to the vertebral instability. Once the disc has failed the intervertebral joint is less well supported and disc space narrowing is inevitable. Whether this fairly subtle change in alignment alters the dynamics of the cervical spine is questionable.

Traction views (see Chapter 15) that attempt to demonstrate whether distraction of adjacent vertebrae will 'improve' the compression over the affected disc space also support the assumption that there are dynamic components to the disease. In most cases the dorsal ligament and annulus encroachment is 'stretched out', alleviating the compression. This view is invaluable in the decision making process for the surgeon (Figure 17.19). Surgical techniques employed centre

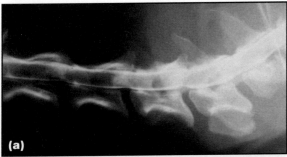

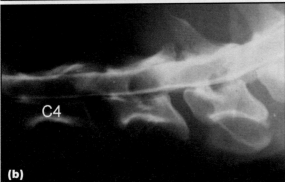

**17.19** Cervical myelogram in an 8-year-old Labrador Retriever. **(a)** The neutral view shows a small ventral compression at C5–6. The affected disc space is narrow. **(b)** After traction the compression was relieved and the disc space re-expanded, suggesting that surgical distraction techniques may be helpful.

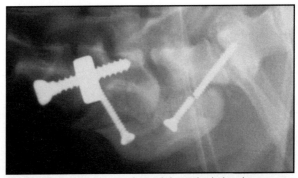

**17.20** Close-up lateral caudal cervical view in a 6-year-old Labrador Retriever shows failure of a screw and fissuring of the bone cement used to stabilize the cervical spine.

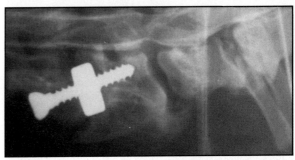

**17.21** Close-up lateral view of caudal cervical region after a myelogram in an 8-year-old Dobermann that previously had been treated by distraction-fusion at C5–6 using a screw and washer. Subsequently, C6–7 has failed causing a further compression; this is the so-called 'Domino effect'.

on dorsal or ventral decompression (laminectomy and ventral slot, respectively) or distraction fusion. Historically fusion techniques without distraction, even compressing the adjacent vertebrae, were employed with moderate success. This concept suggested that static compression was better tolerated than dynamic compression. The fact that some success was achieved, again supports the premise that instability might well be a component of the problem.

It should be noted that many 'Wobblers' deteriorate following myelography. This is usually a temporary effect with the dog returning to the *status quo* within 3–4 days. It is very unlikely that this is a chemical effect of the contrast agent. It is more likely that with the neck relaxed under anaesthesia, and particularly if stressed views are carried out, the dynamic effects of any compression are exaggerated causing temporary cord contusion.

## Postoperative changes

In those procedures that employ metallic implants or cement the usual complications can be expected (e.g. incorrect placement, implant loosening, implant fracture, implant-associated infection and collapse of adjacent vertebral bodies around a metallic implant (washer)) (Figure 17.20). In those procedures that endeavour to stabilize the vertebral segments biomechanical forces within the neck may be transferred to adjacent segments. It is not unusual for the disc space immediately cranial or caudal to the stabilized joint to fail some time later. This may sequentially involve more than one disc and has become known as the 'Domino effect' (Figure 17.21).

## References and further reading

Duval J, Dewey C, Roberts R and Aron D (1996) Spinal cord swelling as a myelographic indicator of prognosis: a retrospective study in dogs with intervertebral disc disease and loss of deep pain perception. *Veterinary Surgery* **25**, 6–12

Fourie SL and Kirberger RM (1998) Relationship of cervical spinal cord diameter to vertebral dimensions: a radiographic study of normal dogs. *Veterinary Radiology and Ultrasound* **39**, 137–143

Jeffery ND and McKee WM (2001) Surgery for disc-associated wobbler syndrome in the dog – an examination of the controversy. *Journal of Small Animal Practice* **42**, 574–581

Kirberger RM, Roos CJ and Lubbe AM (1992) The radiological diagnosis of thoracolumbar disc disease in the dachshund. *Veterinary Radiology and Ultrasound* **33**, 255–261

Kirberger RM and Wrigley RH (1992) Myelography in the dog: review of patients with contrast in the central canal. *Veterinary Radiology and Ultrasound* **34**, 253–258

Lamb CR, Nicholls A, Targett M and Mannion P (2002) Accuracy of survey radiographic diagnosis of intervertebral disc protrusion in dogs. *Veterinary Radiology and Ultrasound* **43**, 222–228

Lu D, Lamb CR and Targett MP (2002) Results of myelography in seven dogs with myelomalacia. *Veterinary Radiology and Ultrasound* **43**, 326–330

McKee WM (2000) Intervertebral disc disease in the dog 1. Pathophysiology and diagnosis. *In Practice* **22**, 355–369

Olby NJ, Dyce J and Houlton JEF (1994) Correlation of plain radiographic and lumbar myelographic findings with surgical findings in thoracolumbar disc disease. *Journal of Small Animal Practice* **35**, 345–350

Schulz KS, Walker M, Moon M, Waldron D, Slater M and McDonald DE (1998) Correlation of clinical, radiographic and surgical localization of intervertebral disc extrusion in small-breed dogs: a prospective study of 50 cases. *Veterinary Surgery* **27**, 105–111

Tomlinson J (2001) *Perspective on cervical vertebral malformation/malarticulation (Wobblers disease)* WSAVA Proceedings

Vite CH and Braund KG (2003) Neuroanatomical localization and syndromes – thoracolumbar syndrome; cervicothoracic syndrome; cervical syndrome. In: *Braund's Clinical Neurology in Small Animals: localization, diagnosis and treatment.* International Veterinary Information Service, Ithaca, New York

# Spine – lumbosacral region and cauda equina syndrome

## Johann Lang

## Indications

Cauda equina compression in small animals is a well known clinical entity. Large-breed dogs are more often affected than small-breed dogs or cats. In fact, degenerative lumbosacral stenosis (DLSS) is the single most important cause of cauda equina syndrome in middle-aged non-chondrodystrophic, large-breed dogs (Figure 18.1). In degenerative disease the clinical signs result from neural compression of the cauda equina in the vertebral canal or the nerve roots in the neural foramina, and are caused by a combination of lumbosacral disc degeneration associated with disc herniation and hypertrophic degenerative changes of the articular facets, ligaments and vertebrae.

The clinical sign most often associated with cauda equina compression is back pain, which is most obvious during climbing stairs or jumping (i.e. during hyperextension of the back). The tail may be weak, and in advanced

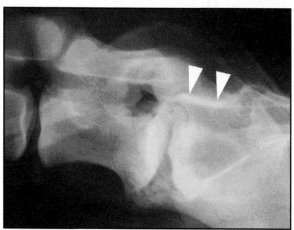

**18.1** Lateral lumbosacral view of a 5-year-old German Shepherd Dog with degenerative lumbosacral stenosis. The sacrum is displaced ventrally with its floor thickened by deposition of new bone. There is a thickened and elongated 'roof' (arrowheads). The lumbosacral disc space is narrowed and irregular, the dorsal part of the sacral end plate is angled caudally and has a large rounded osteophyte protruding into the intervertebral foramen. The end plates and adjacent vertebral bodies appear sclerotic with spondylotic changes ventrally and dorsally. The vertebral canal and lumbosacral intervertebral foramen are obscured by mineralized granular material, the vertebral canal at this level appears narrowed. At L6–7, mineralization within the intervertebral foramen and ventral part of the vertebral canal is also present.

cases the cauda equina compression will lead to paresis of the pelvic limbs and finally to faecal and urinary incontinence. Upon neurological examination, resentment of palpation or hyperextension of the pelvic limbs is present in over 90% of the cases. Occasionally, most often in small-breed dogs (and in cats), paraesthesia or hyperaesthesia of the tail, the digits or the skin innervated by the affected sensory nerves may lead to licking or severe chewing of the hindquarters. Gait abnormalities associated with cauda equina compression may vary from mild unilateral lameness to severe bilateral paresis with muscle atrophy. Paresis is characterized by lower motor neuron signs with decreased cranial tibial muscle reflexes. The bulbo- or vulvo-urethral reflexes may also be decreased in severe cases. In many instances, the patellar reflex remains normal or may even be exaggerated because of weak antagonist function. Rarely, infarction of the sacral spinal cord may evoke similar neurological signs; however, pain is usually not present in these cases.

Animals of both sexes at any age may be affected by cauda equina compression. Cauda equina compression has been reported in 1-year old dogs with congenital vertebral canal stenosis and dogs with large osteochondrotic fragments of S1. However, at the time of clinical onset the typical signalment of cauda equina compression is a male large-breed working dog (there is breed predisposition towards German Shepherd Dogs), between six and seven years of age and suffers from DLSS. Dogs with sacral osteochondrosis, a condition always associated with disc degeneration, are on average two years younger (mean age 4.8 years). There are breed predispositions for osteochondrosis, for congenital conditions (such as transitional lumbosacral vertebrae, agenesis of caudal and sacral vertebrae or spina bifida) and for degenerative conditions (such as the type of disc degeneration and herniation or DLSS).

## Radiography and normal anatomy

### Standard views

Standard radiographic views, including lateral and ventrodorsal (VD) views and the normal anatomy of the lumbosacral junction have been described previously (see Chapter 15). Due to the complex anatomy of the lumbosacral region true lateral views with superimposed wings of the ilia are essential to avoid interpretation problems.

## Special views

### Stressed lateral views

In addition to the standard views, lateral views in hyperflexion and hyperextension may be helpful in assessing the lumbosacral angle and alignment of vertebrae (Figure 18.2). Ventral displacement of the sacrum may occur in neutral, hyperextended and hyperflexed positions, and has been described as static or dynamic malalignment or lumbosacral instability. In the human spine it has been shown that early disc degeneration often leads to segmental instability, whereas with severely degenerated discs motion will be reduced. Although described as a specific entity, it remains possible that the lumbosacral malalignment/instability in the dog also reflects lumbosacral disc degeneration rather than a primary condition. Lumbosacral malalignment/instability has been described in clinically affected and normal dogs, and the benefit of dynamic studies without contrast procedures (myelography or epidurography) remains questionable.

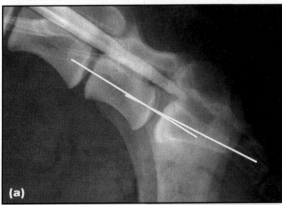

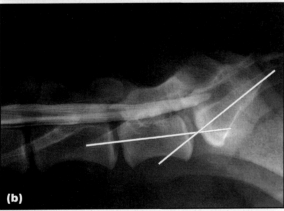

**18.2** Lateral stress views of a normal dog after a cervical myelogram. The lumbosacral angle and vertebral mobility (white lines) are normal. The dural sac does not change position, shape or diameter during flexion and extension. **(a)** Flexion view. **(b)** Extension view.

### Oblique lumbosacral views

Oblique views, such as the ventral 30° left-dorsal right (V30°Le-DRt) and ventral 30° right-dorsal left (V30°Rt-DLe), can help demonstrate abnormalities of the articular facets.

## Lumbosacral angle

The lumbosacral angle is defined as the angle between two lines bisecting L7 and S1 vertebral bodies longitudinally, or the lines marking the floor of the vertebral canal. In the dog the sacrum is slightly angled dorsally at the lumbosacral level, and accordingly the lumbosacral disc space appears wedge-shaped. The mobility of a vertebral motion segment (two vertebrae including the articular facets and the discovertebral junction) has been defined as the angle between maximal flexion and extension (see Figure 18.2).

Mobility increases within the lumbar spine from cranial to caudal with the highest values at the lumbosacral level (L6–7 = 12 ± 3 degrees; L7–sacrum = 37 ± 6 degrees). There is little known about how breed and size of a dog correlate with mobility of the lumbosacral junction. However, the German Shepherd Dog (the breed with the highest prevalence of DLSS) has a range of motion that is lower than the range of motion of other large-breed dogs. Gender also has an influence on mobility with bitches having a higher mobility than dogs, but interestingly, dogs have a two times higher incidence of DLSS than bitches. Excessive motion obviously is not the cause of DLSS. Dogs affected by DLSS were found to have reduced flexion in the lumbosacral junction in one study, while in a second study increased flexion was found. In both studies reduced mobility in the lumbosacral junction was found to be a common feature of DLSS. This reduced motion is an effect of the thinning of the disc due to degeneration and hypertrophic changes of the ligaments.

## Contrast studies

### Myelography

Before computed tomography (CT) and magnetic resonance imaging (MRI) became more readily available in veterinary medicine there were many discussions about the contrast procedure of choice for assessing the cauda equina. Together with others, the author favours cisternal myelography (see also Chapter 15), despite the fact that the dural sac in large-breed dogs often ends at, or cranial to, the lumbosacral junction. In animals with cauda equina syndrome and spinal cord compression at a more cranial level, the more caudal lesion will dominate the clinical presentation. Animals with upper and lower motor neuron lesions, therefore, will present with lower motor neuron disease and the spinal cord lesion may be clinically missed (Figure 18.3). Cisternal myelography is superior to a lumbar injection for two reasons: injecting contrast media at the L5–6 level may be associated with leaking of contrast material into the epidural space, thus making interpretation difficult; and a lesion affecting the cauda equina may not be limited to the L7–S1 disc space and injection of contrast media at the site of a potential lesion should be avoided (Figure 18.4).

In DLSS the compression often has a dynamic component, which will be exaggerated when the lumbosacral junction is hyperextended. Myelograms, therefore, should be performed dynamically. After injecting a suitable contrast medium at 0.3 ml/kg, the table must

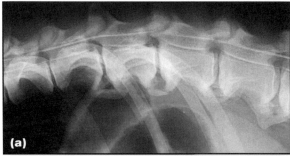

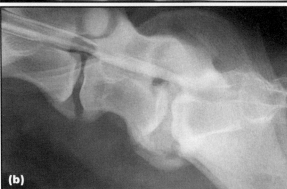

**18.3**   Cervical myelogram in a 9-year-old German Shepherd Dog presenting with clinical signs of cauda equina compression; there is spondylosis from T12 to L3. **(a)** Thoracolumbar region. There is moderate ventral extradural compression at the T13–L1 disc space with similar but milder pathology at the disc spaces cranial and caudal to this level. The thoracolumbar lesion was not apparent clinically. **(b)** Lumbosacral region. There are degenerative changes at the L6–7 and the L7–S1 disc spaces, including spondylosis with mild ventral compression at both sites.

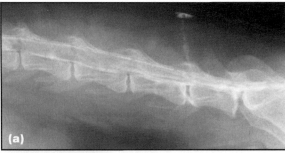

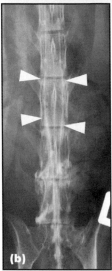

**18.4**   Lumbar myelogram of L6–7 in a cat with intramedullary lymphoma at the lumbosacral intumescence. There is some extradural contrast medium spillage and multiple small radiolucent filling defects caused by iatrogenic air.
**(a)** Lateral view. **(b)** VD view. The thickened intumescence is outlined with white arrowheads.

be tilted (or the head and thorax elevated) and the lumbar spine kept in flexion to promote the flow of contrast medium into the dural end-sac. Flexed radiographs are taken followed by a second hyperextended lumbosacral view. The procedure should be done in lateral and dorsal recumbency (Figure 18.5). Care has to be taken while performing this procedure since the dural end-sac will be compressed and the contrast medium forced in a cranial direction if the pelvic limbs are excessively extended (Figure 18.6).

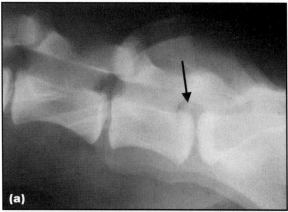

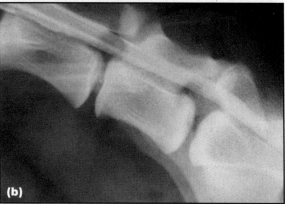

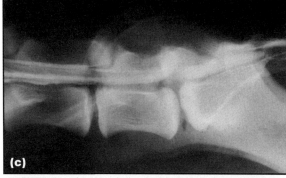

**18.5**   Lumbosacral disc herniation and dynamic lumbosacral stenosis in a 7-year-old Bernese Mountain Dog with right pelvic limb paresis. **(a)** Lateral plain film radiograph showing a narrowed intervertebral disc space, thickened and sclerotic end plates, faintly visible vacuum phenomenon and mineralization overlying the intervertebral foramen (arrowed). **(b)** Lateral flexed view after cervical myelogram. Note the wide dural sac extending far into the sacrum. There is slight dorsal deviation but no compression is visible. **(c)** Lateral extended view shows pronounced ventral compression and accentuation of the vacuum phenomenon, which has been displaced ventrally. (continues) ▶

259

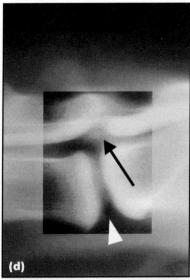

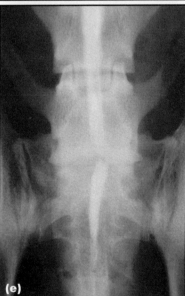

**18.5** (continued) Lumbosacral disc herniation and dynamic lumbosacral stenosis in a 7-year-old Bernese Mountain Dog with right pelvic limb paresis. **(d)** Linear tomogram in extension of the same region. The highlighted area again shows the vacuum phenomenon (arrowhead) and the mineral opacity just ventral to the contrast medium line (arrowed). **(e)** VD view reveals the attenuation and deviation of the dural sac to the left side (the left side of the dog is on the right side of the figure).

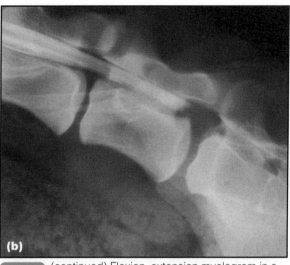

**18.6** (continued) Flexion–extension myelogram in a dog with suspected lumbosacral compression with a false-positive result. **(b)** Lateral flexed view, which is normal.

## Epidurography

In patients with a short or small dural sac a myelogram is unrewarding and other contrast procedures, such as a discogram or epidurogram, may be performed. Epidurography is a technically easy procedure with low morbidity. After placing a spinal needle (23–24 gauge; 4–5 cm long) through an interarcuate space into the vertebral canal, anywhere between the sacrum and Cd3, the contrast medium is injected at a similar dose as for myelography. Flexed and extended radiographs are immediately taken and the continuity and location of the lines of contrast medium are evaluated. Dorsal displacement, filling defects and obstruction to cranial flow are consistent with cauda equina compression (Figure 18.7). However, the diagnosis mainly relies on the lateral view and may be affected by artefacts causing misinterpretation (Figure 18.8).

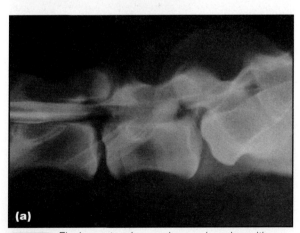

**18.6** Flexion–extension myelogram in a dog with suspected lumbosacral compression with a false-positive result. **(a)** Lateral extended view. Forced extension of the pelvic limbs increased the pressure in the vertebral canal, leading to venous congestion and resulting in diffuse compression of the dural sac. True dynamic compressions are usually seen as a focal lesion at the intervertebral disc space. (continues) ▶

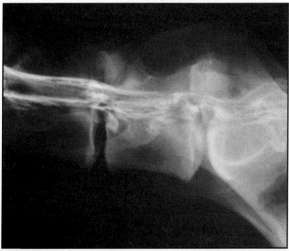

**18.7** Lateral epidurogram in a dog with lumbosacral disc herniation. The hernia is seen as a filling defect in the ventral part of the vertebral canal over the intervertebral disc space. Note the extradural contrast medium with leakage beyond the vertebral canal.

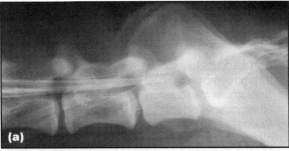

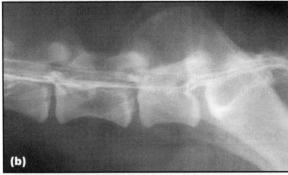

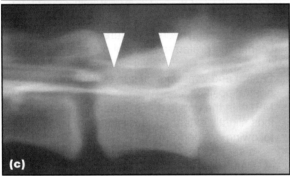

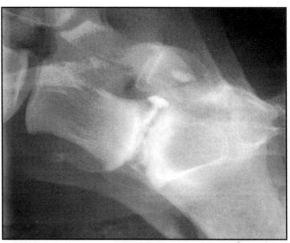

18.9 Lateral view after a discogram, in a dog with lumbosacral disc herniation. The entire area of the disc is opacified by contrast medium and there is leakage into the ventral part of the vertebral canal. The mushroom-like shaped contrast medium has a well delineated dorsal border. This indicates that the annulus fibrosus has probably ruptured with an intact dorsal longitudinal ligament, signifying a 'contained' disc herniation.

18.8 Non-diagnostic contrast studies in a dog with a short dural sac. **(a)** Cervical myelogram; the thin dural sac is positioned in the dorsal part of the vertebral canal and ends at the lumbosacral junction. This study was considered non-diagnostic. **(b)** The same dog after an epidurogram from a caudal intervertebral disc space has been performed. There is a filling defect dorsally in the L7 area. **(c)** Linear tomogram also revealing a large filling defect (arrowheads) in the L7 area. At surgery, this was found to be a large fat pad, which did not compress the cauda equina.

## Discography

Discography and epidurography may be performed as a combined procedure and provide an excellent method of assessing the lumbosacral disc. A 24 gauge spinal needle is placed through the interarcuate ligament, the vertebral canal and the annulus fibrosus (resistance will be met) into the nucleus pulposus. It is necessary to control the placement of the needle tip radiographically or fluoroscopically before injecting the contrast medium. After injecting a small dose the needle is withdrawn into the vertebral canal and an epidurogram can be performed. In a normal disc a resistance to the injection will be present after injecting 0.1 ml of contrast medium. Injection of more than 0.2–0.3 ml of contrast medium is considered a sign of disc degeneration. In cases with a ruptured disc, contrast medium may leak back into the vertebral canal (Figure 18.9).

## Sinus venography

Lumbosacral sinus venography, as an angiographic procedure or by injection of contrast medium into a caudal vertebral body, is the third procedure for assessing the lumbosacral vertebral canal. It is not described here as the procedure is technically demanding and has never gained clinical acceptance in veterinary medicine.

## Alternative imaging techniques

### Linear tomography

Linear tomography or planigraphy is a special type of body section tomography. This type of tomography is an old X-ray technique that blurs out shadows of superimposed structures by moving the tube about a fulcrum and simultaneously moving the imaging system in the opposite direction. It is a process of controlled blurring that leaves the plane of interest at the fulcrum level less blurred than the structures above or below. For example, the vertebral canal of the lumbosacral junction, superimposed by other bony structures, may be displayed without the overlying pelvis (see Figures 18.5 and 18.8).

### Magnetic resonance imaging

MRI, and to a lesser extent CT, have been shown to be the diagnostic imaging procedures of choice for evaluating cauda equina problems (see Chapter 15). The complex anatomy and the often absent or small dural sac at the L7–S1 level limit the value of conventional radiography. In addition to this, pathologies affecting the nerve roots are often located laterally in the area of the intervertebral foramina and invariably will be missed with plain film or contrast radiography. In countries and regions where access to MRI has become easy, this diagnostic gold standard should be the first choice to assess the cauda equina (Figure 18.10).

is often underestimated (Figure 18.13). In addition, fractures of the sacrum may lead to direct trauma to, or encroachment of, the ischiatic nerve at the fracture site; this can also be caused by scar tissue (Figure 18.14). Imaging of these lesions, as for any peripheral nerves, requires MRI.

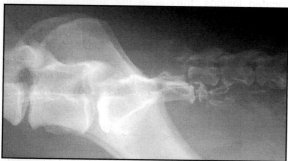

**18.13** Lateral view of a dog with a fracture of the cranial end plate and the transverse processes of Cd1, with dorsal displacement of Cd1. The vertebral canal is totally disrupted. The spinous process of S3 is fractured and the associated lamina is ventrally displaced. Note the bony fragments ventral to Cd1 and Cd2. It was discovered during surgery that there was also avulsion of the cauda equina at the L6–7 level and haemorrhage in the vertebral canal.

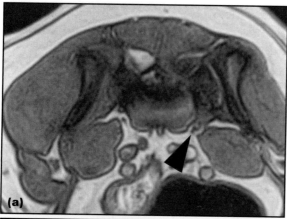

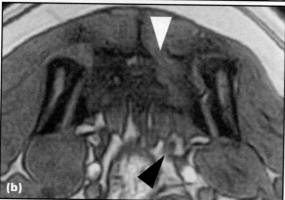

**18.14** Transverse MRI CBASS (high-resolution fluid-sensitive) sequences in an Appenzeller Hound with severe pain and non-weight bearing lameness of the left pelvic limb 10 days after a car accident. **(a)** At the level of the cranial end plate of S1 the ischiatic nerve is normal (arrowhead). **(b)** 12 mm further caudally, at the level of the iliosacral joints, the ischiatic nerve on the left side was encroached by callus formation and scar tissue, and appears thickened where it passes ventral to the fractured sacrum (black arrowhead). The sagittal fracture (white arrowhead) was not readily appreciated on survey radiographs.

## Congenital disorders

A variety of congenital anomalies involving the lumbosacral region have been described (see Figure 18.12). Malformation of skeletal structures is readily assessed with plain film radiographs. Evaluation of malformation of neural structures requires advanced imaging modalities.

### Transitional vertebrae

Lumbosacral transitional vertebrae are commonly described in many breeds. In the German Shepherd Dog transitional vertebrae at this level seem to be an inherited familial condition. A recent study (Julier-Franz *et al.*, 2002) indicated that 6% of German Shepherd Dogs have lumbosacral transitional vertebrae, excluding dogs with an isolated sacral spinous process as the sole Roentgen-sign. Other affected breeds include the Labrador Retriever, Rhodesian Ridgeback, Malinois, Brittany Spaniel and Dobermann.

If S1 is separate or incompletely fused to a short sacrum (S2 and S3), the result is lumbarization of S1. Partial or complete fusion of L7 with the sacrum or ilium is called sacralization of L7. Transitional vertebrae may also occur as fusion of Cd1 to S3. The mildest transitional form in this region is an isolated spinous process of S1. These are of no clinical significance but are important for estimation of heritability of the condition. Complete transitional vertebrae are symmetrical. Sacralization of L7 results in both transverse processes lying in contact with the ileum. Lumbarization of S1 produces a vertebra which is not part of the iliosacral joint but instead has transverse processes. An asymmetrical transitional vertebra is seen as a unilateral fusion or detachment and may lead to rotation of the pelvis with the side of fusion rotated dorsally.

Dorsal rotation of the pelvis around the long axis of the body leads to incomplete coverage of the femoral head and thus favours ipsilateral hip dysplasia (Figure 18.15). Transitional vertebrae usually do not cause stenosis of the vertebral canal and neural compression, but may predispose to DLSS as described by Morgan *et al.* (1993). They are associated with an abnormal intervertebral disc, disc degeneration and spondylosis. In addition there seems to be an association between transitional vertebrae and congenital stenosis of the vertebral canal (Figure 18.16).

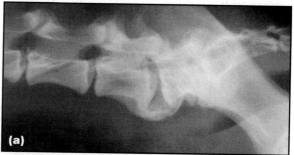

**18.15** Lumbosacral transitional vertebra in a German Shepherd Dog with sacralization of a short L7 and a normal sacrum consisting of three vertebrae. **(a)** Massive degenerative changes of the discovertebral apparatus and articular facets from L6 to the sacrum are present with a markedly decreased ventrodorsal diameter of the L7 vertebral canal. (continues) ▶

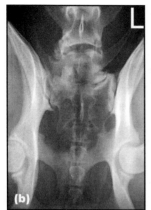

**18.15** (continued) Lumbosacral transitional vertebra in a German Shepherd Dog with sacralization of a short L7 and a normal sacrum consisting of three vertebrae. **(b)** On the VD view the pelvis is rotated to the right side and the ipsilateral hip joint appears dysplastic.

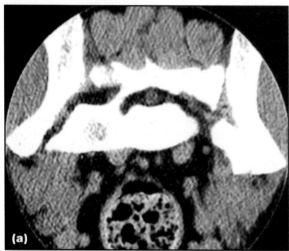

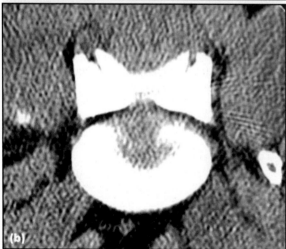

**18.16** Transverse CT images (soft tissue window) of the lumbosacral area in a dog with a transitional vertebra. **(a)** L7 is asymmetrical and the right transverse process (left side of image) articulates with the iliac wing. **(b)** The L6–7 disc protrudes dorsally and compresses fat and neural structures within the vertebral canal.

## Other vertebral abnormalities

Spina bifida, block vertebrae, hemivertebrae, agenesis of sacral and coccygeal vertebrae (see Figure 18.12) are described in Chapter 16 and are readily appreciated on plain film radiographs. Spina bifida may be seen as short or absent spinous processes on lateral radiographs and as a midline cleavage or duplication of the

spinous processes on VD views. Spina bifida may be associated with spinal dysraphism and is most often seen in brachycephalic dogs with screw-tails and in Manx cats. In these animals agenesis of part or all caudal vertebrae, and the sacrum, as well as hemivertebrae and block vertebrae are very common (Figure 18.17).

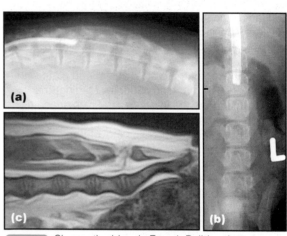

**18.17** Six-month-old male French Bulldog that was presented with paraparesis and urinary and faecal incontinence. **(a, b)** Cervical myelogram demonstrating multiple vertebral malformations, including a butterfly hemivertebra at L1, a missing spinous process of L7 and sacrococcygeal dysplasia. The dorsal contrast medium column is wider than the ventral column and ends bluntly at the level of L3, corresponding with an arachnoid cyst. The subarachnoid space caudal to the cyst is poorly filled with contrast medium. **(c)** MRI sagittal CBASS (high-resolution fluid-sensitive) sequence of the caudal lumbar spine of the same dog also demonstrates spina bifida with meningocele at L7. In this sequence, cerebrospinal fluid and epidural fat are hyperintense, resulting in a myelographic effect. A marked defect of the lamina of L7 continuous with the dorsal intervertebral foramen is seen. The end of the dural sac continues in the direction of the defect and some linear structures of low signal intensity that may represent nerve roots are leaving the vertebral canal through the defect. There is high signal intensity in the dorsal spinal cord at the level of L5 and L6, which could represent oedema.

### Spinal cord abnormalities

The radiological diagnosis of meningocele, myelomeningocele, spinal dysraphism or dermoid sinus requires myelography, CT or MRI (Figure 18.17c). Ultrasonography using a high frequency transducer placed dorsally on the lumbosacral region may also be helpful.

## Developmental disorders

### Osteochondrosis

Osteochondrosis is observed most often at the dorsal aspect of the cranial vertebral end plate of S1, and occasionally also at the dorsal aspect of the caudal vertebral end plate of L7. The aetiology is unclear but a genetic component seems possible in the German Shepherd Dog. Important regional differences exist for the prevalence of this condition. Reports from the USA are sparse, whereas the condition has been described more often in continental Europe as well as in the UK in various large breeds, and particularly in the German Shepherd Dog. Dogs are more often affected than bitches. Osteochondrosis invariably leads to disruption of the intervertebral disc, disc degeneration and carries a very high risk for the development of DLSS. Dogs suffering from osteochondrosis usually manifest clinical signs of cauda equina compression at a younger age (4.8 years) than other dogs (>6 years).

Radiological diagnosis requires precise lateral and VD flexed positioning or linear tomography. The radiological features of sacral osteochondrosis are:

- Deformation of the cranial sacral end plate with the dorsal part angled caudally, leading to a deformation of the intervertebral disc space (i.e. it becomes shaped like a butterfly)
- Apparent elongation or 'lipping' of the craniodorsal border of the sacral vertebral body, leading to a narrowed ventrodorsal diameter of the cranial vertebral foramen of the sacrum
- Sclerosis of the dorsal part of the end plate (always present and can be severe)
- A visible isolated fragment in the vertebral canal or a radiolucent line at the base of the elongated sacral end plate in advanced cases
- In the VD view, an irregular cranial border of the sacrum, with one or more isolated fragments is sometimes seen.

In addition, discography usually shows leaking of contrast medium through the gap between the fragment and the end plate and is an excellent diagnostic method for this condition. CT and MRI are the most sensitive imaging modalities for the condition. The free fragment and the secondary degenerative lesions are easily seen (Figure 18.18).

### Intravertebral disc herniation

Intravertebral disc herniation (Schmorl's node) at the lumbosacral level is a very rare condition described only in dogs. The condition may be associated with pain. The aetiology is unclear but may be similar to osteochondrosis of the sacrum. Schmorl's node can be located anywhere in the end plate of either L7 or S1. The radiological features are sharply defined lucent defects of varying size with sclerotic margins in the vertebral end plate, which may be associated with a narrowed intervertebral disc space.

## Degenerative disorders

### Degenerative lumbosacral stenosis

Degenerative diseases are the most often encountered pathological conditions of the lumbosacral segments and are collectively named degenerative lumbosacral stenosis (DLSS). The pathology originates at the discovertebral apparatus or the articular

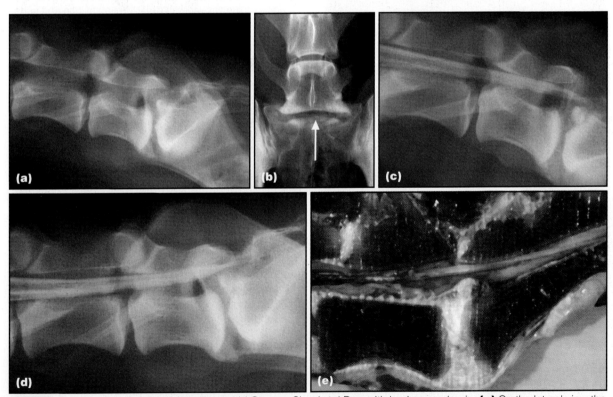

**18.18** Sacral osteochondrosis in a 4-year-old German Shepherd Dog with lumbosacral pain. **(a)** On the lateral view the intervertebral disc space appears narrowed and butterfly-like. The dorsal part of the sacral end plate is angled caudally and a large detached bone fragment can be seen in the vertebral canal. The end plates of L7 and the sacrum and adjacent vertebral bodies appear sclerotic. **(b)** On the VD view the cranial border of the sacrum appears irregular; the free fragment is to the left of the midline (arrowed). Note also the bilateral spondylosis at the caudal end plate of L7. The **(c)** flexion and **(d)** extension cervical myelograms reveal no clear compression. **(e)** Post-mortem sagittal section through the lumbosacral spine in another German Shepherd Dog with sacral osteochondrosis, showing the abnormal intervertebral disc, the defect in the dorsal part of the sacrum and the fragment (mainly cartilage) protruding into the vertebral canal.

facets, which leads to hypertrophic changes of the dorsal longitudinal and flaval ligaments, and to apposition of bone at the borders of the vertebral canal and the articular facets, resulting in narrowing of the vertebral canal and the intervertbral foramina. The end result is compression or encroachment of the cauda equina.

Anatomical conformation, especially the orientation of the articular facets, varies amongst breeds and may, together with the dimensions of the disc and high mechanical load in working dogs, play an important role in the pathogenesis of DLSS. The diagnosis usually can be made radiologically (see Figure 18.1). However, the diagnosis of cauda equina and nerve root compression requires myelography, epidurography or CT and MRI, with MRI currently being the most sensitive diagnostic imaging modality. Since the correlation of the abnormalities found with MRI and clinical signs is poor, care has to be taken not to over interpret degenerative disease. It has to be emphasized that neither MRI nor CT replaces a thorough clinical examination. Only the clinical signs (including pain) or neurological deficits will decide whether CT or MRI changes are of clinical importance.

Intervertebral disc degeneration with disc herniation is the single most important cause leading to DLSS (Figure 18.19). Dogs with transitional vertebrae or osteochondrosis seem to be predisposed. Any medium to large-breed dog can be affected by DLSS. However, German Shepherd Dogs are clearly predisposed, making up 50% of cases. In this breed, the lumbosacral disc at a young age more often shows degeneration, compared with other breeds, and has a higher degree of disc degeneration.

Depending on the underlying cause and breed affected, dogs at almost any age may be affected; the mean age of clinical onset or diagnosis varies between 4.8 years in dogs with osteochondrosis and 7 years.

The radiological signs of intervertebral disc degeneration are described in Chapter 17. Disc degeneration may be associated with disc mineralization, vacuum phenomenon, spondylosis and hypertrophy of the longitudinal and flaval ligaments, as well as degenerative disease of the articular facets. Disc degeneration may lead to disc herniation with protrusions more common than extrusions in the lumbosacral region (see Figures 18.1, 18.5, 18.9 and 18.20). Disc herniation may be central in the direction of the vertebral canal, usually causing bilateral signs, paresis of the tail and, with pronounced compression, signs of pudendal nerve compression. Dorsolateral herniation into the lateral aspects of the vertebral canal or intervertebral foramen will lead to unilateral signs. Degenerative changes with vertebral canal stenosis can occur at any level between L5 and the sacrum with similar neurological signs. Depending on the segment affected, the clinical signs may be related to L6, L7 or S1 nerve root signs (Figure 18.21).

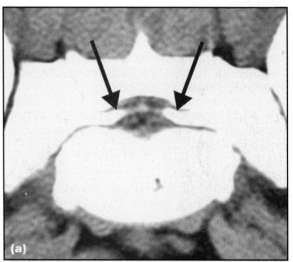

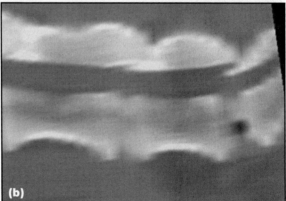

**18.20** Intervertebral disc degeneration and vertebral canal stenosis. **(a)** Transverse CT image (soft tissue window) and **(b)** sagittal reconstruction (bone window) of the lumbosacral region in a dog reveals a vacuum phenomenon in the L7–S1 intervertebral space, presenting as a discrete well defined area of hypoattenuation. The elongated and thickened dorsal lamina of S1 (arrowed) reaches too far ventrally, causing dorsal stenosis of the vertebral canal. Mild spondylosis is also present. No ventral displacement of the sacrum can be seen. (Courtesy of F Rossi and M Vignoli.)

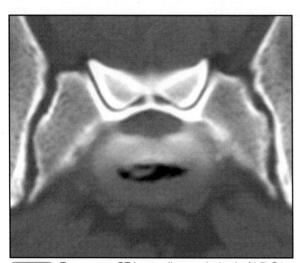

**18.19** Transverse CT image (bone window) of L7–S1 in a dog with a fusiform hypoattenuating structure in the centre of the intervertebral disc, consistent with a vacuum phenomenon and severe disc degeneration. (Courtesy of F Rossi and M Vignoli.)

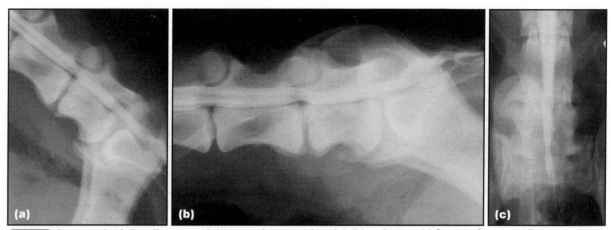

**18.21**  Intervertebral disc disease and degenerative stenosis at L6–7 in a 5-year-old German Shepherd Dog.
Radiologically, a narrowed intervertebral disc space at the L6–7 level with sclerotic end plates and vertebral
bodies and mild ventral spondylosis is present. At the level of L7–S1 moderate spondylotic changes can be seen.
The **(a)** flexion and **(b)** extension myelogram studies reveal dynamic vertebral canal stenosis dorsally at the L6–7 level,
caused by a thickened dorsal lamina of L7. **(c)** The VD view demonstrates marked lateral spondylosis bilaterally at the
L6–7 disc space, with mild left lateral compression (the left side of the dog is on the right side of the image) of the cauda
equina at this level, as well as mild bilateral compression at the lumbosacral junction.

## Articular facet changes

Hypertrophic degenerative changes of the articular
facets are common and may cause stenosis of the
intervertebral foramen (see Figure 18.15). Radiological diagnosis of osteoarthrosis of the articular facets
(spondyloarthrosis) is made using the standard views,
with oblique views sometimes being helpful. Severe
osteophyte formation may be present, which can
impinge upon the nerve roots and cause radiculitis or
root compression.

## Juxta-articular cysts

Juxta-articular (facetal) synovial or ganglion cysts may
be considered as a specific sign of articular facet
osteoarthrosis. Synovial cysts are lined by an epithe-
lium and filled with synovial fluid, whereas ganglion
cysts are not. Macroscopically, they can not be distinguished from each other. Juxta-articular cysts may be
solitary or multiple. The lower lumbar and lumbosacral
area seems to be a preferred location. Since the cysts
are located at the ventral margins of the articular
facets, and grow into the lateral aspects of the vertebral
canal (where the nerve roots leave the vertebral canal),
they may contribute to or cause nerve root compression (Figure 18.22). Diagnosis with conventional radiography is not possible and requires advanced imaging
modalities. MRI is the diagnostic modality of choice,
since fluid-sensitive sequences can clearly distinguish

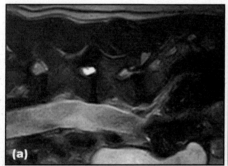
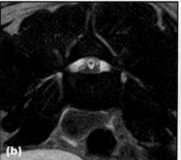
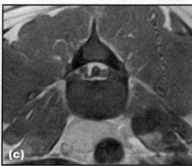

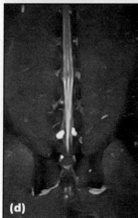

**18.22**  Multiple juxta-articular cysts at the lumbosacral area in a 6-year-old German
Shepherd Dog. The clinical signs were thought to be caused by nerve root
compression induced by the cysts at the L6–7 level. **(a)** The left parasagittal MRI T2-
weighted image reveals a lesion with a high signal intensity (fluid) in the right L6–7 foramen.
**(b)** T2-weighted and **(c)** post-contrast T1-weighted transverse sections at the L6–7 level
reveal bilateral juxta-articular cysts with a typical high signal intensity in T2-weighted and a
low signal intensity in T1-weighted sequences. The borders of the cysts showed only minimal
contrast enhancement. **(d)** The dorsal fat suppressed sequence (STIR) demonstrates the two
large cysts at the L6–7 level, a small cyst at the lumbosacral level, and is suggestive of a
small cyst at L5–6 (right side).

between soft tissue and cystic structures. On T1-weighted images, cysts have a low signal intensity; in T2-weighted and fat suppression sequences they are round to ovoid structures with a high signal intensity. Rim enhancement may be observed in T1-weighted sequences after administration of a paramagnetic contrast medium.

### Spondylosis deformans

In middle-aged to older dogs, spondylosis deformans is a very common finding at the lumbosacral junction. Spondylotic changes may be located anywhere at the level of the intervertebral foramina, or the lateral or ventral aspect of the vertebral end plate where it meets the cortex of the vertebral body. The presence of spondylosis correlates poorly with clinical signs. Occasionally, if located near the intervertebral foramina the nerve roots may be impinged, causing signs of radiculitis (Figure 18.23). As in other locations, spondylotic lesions may be a sign of intervertebral disc degeneration or chronic inflammation, but are very often idiopathic.

extension of the pelvis. This condition has been named lumbosacral instability and is discussed as a specific entity and possible cause of DLSS. Biomechanically, ventrodorsal gliding of two vertebral bodies against each other is termed translation and is normal to a certain degree, since normal flexion–extension is composed of both rotation and translation. Since translation also occurs in clinically normal dogs, and the correlation with cauda equina compression is poor, non-contrast flexion–extension radiographs are of little diagnostic importance. It is equally questionable whether primary instability really exists. In the author's opinion translation to a noticeable degree does not occur in dogs with a normal lumbosacral disc, as assessed by MRI. Lumbosacral 'instability' very likely occurs secondary to a loss of intradiscal pressure (allowing disc gliding) and thus may be considered as a sign of intervertebral disc degeneration (Figure 18.24).

Fractures or surgical removal of the articular processes will always result in true lumbosacral instability and this is always associated with disc pathology.

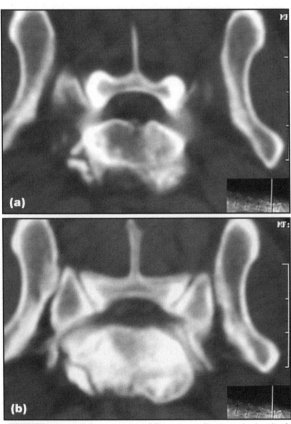

**18.23** **(a, b)** Transverse CT images (bone window) of a Boxer with severe spondylosis at the lumbosacral level. Osteophytes obliterate the neuroforamina bilaterally, leading to encroachment of the L7 nerve roots. Images made 2 mm apart. (Courtesy of F Rossi and M Vignoli.)

### Lumbosacral instability

In many dogs, clinically affected or normal, a step can be observed between the dorsal border of the vertebral bodies of L7 and the sacrum, with the sacrum displaced ventrally. Ventrodorsal displacement of the sacrum can be exaggerated or induced by flexion and

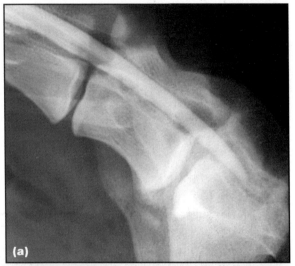

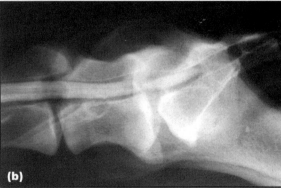

**18.24** Flexion–extension myelography in a dog with the dural end-sac ending at S1–2 and dynamic lumbosacral 'instability' and stenosis. **(a)** In flexion there is good alignment of L7 and S1 and no sign of compression of the dural end sac. Note the slight spondylotic changes ventral to the caudal end plate of L7 and the cranial end plate of S1. The end plates are sclerotic and thickened. **(b)** In extension there is ventral subluxation of the sacrum with dorsoventral narrowing of the dural end sac due to folding of a thickened flaval ligament. The instability is caused by disc gliding due to a degenerated disc.

Similar to spondylolisthesis in humans, the sacrum will move in a dorsal direction, resulting in an abnormal alignment of L7 and the sacrum. In chronic cases the sacrum will be almost fixed in this abnormal location and flexion/extension will be reduced. The L7 nerve roots are usually not as severely affected as those of the sacrum; ventral displacement of the sacrum results in the narrowing of the intervertebral foramina.

## Infection

The lumbosacral junction is a common location for discospondylitis (see Chapter 16). In contrast to other sites, soft tissue swelling ventral to the lumbosacral disc is readily appreciated radiologically (see Figures 18.25 and 18.28). In the acute stage, ventral vertebral ultrasonography and scintigraphy can be sensitive imaging modalities.

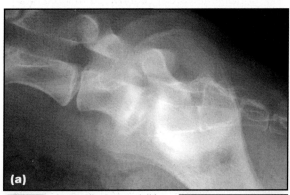

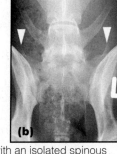

**18.25** Acute discospondylitis in a Labrador Retriever bitch. **(a)** On the lateral view there is mild soft tissue swelling ventral to the lumbosacral disc space. The end plates are lytic, bordered by sclerotic walls in the adjacent vertebral bodies. At the ventral border irregular periosteal reactions are present. The sacrum is displaced ventrally. **(b)** In addition to the lytic end plates the VD view also shows an incomplete lumbosacral transitional vertebra with an isolated spinous process and incomplete sacralization of the transverse processes of L7 (arrowheads).

## Neoplasia

There are no primary neoplasms affecting specifically the bone or neural tissue in the lumbosacral area, and the pathology described in Chapter 16 also applies to the lumbosacral region. Nerve root and lumbosacral plexus neoplasms do occur and have similar features as brachial plexus neoplasms. The close proximity of the lumbosacral region to the sublumbar lymphatic centres, responsible for the drainage of the perineal area, the prostate, uterus and bladder, as well as the pelvic limbs, make this area a preferred location for metastasis. Sublumbar lymphadenopathy can readily be seen on survey radiographs but ultrasonography is the method of choice for assessment. Palisade-like periosteal reactions along the ventral borders of the lumbosacral vertebrae, and occasionally the pelvic border and transverse processes, are suggestive of metastatic neoplasia. This

bony reaction is most commonly associated with prostatic carcinoma, although it can be seen with other neoplastic conditions as well. In contrast to discospondylitis, the intervertebral disc spaces are usually not affected (Figures 18.26 and 18.27).

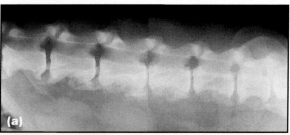

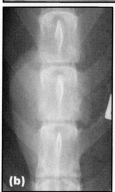

**18.26** Eight-year-old dog with a metastatic adenocarcinoma (prostate) in the sublumbar region. **(a)** In this image (composed of two lateral views) irregular bony proliferations are present ventrally on the vertebral bodies from L2 to the sacrum. Neither soft tissue swelling nor bone lysis can be seen. The intervertebral disc spaces are normal. **(b)** On the VD view the bony proliferations can be seen bilateral to the vertebral bodies but to a lesser extent.

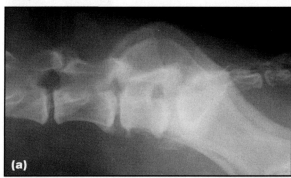

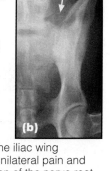

**18.27** Chondrosarcoma of the left iliac wing in a 9-year-old mixed-breed dog with left-sided lameness and pain. **(a)** Lateral view of the lumbosacral area with relatively short L7 and extensive spondylotic changes at the L6 to S1 disc spaces. The vertebral canal and intervertebral foramina are obscured by overlying bony reactions. **(b)** VD view: the degenerative changes also affect the lateral aspect of the L6 to S1 disc spaces. Note the aggressive bone lesion in the left iliac wing and the mineralization of the soft tissues between the left neural foramen and the iliac wing (arrowed). The neurological signs of unilateral pain and lameness were caused by compression of the nerve root lateral to the foramen (determined on post-mortem examination).

## Metabolic disorders

Metabolic disorders are not usually restricted to the lumbosacral area and are discussed in Chapter 16.

## Miscellaneous disorders

If cauda equina disease is suspected, it is important to consider possible differential diagnoses. Orthopaedic disease, such as bilateral cruciate or patellar ligament rupture, can mimic cauda equina compression. Since middle-aged to older dogs are more often affected by cauda equina problems, concomitant osteoarthrosis of the hip or stifle joints may be present. In such cases it can be very difficult, even for an experienced clinician, to distinguish between neurological and orthopaedic disease.

Thrombosis or thromboembolism in the caudal aorta and iliac arteries has been described in cats with cardiomyopathy, in dogs with hyperadrenocorticism, and with other disease conditions. This may lead to severe pain and pelvic leg paresis and has to be clinically distinguished from neurological disease. Non-selective angiography or ultrasonography will usually be able to identify the vessel obstruction.

Masses in the pelvic canal (e.g. paraprostatic cysts, primary or metastatic neoplasms or abscesses) may also cause neural disease due to compression of the ischiatic nerve. A thorough clinical examination and diagnostic imaging may be very helpful in differentiating such a condition from any neural canal stenosis (Figure 18.28).

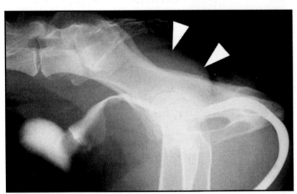

**18.28** Lateral view of retrograde urethrocystogram in a male mixed-breed dog with a caudal prostatic abscess and chronic discospondylitis. The pelvic urethra is displaced ventrally by a large space-occupying abscess (arrowed) in the pelvic canal. Note the narrowed intervertebral foramen, collapsed lumbosacral intervertebral disc space with irregular borders, and the sclerotic end plates and adjacent vertebral bodies.

## References and further reading

Adams WH, Daniel GB, Pardo AD and Selcer RS (1995) Magnetic resonance imaging of the caudal lumbar and lumbosacral spine in 13 dogs (1990–1993). *Veterinary Radiology and Ultrasound* **36**, 3–13

Barthez PY, Morgan JP and Lipsitz D (1994) Discography and epidurography for evaluation of the lumbosacral junction in dogs with cauda equina syndrome. *Veterinary Radiology and Ultrasound* **35**, 152–157

Blevins WE (1980) Transosseous vertebral venography: a diagnostic aid in lumbosacral disease. *Veterinary Radiology and Ultrasound* **21**, 50–54

De Haan JJ, Shelton SB and Ackerman N (1993) Magnetic resonance imaging in the diagnosis of degenerative lumbosacral stenosis in four dogs. *Veterinary Surgery* **22**, 1–4

De Risio L, Thomas WB and Sharp NJ (2000) Degenerative lumbosacral stenosis. *Veterinary Clinics of North America: Small Animal Practice* **30**, 111–132

Fardon DF and Milette PC (2001) Nomenclature and classification of lumbar disc pathology. Recommendations of the combined task forces of the North American Spine Society, American Society of Spine Radiology and American Society of Neuroradiology. *Spine* **26**, E93–E113

Jones JC, Sorjonen DC, Simpson ST, Coates JR, Lenz SD, Hathcock JT, Agee MW and Bartels JE (1996) Comparison between computed tomographic and surgical findings in nine large-breed dogs with lumbosacral stenosis. *Veterinary Radiology and Ultrasound* **37**, 247–256

Julier-Franz CH, Tellhelm B and Schimke E (2002) Dissertation: Der lumbosakrale Uebergangswirbel beim DSH – Formen, Häufigkeit, Genetik. Referatesammlung 48. Jahrestagung der FK-DVG, Magdeburg

Lang J (1988) Flexion–extension myelography of the canine cauda equina. *Veterinary Radiology and Ultrasound* **29**, 242–257

Lang J, Häni H and Schawalder P (1992) A sacral lesion resembling osteochondrosis in the German Shepherd Dog. *Veterinary Radiology and Ultrasound* **33**, 69–76

Leipold HW, Huston K, Blauch B and Guffy MM (1974) Congenital defects on the caudal vertebral column and spinal cord in Manx cats. *Journal of the American Veterinary Medical Association* **164**, 520–523

Lenehan TM (1983) Canine cauda equina syndrome. *Compendium on Continuing Education for the Practicing Veterinarian* **5**, 941–951

Morgan JP, Atilola M and Bailey CS (1987) Vertebral canal and spinal cord mensuration: a comparative study of its effect on lumbosacral myelography in the Dachshund and German Shepherd Dog. *Journal of the American Veterinary Medical Association* **191**, 951–957

Morgan JP, Bahr A, Franti CE and Bailey CS (1993) Lumbosacral transitional vertebrae as a predisposing cause of cauda equina syndrome in German Shepherd Dogs: 161 cases (1987–1990). *Journal of the American Veterinary Medical Association* **202**, 1877–1882

Morgan JP and Bailey CS (1990) Cauda equina syndrome in the dog: Radiographic evaluation. *Journal of Small Animal Practice* **31**, 69–77

Ness MG (1994) Degenerative lumbosacral stenosis in the dog: a review of 30 cases. *Journal of Small Animal Practice* **35**, 185–190

Palmer RH and Chambers JN (1991) Canine lumbosacral diseases. Part I. Anatomy, pathophysiology and clinical presentation. *Compendium on Continuing Education for the Practicing Veterinarian* **13**, 61–79

Schmid V and Lang J (1993) Measurements on the lumbosacral junction in normal dogs and those with cauda equina compression. *Journal of Small Animal Practice* **34**, 437–442

Selcer BA, Chambers JN, Schwensen K and Mahaffey MB (1988) Epidurography as a diagnostic aid in canine lumbosacral compressive disease. *Veterinary and Comparative Orthopaedics and Traumatology* **2**, 97–103

Sisson A, Lecouteur R, Ingram J, Park R and Child G (1992) Diagnosis of cauda equina abnormalities by using electromyography, discography and epidurography in dogs. *Journal of Veterinary Internal Medicine* **6**, 253–263

Wheeler SJ (1992) Lumbosacral disease. *Veterinary Clinics of North America: Small Animal Practice* **22**, 937–950

# Appendix

# Abbreviations

| Abbreviation | In full |
|---|---|
| 3D | Three dimensional |
| ACTH | Adrenocorticotrophic hormone |
| CCL | Cranial cruciate ligament |
| CCM | Caudal cervical malformation |
| CCO | Caudolateral curvilinear osteophyte |
| CdCr | Caudocranial |
| CdMCrLO | Caudomedial-craniolateral oblique |
| CdR | Caudorostral |
| CPDD | Calcium pyrophosphate deposition disease |
| CrCd | Craniocaudal |
| CrDi-CrPrO | Craniodistal-cranioproximal oblique |
| CrLCdMO | Craniolateral-caudomedial oblique |
| CrMCdLO | Craniomedial-caudolateral oblique |
| CrPr-CrDiO | Cranioproximal-craniodistal oblique |
| CSF | Cerebrospinal fluid |
| CT | Computed tomography |
| DAR | Dorsal acetabular rim |
| DAWS | Disc-associated 'Wobbler syndrome' |
| DI | Distraction index |
| DiMPrLO | Distomedial-proximolateral oblique |
| DISH | Diffuse idiopathic skeletal hyperostosis |
| DL | Dorsolateral |
| DLPaMO | Dorsolateral-palmaromedial oblique |
| DLSS | Degenerative lumbosacral stenosis |
| DM | Dorsomedial |
| DMPaLO | Dorsomedial-palmarolateral oblique |
| DPa | Dorsopalmar |
| DPl | Dorsoplantar |
| DV | Dorsoventral |
| FeLV | Feline leukaemia virus |
| FFD | Focal film distance |
| FIV | Feline immunodeficiency virus |
| FMCP | Fragmented medial coronoid process |
| GH | Growth hormone |

| Abbreviation | In full |
|---|---|
| GME | Granulomatous meningoencephalomyelitis |
| HOD | Hypertrophic osteodystrophy |
| LeD-RtVO | Left dorsal-right ventral oblique |
| LeR-RtCdO | Left rostral-right caudal oblique |
| LeV-RtDO | Left ventral-right dorsal oblique |
| ML | Mediolateral |
| MPS | Mucopolysaccharidosis |
| MRI | Magnetic resonance imaging |
| OC | Osteochondrosis |
| OCD | Osteochondritis dissecans |
| PaL | Palmarolateral |
| PaM | Palmaromedial |
| PaMDLO | Palmaromedial-dorsolateral oblique |
| PlD | Plantarodorsal |
| PlL | Plantarolateral |
| PlLDMO | Plantarolateral-dorsomedial oblique |
| PlM | Plantaromedial |
| PlMDLO | Plantaromedial-dorsolateral oblique |
| PTH | Parathyroid hormone |
| RCd | Rostrocaudal |
| RtD-LeVO | Right dorsal-left ventral oblique |
| RtR-LeCdO | Right rostral-left caudal oblique |
| RtV-LeDO | Right ventral-left dorsal oblique |
| RV-CdDO | Rostroventral-caudodorsal oblique |
| TMJ | Temporomandibular joint |
| TPO | Triple pelvic osteotomy |
| UAP | Ununited anconeal process |
| VCd-DCr | Ventrocaudal-dorsocranial |
| VCr-DCd | Ventrocranial-dorsocaudal |
| VD | Ventrodorsal |
| VLe-DRtO | Ventral left-dorsal right oblique |
| VR-DCdO | Ventral rostral-dorsocaudual oblique |
| VRt-DLeO | Ventral right-dorsal left oblique |

# Index

# Index

# Index

# Index

# Index

# Index

# Index

Tendinopathy *161*
Tendons
  damage 160–1
  intra-articular 72
  ultrasonography *3, 91*
Thoracic vertebrae, anatomy *221, 222*
Thyroid hormone, role in bone metabolism 20–1
Tibetan Mastiff, hypertrophic neuropathy 233
Tibia/fibula
  fibrosarcoma *44*
  fractures
    complete *52*
    delayed union *63*
    fixation *62*
    healing *60*
    oblique *52*
    osteomyelitis *68*
    physeal *50*
    scintigraphy *38*
    spiral *52*
    transverse *52*
  hypertrophic osteopathy *46*
  neoplasia *45, 69*
    dog/cat 37
  normal appearance, dog/cat 37
  normal development *20*
  osteomyelitis *41*
  osteopetrosis *47*
  osteosarcoma *43*
  popliteal sesamoid 37
  radiographic views
    caudocranial 35
    craniocaudal 35
    mediolateral 34
  tibial tuberosity avulsion *53*, 141–2
Tibial plateau angle, measurement *139*
Tibial tuberosity avulsion 141–2
TMJ *see* Temporomandibular joint
Total hip replacement 131
Transition zone, neoplasia *versus* osteomyelitis *45*
Trauma *see* Avulsion; Fractures; Luxation; Subluxation
Tympanic bulla *see* Ear

UAP *see* Ununited anconeal process
Ulna see Radius/Ulna
Ultrasonography
  Achilles tendon *163*
  biceps tendon *75*
    rupture *93, 99*
  distal limb 160
  ear 190
  foreign bodies 185
  fractures 49
  hip 123
  joints 74–5
  larynx 179
  long bones
    adults 38
    juveniles 21
  masses 3, 8
  muscle 3
  nasal cavity 196

  orbit 179, *184*
  osteochondrosis dissecans 96, *97*
  persistent fontanelle 179
  shoulder 91
  soft tissues 2–3
  spine 232, 262
  stifle 141
  tendons *3*
Ununited anconeal process 84, 112–13
Ununited medial humeral epicondyle 116

Vacuum phenomenon 80
  hip *81*
  shoulder *95*
  spine 251, *267*
Vascular occlusion 8
Vertebrae
  alignment 225
  anatomy 221, 222
  articular facet abnormalities 237, 250, 254–5
  atlantoaxial instability 236–7
  block 235
  breed-related conditions 237
  butterfly 236
  hemivertebrae 235–6
  ossification centres 225
  radiographic abnormalities 250
    'Wobbler syndrome' 253–6
  transitional 124, 235, 264–5
  (*see also* Cervical vertebrae; Lumbar vertebrae; Sacrum;
    Spine; Thoracic vertebrae)
Vertebral canal abnormalities 249
  stenosis 254
Villonodular synovitis 85
Vitamin A, role in bone metabolism 20–1
Vitamin D
  deficiency 28
  role in bone metabolism 20–1

Weber–Cech classification 64
Weight loss *4*
Weimaraner
  metaphyseal osteopathy 30
  myelodysplasia 237
Welsh Springer Spaniel, juvenile polyarteritis syndrome 243
West Highland White Terrier, craniomandibular osteopathy
  30, 187
Whippet
  intervertebral disc disease 252
  sporting injuries 39
'Wobbler syndrome' 253–6
  dog breeds 232, 253
  dynamic changes 255–6
  postoperative changes 256
  soft tissue changes 255
  synonyms 253
  vertebral changes 254–5
Wounds 7

Yorkshire Terrier, proximal ulnar luxation 109

Zygomatic arch *209*

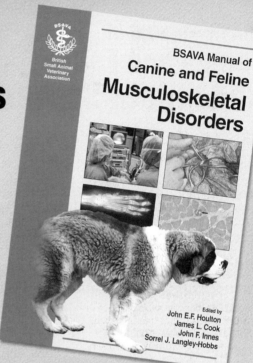
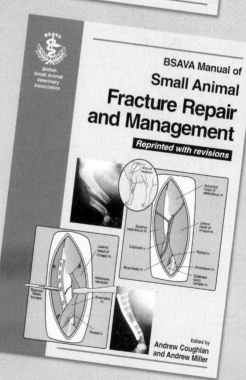

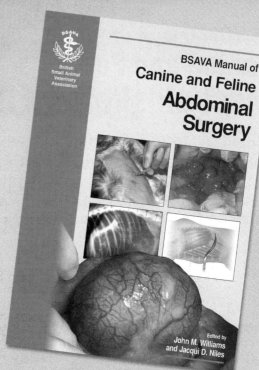
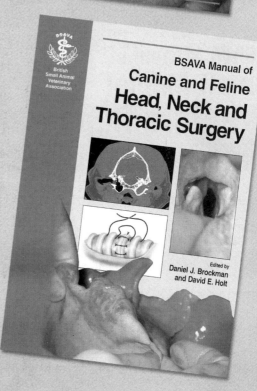